Reproductive Health and
Human Rights

Reproductive Health and Human Rights

The Way Forward

Edited by Laura Reichenbach and Mindy Jane Roseman

PENN

University of Pennsylvania Press

Philadelphia

Published by
University of Pennsylvania Press
Philadelphia, Pennsylvania 19104-4112

Printed in the United States of America on acid-free paper
10 9 8 7 6 5 4 3 2 1

Library of Congress Cataloging-in-Publication Data
Reproductive health and human rights : the way forward / edited by Laura
Reichenbach and Mindy Jane Roseman.
    p.   cm.—(Pennsylvania studies in human rights)
  ISBN: 978-0-8122-4152-5 (alk. paper)
  1. ICPD Programme of Action. 2. International International Conference on
Population and Development (1994 : Cairo, Egypt). 3. Human rights. 4. Reproductive
health. 5. International cooperation. 6. Right to health care. 7. Reproductive Medicine.
8. International Cooperation. 9. Reproductive Rights. 10. Women's Health.
I. Reichenbach, Laura. II. Roseman, Mindy Jane
HQ766.G56   2009
362.1—dc22   2008035360

Contents

Preface

Reproductive Health and Rights: The Way Forward is an edited collection of critical essays by leading scholars and practitioners in this protean field. The United Nations held the International Conference on Population and Development (ICPD) in Cairo, Egypt, from 5 to 13 September 1994. Its resulting Programme of Action represented a consensus agreement among 179 governments, UN agencies, and NGOs, intended to guide the next twenty years of efforts concerning population and development—reinterpreted as "reproductive health." Although many critics of ICPD blame its lack of progress on the diffuse concept of "reproductive health" or on the effect of successful fertility decline in much of the world, among other explanations (Sinding 2006; Blanc and Tsui 2005), this book contends that the Programme of Action still has great merit. The essays in this book examine the diversity of interpretations and applications of ICPD that have flourished since its original passage in 1994. These essays consider how the understanding of reproductive health has evolved and provide a vision of how reproductive health and rights continue to be vital to the achievement of international population and development goals.

Understanding where reproductive health and rights fit at the global policy level requires addressing fundamental questions about the relationship between population, reproductive health and rights, and development. What are the underlying arguments for rights or rights-based approaches to reproductive health? What has been the nature of the relationship among population, reproductive health, and poverty reduction, and what are its implications for achievement of the subsequently approved UN millennium development goals (MDGs), which did not explicitly address reproductive health as a goal; and what becomes the role for population policy given the current decline in fertility rates to below replacement levels in some countries? Answering these questions requires attention to the various arguments—demographic, public health, human rights-based, and economic—that work both for and against ICPD today.

This collection of essays provides an assessment of the state of the arguments for reproductive health and rights and aims to supply policymakers, scholars, and activists with a better understanding of how reproductive health and rights have developed, how they fit on the global policy agenda, and how they might evolve most effectively into the future. While the majority of essays in this book reflect a U.S.-based perspective, many of their conclusions and strategies have relevance to national contexts around the world. That is to say, while some of the political vagaries that have made the concept of reproductive health vulnerable to distortion may be peculiar to the United States, the current specific context that affects reproductive health (for example, a growing HIV epidemic and a strong policy focus on poverty alleviation) are relevant across nations. Proponents of ICPD will have to respond to interrelated health and development challenges such as these, regardless of the political leanings of their governments. These essays were written during a time when the political environment was particularly hostile towards reproductive health and rights issues—especially in the U.S. While the political climate may change with a new U.S. administration, the conclusions of the chapters in the book remain salient.

The sixteen chapters consider the strengths and weakness of the ICPD idea of reproductive health, largely from the perspective of scholars and advocates located in the United States. What connects the diverse essays in this book is their focus on ICPD. We challenged the authors of these chapters to be "offensive" rather than "defensive" in their analysis of ICPD. While no essay treats ICPD as a sacred text or set of principles that need to be defended at any cost, all the contributors agree that reproductive health matters still as a primary concern of global health. Through descriptive analysis, the chapters bolster arguments for the continued relevance of ICPD, while pointing out important shortcomings and suggesting ways to strengthen the ICPD approach. Each author speaks in his or her own voice, sometimes in the first person. Some of the authors diverge in their analysis; sometimes there is consensus. Where there is overlap in the chapters, we as editors interpret it as reinforcing common interpretation rather than as mere repetition. Throughout this book, the editors use the terms ICPD and reproductive health to stand for the range of concepts commonly associated with improving health outcomes related to sexuality, reproduction, and social inequalities. Not all the contributors in this book necessarily use ICPD or reproductive health in the same way; nor should they, given their differences in discipline and orientation. As a theme throughout this book, the terms are less important than the validity and continued resonance of the ideas.

Part I
Global Agendas and Population and Development Perspectives

Chapter 1
Global Reproductive Health and Rights: Reflecting on ICPD

Mindy Jane Roseman and Laura Reichenbach

More than a decade after the enthusiasm that launched the 1994 International Conference on Population and Development (ICPD), there is growing concern about the status of ICPD. Does it have the same purchase today as it did in the immediate post-Cairo period? While many gains have been achieved because of ICPD (Countdown 2015 2007; UNFPA 2004a, b; Haberland and Measham 2002; UNFPA 1999), the health and development issues that brought the nations of the world to consensus persist. Approximately half a million women die in child-birth annually; the AIDS epidemic is increasing in both scale and scope; declining fertility rates in much of the world have not translated into improved standards of living. Over one billion people live in extreme poverty and have inadequate access to health care. The post-ICPD world is still one where women do not exercise control over their bodies. Women and girls are forced into marriages and into sexual relations. Their spouses and families make decisions about when and whether they can leave the home, be it to go to work or to obtain health care. Their governments do not protect them from domestic violence. And in too many places women who belong to ethnic or other minorities are subjected to involuntary sterilization and other forms of violence.

Should more have been accomplished, more than halfway through ICPD's twenty-year Programme of Action? And in looking toward its fifteen- and twenty-year reviews, how might ICPD's potential be finally realized? The Programme of Action laid out an innovative and broad framework for population and development. Following the Cairo conference, 179 nations agreed to the Programme of Action's sixteen chapters (UN 1995). The Programme explicitly addressed a comprehensive set of population and development goals and objectives to be achieved through universal provision of a range of reproductive health services by 2015.[1] Specifically, the consensus document called for "sustained economic growth in the context of sustainable development; education, especially for girls; gender equity and equality; infant, child and maternal mortality reduction; and the provision of universal access to reproductive health services, including family planning and sexual health" (para. 1.12). Prior to ICPD, the international lexicon and national policies addressing population focused on the control of fertility, understood entirely as women's fertility (Hartmann 1998), and births averted and reductions in family size were important measures.

The Programme of Action was fundamentally important because it laid out a radically different approach to the population "problem," stating that population concerns could not be separated from other economic and social development agendas, particularly the need for women's empowerment. ICPD transformed population and development into reproductive health, defining it as

a state of complete physical, mental and social well-being and not merely the absence of disease or infirmity, in all matters relating to the reproductive system and to its functions and processes. Reproductive health therefore implies that people are able to have a satisfying and safe sex life and that they have the capability to reproduce and the freedom to decide if, when and how often to do so. (para. 7.2)

Reproductive health, it stated, should be delivered by services through the primary health care system and also by advancing gender equality and ensuring a woman's ability to control her own fertility. In other words, beyond reflecting a range of multidisciplinary perspectives and promoting ambitious goals, the ICPD contained what has come to be known as the "Cairo Paradigm," which shifted population policy away from fertility regulation and toward the notion of reproductive health, predicated on the exercise of reproductive rights and women's empowerment. The extent to which this paradigmatic shift still resonates is an important measure of ICPD's relevance.

In addition to a paradigm, ICPD is also referred to as a "consensus" as well as a "compromise." As we argue in this chapter, we believe all of these dimensions are contained in ICPD and contribute to its endurance, but also to its vulnerabilities. ICPD is an innovative model for understanding the connections between health, human rights, population, and development. It was produced out of consensus forged after two years of local, national, regional, and international preparatory meetings. And it is a product of a compromise among different groups—feminists, public health professionals, development economists, demographers, environmentalists, faith communities, donors, and governments.

Some of these differing perspectives can be understood by appreciating the words that circumscribe and define the "field" of reproductive health and rights. Sexuality and reproduction sit, after all, at the intersection of health and human rights. Political and programmatic tensions run through the vocabulary used throughout all discussions of "reproductive health," "sexual health," "reproductive rights," "sexual rights," gender, population, and even development. While examination of how these different terms play out is beyond the scope of this book, we recognize the importance that language and terminology have had in creating both consensus and division in policy making related to reproductive health. According to Sonia Correa, one of the architects of ICPD, the terminology "reproductive health" and "reproductive rights" reflects agreed-to compromises within the global women's health movements (Correa 1997). She notes that "in a number of . . . contexts, reproductive health policies since 1995 may simply be semantic re-interpretations or refinements of conventional maternal and child health or family planning programs" (Correa 1997: 110). However for progressive advocates, sexual and reproductive health and rights are a political and transformative platform that seek to redefine "the spheres where sexual and reproductive needs are defined . . . the domains in which gender power relations are played out, and . . . subjective views of women's bodies and reproduction" are negated (110). As such, redress of power imbalances through the identification of women's subjection based on sexual difference (and the social significance that was made of that difference) has been a common point of departure for women's health and rights activists, among others.

A striking example of the implications of language in the realm of reproductive health has to do with understandings of sexual health, sexual rights, and sexuality. Although ICPD does not include any explicit mention of sexual rights, the notion of sexual health and rights has gained renewed attention since 1994, particularly as AIDS became a feminized epidemic and international movements organized around issues like female genital mutilation (Klugman 2005; Miller 2000). There remains no consensus around the meaning of sexual rights—it includes identity politics and choice of sexual partner but also embraces notions of inherent rights to sexual pleasure—but recent efforts by WHO have helped to delineate working definitions for sex, sexuality, and sexual health (WHO 2006a).

Efforts to interpret the meaning of sexual health as it relates to reproductive health will continue to be circumscribed by and influenced by political and social constraints. For many countries, the very notion of "sexual health" remains too political to contemplate despite the real public health pressures of the global HIV/AIDS epidemics. Whether and how reproductive health embraces sexuality and sexual health is an ongoing challenge for ICPD, although not necessarily an unmovable obstacle (see Gruskin, this volume).

Language and terminology aside, there is general consensus about the paradigm shift that reproductive health generated. However, despite its promise and some demonstrated achievements in promoting women's education, development, health, and rights (Countdown 2015 2007; UNFPA 2004b), ICPD and the field of reproductive health have fallen short of what its supporters had hoped the field would accomplish (World Bank 2007). Concerns about the relevance of ICPD are warranted given the broader health and development environment, which has created a challenging set of conditions in which reproductive health must operate. In particular, the conservative political environment emanating from the United States, a prioritization of poverty reduction on the development agenda, and the increasing shift to global health approaches challenge the continued implementation of ICPD. ICPD faces new tests, perhaps even threats to its continued international political salience. The reservations expressed in 1994 by the Holy See and a few Islamic states have come back to bite with a vengeance, when coupled with the changed position of the U.S. government—ICPD's major supporter in 1994 and its major backtracker in 2004. The trend toward more conservative politics in the United States and elsewhere has had major implications for how the international community prioritizes reproductive health issues, including the most contentious ones of abortion and sexuality. The prevailing neoliberal approach to international economic policy has thrust the eight Millennium Development Goals (MDGs), launched by the UN in 2000 to first place, subsuming and replacing the range of international development targets and goals set at the various UN conferences, such as ICPD, which took place during the 1990s. In addition, the large-scale and generalized epidemics of HIV have contributed to a waning of interest in the broad, comprehensive approach of ICPD. These developments are salutary reminders that Cairo's much lauded "paradigm shift" might be exaggerated in certain contexts.

These changes in international policy and political environments contribute to the perception by many in development circles that reproductive health and rights are increasingly fragmented and marginalized (El Feki 2004; Sinding 2005a; Gillespie 2004a). In addition, the field of reproductive health and rights faces important questions related to its programmatic agenda, the status of its implementation, and how it connects with other development goals. These questions and concerns are

worthy of more careful examination. Critical reflection on this field is timely and important not only because of upcoming progress reviews of ICPD for 2010 and beyond, but also because of recent changes in the broader policy environment that may have continued impacts on the ability to achieve the goals of ICPD.

It has become apparent that when understood conceptually, ICPD has had much enduring success. Yet when viewed operationally it faces serious challenges. This chapter considers ICPD from the perspectives of its conceptual underpinnings and in terms of operationalizing some of the issues contained in the Programme of Action. We first discuss the conceptual foundations, such as human rights, development, and empowerment that strengthen ICPD. In the next section we lay out the issues and challenges that have tested these foundations and created obstacles to its operationalization. These obstacles include the political environment in which ICPD operates, stronger focus on poverty reduction, and increased importance of global health. Finally, the chapter explores the future of reproductive health and rights and suggests strategies for ensuring that reproductive health and rights remain on the global agenda—both on their own merits and as a means toward other goals related to population and improved health for all.

ICPD and Its Conceptual Foundations

The concept of "reproductive health" was not newly minted at ICPD. The term was first coined by Dr. Mahmoud Fathalla when he was working at the Human Reproduction Programme of the World Health Organization. His initial definition, the basis for the ICPD definition, was based on the WHO Constitution's description of health as a "state of complete physical, mental and social well-being and not merely the absence of disease or infirmity." Fathalla proposed that "Reproductive health, in the context of this positive definition, would have a number of basic elements. It would mean that people have the ability to reproduce and the ability to regulate their fertility; that women are able to go safely through pregnancy and childbirth; and that reproduction is carried to a successful outcome through infant and child survival and well-being. To this may be added that people are able to enjoy and are safe in having sex. In all of these elements, from a global perspective, health in human reproduction seems to be an impossible goal" (Fathalla 1988: 7).

"Reproductive health" emerged out of the women's health and rights movements that preceded ICPD by at least two decades (Correa and Reichmann 1994). Women's health and rights movements in North America, Europe, Latin America, subcontinental Asia, Africa, and the Asia/Pacific region had been galvanized to varying degrees by the abuses of population control, discrimination against women, lack of concern for abortion rights and safe motherhood, and women's exclusion from the development agenda (Keck and Sikkink 1998). Forced sterilization to keep poor or otherwise "undesirable" women from having "too many" children has at various times been official policy in countries as varied as India, Peru, Sweden, and the United States. Often governments would set targets (if not quotas) for the identified population. Incentives were paid to women and health workers who "agreed" to permanent forms of contraception; disincentives, such as withholding government benefits or pay, were meted out to those who rejected offers of oral contraception or IUDs (Garcia-Moreno and Claro 1994). Women's health and rights movements analyzed these and other abuses as resulting from society's systematic devaluation and oppression of women. The global women's health and rights movement—complex and at times divided[2]—was and is rightly credited with moving ICPD's agenda forward (Garcia-Moreno and Claro 1994; Dixon-Mueller 1993). Reproductive health focused on power inequalities—the subordination of women—and the ill consequences for their health that ensued.

Because this analysis focused on the injustice and unfairness done principally to women due to their biological and social status as "reproductive," reproductive health as defined in the Programme of Action was to be realized through the promotion and protection of reproductive rights. Prior to ICPD, feminist scholarship influenced national courts and international human rights institutions and helped establish norms around women's human rights that related to their health, particularly their reproductive and sexual health (Cook 1994). Reproductive rights were identified as a set of human rights enumerated in international human rights treaties, including, among others, the right of individuals and couples to decide on the timing and spacing of their children, and the right to have the information and means to do so, free from coercion, discrimination, and violence. Because women's exercise of their autonomy in relation to childbearing in particular so profoundly affects their health, the logical tie between rights and health was easily forged. For example, pregnancies that are not well spaced place a burden on the woman as well as compromising the well-being of her children; lack of control over when and whether a woman will have sex, or whether she or her partner uses effective contraception, directly contributes to poorly spaced pregnancies (Ravindran and Balasubramanian 2004). Similarly, lack of provision of comprehensive information about sex has led to increasing rates of sexually transmitted infections (STIs) and unintended pregnancies among adolescents in parts of the United States (Human Rights Watch 2002).

The innovation of tying health outcomes to rights promotion and protection was twofold. First, human rights are not abstract aspirational wishes, but concrete obligations governments assume when they ratify international human rights treaties.[3] At a minimum, governments are supposed to ensure that their national laws and policies are in accord with the rights contained in the treaty and to promote and protect the human rights contained therein. Second, human rights directly address power imbalances. Denying or neglecting to provide women access to information and services that contribute to their health, for example, or failing to intervene in a father's decision to marry off his preteen daughter, are understood to be violations of women's human rights (Bunch 1995). The effort to stake out human rights as they directly relate to women's lives led to international human rights norms on government action and inaction around the provision of health information and services, as well as around the conditions under which women can exercise their agency with regard to health care. These rights were then explicitly extended to an analysis of reproduction. ICPD built on this to articulate women's reproductive rights—as already existing human rights applied to women's experiences related to reproduction. Human rights, therefore, provided a tangible, legitimate methodology as well as an agenda for social transformation, through which international and national health policies and programs could be revised in ways that would improve health and its underlying social determinants (see Roseman, this volume).

Another major accomplishment of ICPD has been expanding the concept of reproductive health to mean human rights and empowerment of women as much as it means delivery of health care services or achievement of health outcomes. There is little doubt that ICPD has been a major, if not proximate, factor in promoting the use of law, policy, and international human rights mechanisms in the service of reproductive health. A number of leading scholars have articulated both the novelty and importance of ICPD in its ability to forge a connection between health and human rights:

Broadly and simply stated, the essence of [ICPD's paradigm change] is this: previous governmental and nongovernmental statements, as well as maternal-child health/family planning programs and policies themselves, regularly conceptualized and treated women . . . as tools through which to implement population control policies, child survival strategies, nationalist or fundamentalist agendas, development schemes, or patriarchal family values and structures. By contrast, the reproductive health and rights approach adopted at ICPD is premised on a view of women as valuable intrinsically, as well as for the contribution they make to a broader society. (Freedman 2005: 532–33)

Research supports the observation that women's poor reproductive health outcomes are not only correlated with gender discrimination, but they are sometimes caused by such gendered ideologies (Sen, George, and Östlin 2002). Cultures that praise motherhood nonetheless can also propound discriminatory ideologies that consign women to roles of childbearing and rearing; women living in these cultures often have higher rates of maternal mortality and reproductive morbidity (Doyal 1995). Although reproductive rights have been solidified as a core component of the strategy to achieve ICPD's goals, significant gaps exist more than ten years after ICPD to move beyond rhetoric with clear evidence that gender discrimination is a causal factor linked to women's health outcomes, and to show that attention to women's human rights and equality improves health outcomes (see Roseman, this volume).

ICPD also systematized the longstanding idea that reproductive health is instrumental to achieving economic development—either through its role in increasing income growth or in improving social development. The relationship and connections between reproductive health and economic development and poverty reduction have a long history with origins in neo-Malthusian arguments about population growth and its impacts on economic growth. The argument that high fertility rates do impede economic growth was later criticized and questioned (National Research Council 1986) and has since been revitalized by economists examining the impact of the population age structure on a country's economic growth (Bloom, Canning, and Sevilla 2003). Population policy has also historically been tied to policy about environmental degradation and global insecurity (Hartmann 2005):

> Degradation narratives link population pressure to poverty and degradation of the environment. . . . In the 1990s this narrative extended to include security concerns: the cycle of poverty leads to conflict and to a rise of migration to urban areas, the creation of slums and the youth bulge—a high proportion of young men in urban populations is blamed for escalating crime, political violence, and terrorism. . . . It is not surprising that some population and environmental organizations feel the need to use national security arguments to win support from legislators . . . for international family planning assistance. (Ashford 2001: 16–17)

Linking reproductive health and rights to development and poverty reduction helped forge an initial consensus on ICPD, and improving understandings about the relationship between reproductive health and poverty reduction has been an important focus of many policymakers since the UN Millennium Summit in 2000, during which participating nations identified the first of eight major international development goals to be poverty reduction. Since universal access to reproductive health information and services was not included as a separate MDG during that summit, the close relationship between population control/ reproductive health and economic development has been stressed even more as advocates scramble to present evidence and arguments for how the provision of reproductive health is critical for the achievement of the MDGs (Freedman et al. 2005a; see Bloom and Canning and Girard, this volume).

Although the impact of dropping reproductive health as a specific goal has yet to be determined, to a certain measure, this argument has been mostly resolved. The five-year review of the MDGs during the 2005 World Summit resulted in new commitments by governments to work toward universal access to reproductive health by 2015 (UN 2005a, para. 57(g)). The UN General Assembly endorsed that target in 2006 (UN 2006a).

Population control has long been the rationale for reproductive health, and ICPD reflected both that ideological tradition and its evolution. The literature on reproductive health as demography and population policy is vast. Demography became the social science and methodology of choice to understand population dynamics and devise interventions and strategies for addressing neo-Malthusian concerns about resource depletion and other presumed effects of overpopulation. Birth control through modern contraceptive technology became the preferred tool to achieve demographic objectives of reducing population and increasing per capita wealth.

From this platform came at least two sets of responses that contributed to the articulation of the ICPD reproductive health and rights approach. On the one hand, researchers questioned the hypothesis that poverty was caused by large family size; rather, evidence emerged that people chose to have large families because they were poor (Mamdani 1972), reflecting the motto "development is the best contraceptive."[4] Over time, U.S. and other support for population programs diminished. On the other hand, recent interest in population control in some local areas has led to a surge in interest in reproductive health programming (Chatterjee 2005), but the tendency is to focus on family planning alone, reflecting a belief that a technical/vertical intervention can achieve what ICPD's horizontal/holistic/rights-based approach could not (see Zeidenstein and Bloom and Canning, both in this volume). Like the yearning to reduce provision of reproductive health services to the provision of family planning, there is a desire on the part of some to revive demography and population policy as the principal rationale for reproductive health (Sinding 2006, 2005b).

As a concept that relates human rights, development, and health together through the social (gendered) and biological aspects of reproduction, reproductive health has, as nearly all the chapters in this volume acknowledge, made considerable inroads. The number of UN conferences and international policy documents that contain explicit or implicit reference to ICPD is evidence of this. However, the experiences of implementing and operationalizing the concept of ICPD into policies and programs have brought challenges.

ICPD and Its Operational Issues

The concept of reproductive health was born out of a compromise. Population planners and demographers who previously maintained that targets and quotas had to be met by any means relented when confronted with the harm such coercive policies had for women. This compromise has brought with it both strengths and weaknesses when it comes to operationalizing the ICPD reproductive health agenda. Central to the alliance that helped forge the compromise was the role of family planning and population professionals who were convinced that empowering women and fostering their human rights was a more efficacious strategy for achieving reduced family size and better spaced births (Presser and Sen 2000). Development economists were persuaded that investment in reproductive health and girls' education could lead to economic growth. Joining them were women's health and rights activists, who were content to strike a bargain, even if they might part company with those who viewed women's reproductive capacities in instrumental ways. Women and social activists from the Global South agreed to relax their demands that neoliberal policies be rescinded; feminists accepted that abortion rights were not going to be agreed to at ICPD.

The debate over inclusion of the terms "sexual health" and "sexual rights" illustrates how compromise occurred—and points to both its strengths and weaknesses. The initial draft of ICPD's Programme of Action did not contain any mention of sexuality. For largely tactical reasons, the Norwegian and Swedish delegations added "sexual health" to the text during one of the preparatory meetings, and some feminists lobbied for the inclusion of the term "sexual rights." The idea was advocating for a more radical position would make "reproductive rights" (then, as now, a contentious notion) appear more moderate and become a consensus choice. The ultimate omission of "sexual rights," from the final text of ICPD was therefore "not exactly considered a defeat" (Correa 1997: 110).[5]

ICPD could have been an anomaly—the product of a unique convergence of people and countries with divergent opinions about the meaning of "reproductive health" who united temporarily for short-term gains. That the Programme of Action was to be extended over twenty years suggests, however, that those involved in the Cairo consensus were interested in more than a momentary compromise. Even in debate over particularly sensitive issues such as sexual health and sexual rights, the governments, organizations, and individuals involved in the ICPD process worked together to achieve a common set of agenda points and did not let areas of disagreement derail overall progress. In the end, this process of compromise produced a document far bigger than the sum of its parts, giving strength and purpose to the concept of reproductive health.

Yet only five years after it was created, the ICPD consensus started to show signs of strain, bending under the weight of unanticipated changes in the political, health, and development spheres. By 2000, global health issues such as HIV and AIDS dwarfed other perennial international health concerns (e.g., water-borne diarrheal diseases affecting children). Poverty reduction through meeting the eight MDGs would drive UN, multilateral, and certain bilateral assistance programs. Both shifts would bring to the surface weaknesses in ICPD's conceptualization of reproductive health in regard to its implementation, namely, its holistic focus and lack of agreed upon measures of progress. Furthermore, the 2000 U.S. presidential election heralded a profound and hostile change, creating a uniquely challenging environment for operationalizing ICPD. The overtly conservative politics of the United States, some Islamic states, and the Vatican made abortion and adolescent reproductive and sexual health particularly stubborn areas of ICPD and affected implementation in other areas of reproductive health as well (see Berer, Shepard, and Kissling, all in this volume). The inherent conservatism in part of the reproductive health community itself, among other factors, delayed the implementation of services that integrate HIV prevention and treatment with more general reproductive health care (see Gruskin, this volume).

However, it is not merely a fracturing of the political compromise that has made implementation of reproductive health a challenge. Implementation has been uneven, and this variation can be traced back to underestimation in the Programme of Action about how contentious (or difficult in practice) certain aspects of the ICPD agenda would be to operationalize (UNFPA 2004b). Because there was no agreed upon strategy at Cairo for implementing ICPD, the unforeseen challenges presented by the HIV epidemic and the MDGs in 2000 illustrate how additional pressures on ICPD's already existing compromises further challenge its implementation. ICPD argued for the delivery of reproductive health services through the primary health care system, but it did not and could not specify the best mechanisms for implementing such a plan. Since ICPD, there have been arguments for different approaches to implementing reproductive health services, although they predate the present concerns of global epidemics and poverty alleviation. Instead the first issue facing ICPD implementers was attracting individuals—usually women—to use available services. Quality of care became an intense area of interest for reproductive health programs; this inquiry grew out of early experiences in the implementation of family planning programs when the programs were under pressure to use any means necessary—including coercion and violence—to achieve their goals. Proposed alternative mechanisms include adopting a human rights approach (Cook and Fathalla 1996), policy and legislative reform, advocacy and community involvement, and restructuring of health services (de Pinho 2005). While there is no single mechanism for implementing reproductive health services, there are examples of successes from each of these approaches. For example, efforts to pass national legislation banning female genital mutilation or increasing the legal age for marriage have been successful in some countries, and a combination of these implementation approaches may be appropriate depending on the setting.

The provision of comprehensive reproductive health services through the integration of previously separate activities was part of the ICPD goals to "encourage greater use of services" and maximize service efficiency. To this end, efforts have generally focused on integrating some combination of family planning, maternal and child health, and HIV/AIDS services in different health care settings (Lush 2002; Mayhew et al. 2000). The reasons for integrating or linking reproductive health services are not only technical (increased coverage and greater efficiency) but may also be strategic in nature. For example, a purported benefit of linking reproductive health and HIV services is to ensure continued funding of reproductive health services when politics mean that HIV services garner greater resources. However, service integration efforts present practical challenges, including determining which services to integrate and at which level of the health system, tracking and reporting donor funding, and measuring results, and also raise the larger question whether the ICPD goal of delivering an expanded set of services can be achieved in the absence of integration. It remains unclear whether current efforts to link rather than integrate services will address some of these concerns (WHO 2006b). Debate about the extent to which implementation and integration of reproductive health services has taken place continues, but the underlying need for increased resources (from both donors and national governments) and ensuring accountability remain areas of concern.

There is also resistance to integration. In a telling contretemps, some policy notables who previously embraced ICPD and reproductive health have called for a return to the good old days of family planning when success meant ensuring that couples had their contraceptive needs met. Health advocates and academics have published articles in leading medical and health policy journals, such as the *Lancet*, advocating a "break from the prevailing international discourse that cloaks family planning in the term reproductive and sexual health," arguing that conflating the two "obfuscates rather than clarifies priorities" (Cleland et al. 2006: 14–15).

Such a repudiation of "reproductive health" in favor of family planning (also known as contraception) speaks volumes in the current context of global health (Brown, Cueto, and Fee 2006).[6] This approach to global health has brought with it a tendency to favor disease-specific or intervention-specific approaches to public health—such as addressing the global HIV epidemics with a dedicated fund and a campaign for vaccine development (or more recently universal access to treatment) (Birn 2005; Katz 2005). Vertical approaches to health are not new (Brown, Cueto, and Fee 2006). However they are antithetical to ICPD's comprehensive, life cycle and public health approach. ICPD considers the range of social, cultural, political, and economic contexts that disempower women and make it difficult for them to exercise meaningful decision making about their reproduction. In many ways, family planning is the technical fix reproductive health has to offer; it is more amenable to the vertical approach and is more easily measured than other reproductive health approaches. Yet a basic critique of vertical approaches remains that while these targeted efforts may be relatively efficient and amenable to measurement, they do not address the underlying factors such as poverty and discrimination that directly affect the health and well-being of women and men in developing countries, and which more basically affect people's decisions about family planning. ICPD, through its explicit incorporation of human rights as an essential component, provides a framework to approach these fundamental causes.

Global health issues have been able to capture funding with remarkable speed and scope, particularly in comparison to resources for ICPD. An analysis of donor funding from 2000 to 2004 found that funding for "global health," as opposed to "international health" or any other collective heading, has been steadily increasing since 2000 and approached $14 billion in 2004 (Kates, Morison, and Lief 2006). This increased funding comes from several sources, and global health is commanding an increasingly large portion of official development assistance as well. The World Bank's spending on health reached a peak of $3.4 billion in

2003 "before falling back to $2.1 billion in 2006, with $87 million of that spent on HIV/AIDS, TB, and malaria programs and $250 million on child and maternal health" (Garrett 2007: 4, online version). Private foundation spending also increased. "Between 1995 and 2005, total giving by all U.S. charitable foundations tripled, and the portion of money dedicated to international projects soared 80 percent, with global health representing more than a third of that sum" (Garrett 2007: 3, online version). ICPD was unique in its preparation of cost estimates for implementation of a package of reproductive health services. These estimates, used to mobilize financial resources for reproductive health from both donor countries and developing countries, have not been met by either donors or national governments. After a peak in funding for reproductive health and population in 1995, resources for reproductive health remained relatively flat until 2002, when there was a jump, mainly due to increased global funding for HIV/AIDS (see Merrick and Reichenbach, both in this volume).

It is our contention that the prevailing enchantment with vertical global campaigns and emphasis on funding only specific health issues considered relevant to "global health" disadvantages ICPD's holistic approach.[7] Concepts of market rationality, benchmarks, and targets imported from business and management do not reflect the complex realities in which we live. For instance, it is a challenge to account both financially and politically for efforts to reform laws and policies; it is relatively simpler to account for how many bed nets have been purchased and distributed. But much of reproductive health is not a single disease or health intervention amenable to this type of vertical approach. Although critical for ensuring accountability and assuring donors that their money is being well spent, measurement of reproductive health indicators are uniquely challenging (see Kaufman, Reichenbach, and Bloom and Canning, all this volume). ICPD emphasized the role that underlying social conditions play in health, especially those that foster women's capacities to make decisions about when and whether to have children, to access qualified medical care when necessary, to live free from coercion and violence, and to control their own sexuality. One cannot develop a vaccine to accomplish this: addressing underlying social conditions is slow, costly, often difficult to achieve, and not solely one sector's responsibility.[8] A broader understanding is required of what the "global health agenda" is. How reproductive health and rights fit both retrospectively and prospectively into this agenda is also necessary, in order to hold onto the conceptual gains of the Cairo paradigm and shore up the weak points (see Reichenbach, this volume).

ICPD: Expanding and Strengthening the Networks

The various conceptual and programmatic approaches used to address reproductive health and rights have not occurred in a static world. Whether in the euphoria following the 1989 fall of the Berlin wall, when human rights expanded around the globe, or during the period of fear and defensiveness kicked off by 9-11, interpretations of ICPD have evolved in a changing world. The prevailing international tendency— what we have called neovertical approaches to global health—presents a potentially competing paradigm of health care delivery and outcomes to the comprehensive and inclusive approach of ICPD. Where and how does reproductive health fit into this new paradigm, particularly when the concepts guiding "global health" challenge or even contradict the rights-and-health approach of ICPD? Are global health and ICPD irreconcilable?

Currently, the major new global health funds (e.g., Global Fund to Fight AIDS, Tuberculosis and Malaria), important bilateral donors such as the U.S. government, and large private foundations such as the Bill and Melinda Gates, John D. and Catherine T. MacArthur, and Rockefeller Foundations fragment ICPD. They tend to fund only specific elements of the ICPD Programme of Action—HIV/AIDS or maternal mortality, for example, rather than the range of underlying conditions that contribute to reproductive health. Although technical approaches have always been an important part of public health solutions (Brown, Cueto, and Fee 2006), the new funding environment challenges the ability to fund intersectoral and integrated sexual and reproductive and rights health interventions as envisioned by ICPD. A good example comes from the United States, where recently social and cultural conservatives have been able to undermine the entire concept of reproductive rights. It is particularly prevalent in the United States, and worrisome, because in absolute terms the U.S. contributes the most toward global reproductive health issues (PAI 2004a).

The rejection of human rights in relation to health can be seen in current U.S. Agency for International Development (USAID) health policies and programs.[9] Now part of the Department of State, USAID's "commitment to improving global health . . . includes child, maternal, and reproductive health, and the reduction of abortion and disease, especially HIV/AIDS, malaria, and tuberculosis" (USAID 2006a). That USAID considers as one joint goal addressing child, maternal, and reproductive health and reducing abortion suggests a distancing of its program from the broader formulation of reproductive health as defined by ICPD. Moreover, the USAID website link from the word "reproductive health" takes readers to the page entitled "Family Planning." Family ng—and only family planning, states USAID—is reproductive health; family planning provides direct health benefits for women (reduces high risk pregnancies, fights HIV/AIDS, reduces abortion), children (longer spaced intervals), and the environment (USAID 2006b). What is lost when policies transition from a focus on "reproductive rights"—as stated in ICPD—to "family planning"—USAID's wording— is support for women's rights, opportunities for employment, and full participation in society. The entire point of ICPD was that picking and choosing among services and approaches would not achieve the development gains and health improvements that governments so desired for their populations. To leave off the delicate agenda points (for instance, adolescents' access to reproductive health services) because they contradicted deep-seated cultural views was precisely what ICPD counseled against. Setting priorities among areas was anticipated, not wholesale sidestepping.[10]

The gains of ICPD are not all lost, however. There appears to be an increasing recognition that although health improvements may be achieved through technological approaches, they will not be sustainable unless underlying political, social, cultural, and economic determinants are addressed as well (Boseley 2006; Birn 2005; Katz 2005). In addition, reproductive health as defined and conceptualized at ICPD has been adopted as part of the "global health agenda" of international organizations such as WHO, bilateral donors such as DFID (Department for International Development, the UK bilateral overseas development agency) and SIDA (the Swedish International Development Agency), and private foundations such as the Ford Foundation. WHO, for example, places "promoting universal coverage, gender equality, and health-related human rights" as the third agenda item (out of seven) on its general program of work on global health. In its elaboration of this point, WHO states that "Ensuring everyone's right to the enjoyment of the highest attainable standard of health entails expanding access to sexual and reproductive health care for all" (WHO 2006a: 15).

The viability and utility of ICPD, however, has evolved differently in different parts of the world. The perception of ICPD and its place in the global health agenda differs widely whether viewed from Peru, Bangladesh, Uganda, or the United States. The ownership and design of the global health agenda may occur at the level of international institutions, multilaterals, and bilateral agencies, but the implementation of the priorities that emerge from that agenda takes place at regional, national, and community levels. This distinction between the global health agenda and what transpires at the national levels is seen by some as a detriment to furthering the reproductive health agenda. Many advocates are concerned that if reproductive health is not prominently on the agenda (designated as a separate MDG, for example), then it will be left behind while global health moves forward. In others' eyes, however, the opportunity to operate out of the glare and distraction of international politics allows countries or communities to "just get on with it" and continue to implement reproductive health and rights. How this will turn out will obviously vary from context to context, and the future is far from sure. While there are differences in how ICPD plays out at the international and national levels, the discussion at the international level shapes the language and strategies of women's health advocates and policymakers in implementing reproductive health programs at the national level. A current example is the need to describe the importance of reproductive health in terms of poverty reduction to maintain national funding for reproductive health activities.

Despite these uncertainties in a time of flux, there is no question that the fundamental concepts embodied in ICPD continue to buttress global public health arguments. For scholars and practitioners, women's health and rights activists, and researchers, the theoretical and actual gains of ICPD have been enormous, and ICPD has been the framework that joined together underlying social determinants, health systems, policies, laws, and human rights related to reproductive health. The architecture of global health may have fragmented the ICPD framework. But this fragmentation need not be one of splintering; it may be one of fostering networked nodes—perhaps no longer organized according to the numbered paragraphs of the Programme of Action, but geometrically strengthened and connected in more efficient ways (Valente and Davis 1999). It should be recalled that ICPD is the product of a network of transnational actors. Transnational advocacy groups are networks of people that include both experts and activists with a common value or principle that motivates them to work in a particular issue area. Transnational networks, because they are dispersed locally, nationally, regionally, and internationally, have inherent dynamism and flexibility, even as they are united by common ideas (Keck and Sikkink 1998). They have been able to put issues such as domestic violence on international agendas by appealing to common concerns and taking advantage of political opportunities to generate attention to issues. These transnational networks were critical for ICPD and these networks still have salience today. Whether reproductive health today resembles the way ICPD articulated it may be less important than ensuring that the connections between gender, rights, health, and development are maintained and strengthened. Creating alliances and building coalitions with new actors beyond the field of reproductive health and rights is the way forward for reproductive health and ICPD in the current context framed by "global health." The chapters in this book suggest that reproductive health still matters but less as a framework and more as a network for exploring complex relationships—institutional, individual, and conceptual—necessary for the achievement of ICPD in the larger context of global health. Reproductive health, viewed as a network of related concerns and bound together by the conviction that human rights, equality, nondiscrimination, participation, and accountability are inseparable elements of health and health systems, can thrive in this new global health framework.

Chapter 2
The Global Reproductive Health and Rights Agenda: Opportunities and Challenges for the Future

Laura Reichenbach

There is mounting suspicion among many in the field of reproductive health that reproductive health and rights have become increasingly marginalized on the global policy agenda since the 1994 ICPD conference (El Feki 2004; Gillespie 2004a,b; Sinding 2005a, 2006). An editorial in a *Lancet* series on sexual and reproductive health claims that reproductive health "has been utterly marginalized from the global conversation about health and wellbeing during the past decade" (Horton 2006: 1549). Another article in the same series refers to the last twelve years of reproductive health as a "sorry tale," in part because "sexual and reproductive health has dropped down the international development agenda" (Glasier and Gulmezoglu 2006: 1550). However, not everyone shares such pessimistic views on the state of the reproductive health agenda. Others in the field, particularly those in the women's health movement who were architects of ICPD, are trying to fuel optimism about the state of reproductive health and rights, referring to ICPD as "vigorously alive" and arguing that, when it comes to reproductive health, the glass is "half-full" rather than "half-empty" (Germain and Kidwell 2005; Germain and Dixon-Mueller 2005).

So which of these perspectives most accurately reflects the reality of the reproductive health agenda today? Is there evidence that reproductive health has "fallen off" the global agenda? And if so, what explains this decline and what are the implications for the future? Most important, what are some strategies for ensuring that sexual and reproductive health maintain or increase its visibility on the global policy agenda? This chapter addresses these questions based on a critical analysis of the recent literature on reproductive health. It examines evidence as to where reproductive health is or is not on the global policy agenda and how that may have changed over time; it highlights some major influences affecting the global reproductive health agenda since ICPD; and finally, it suggests strategic areas where the field might maintain as well as improve the status of reproductive health on the global policy agenda.

The Global Policy Agenda and Reproductive Health

For the purposes of this chapter the term "global policy agenda"[1] refers to the myriad health and development issues that the international policy community (which includes international institutions, multilateral and bilateral agencies, and funding and donor agencies) are attending to at any one time. This adapts Kingdon's (1984) definition of agenda, "the list of subjects or problems to which governmental officials, and people outside the government closely associated with those officials, are paying some serious attention at any given time" (1984: 3). This definition allows that the global policy agenda is not encapsulated in a single or set of written documents that guide officials and policy makers as to which issues to assign priority and allocate resources. Rather, it considers the agenda to include the range of health and development issues that decision makers and those who influence them consider.

The global policy agenda as conceived of in this chapter is fluid and influenced, at times unpredictably, by politics, economics, and evidence that persuade policy makers an issue is a problem that requires attention. These influences may come indirectly (e.g., media attention associated with a celebrity) or through the mechanism of bureaucratic machineries or institutional politics (e.g., international meetings or the UN conference process).

An effort to examine and better understand the intersections of reproductive health and ICPD with the global policy agenda is worthwhile given the concern expressed by some in the field, especially practitioners and policy makers, that reproductive health has lost its cachet and is no longer part of the lexicon of international policy makers. If this is so, the hard-earned gains of ICPD may be diminished, or even lost. Policy makers must allocate limited money, time, and attention among a host of competing health and development issues. Issues that are firmly situated on the global policy agenda are more likely to garner resources, not just financial, but political and institutional as well.

These concerns are based on a presumption that the global policy agenda affects national and subnational policy agendas. However, this influence is not straightforward (Lee and Walt 1995); several factors influence the agenda setting process at the national level, including local culture and politics.

Examining the Reproductive Health Agenda

Determining the status of reproductive health on the complex global policy agenda depends on how the reproductive health agenda itself is defined. It is not a single agenda that all stakeholders agree upon. For policy makers and practitioners in the field, the reproductive health and rights (or sexual and reproductive health) agenda is often defined as the individual components outlined in the ICPD Programme of Action (UN 1995). For others, including women's health activists and feminists, the reproductive health agenda is primarily defined by the fundamental concepts and arguments of ICPD—addressing the health and social interventions required to achieve gender equality and equity in the context of human rights and reproductive rights. As the reproductive health agenda is not clear cut, identifying points of intersection with the larger global health agenda is not a straightforward process.

The situation is further complicated because the reproductive health agenda is defined and implemented at several levels—international, national, and subnational. Each country implements ICPD according to its specific political, economic, and social contexts. In many countries, particularly those that have undergone decentralization processes, subnational (provincial or district level) reproductive health agendas may differ from the national one. For the purposes of the arguments here, this chapter focuses on the reproductive health agenda at the global level and defines reproductive health as the underlying cross-sectional components of the ICPD Programme of Action that address gender equality, equity, women's empowerment, and reproductive health and rights. The chapter considers their treatment by the international community, which includes international institutions, multilateral and bilateral agencies, and funding and donor agencies including private foundations.

Is Reproductive Health on the Global Policy Agenda?

Determining whether something is on or off the agenda is not an objective process in which a certain threshold is met. Yet there are several types of evidence that can help to determine an issue's status on the policy agenda. This chapter suggests assessing three areas to determine an issue's agenda status: (1) visibility of the issue on the global political and policy stage; (2) level of resources being spent on the issue; and (3) whether explicit solutions or interventions to address the problem exist and are advocated.

One area of evidence is the level of attention paid by policy makers and other influential people. This can be determined by examining policy documents, conference proceedings, political statements, and media attention. Cumbersome though this may be, it is useful for determining whether an issue is a priority on the agenda (Reichenbach 2002).

Examining the financial resources allocated to a particular issue is a more objective way to assess and compare the level of international attention. Expenditure of funds helps promote accountability and ownership of an issue. Collecting data on resource allocation, while relatively straightforward, is not always easy, particularly for the many interventions of ICPD that are both cross-sectoral (e.g., improving educational opportunities for girls) and highly individualized (e.g., providing maternal health services in a maternal and child health setting) (Ethelston and Leahy 2006; Powell-Jackson et al. 2006).

A final indicator of attention to an issue is whether a specific solution or intervention is associated with it. This affects the status of an issue on the policy agenda by increasing the likelihood that there will be advocacy for an issue by a group or community that takes ownership of an issue and shepherds it onto a policy agenda. Moreover, a clearly stated intervention for a problem increases the likelihood that policy makers will take action on it.[2] The next section briefly reviews the reproductive health agenda from these three perspectives over three time periods: pre-ICPD (1970s and 1980s), during the ICPD preparatory process and at ICPD (early 1990s), and post-ICPD (1995–present).

Reproductive Health and the Global Policy Agenda Prior to ICPD

Reproductive health today, thanks to ICPD, is commonly understood as more than population and family planning or safe motherhood. Prior to ICPD, however, reproductive health was primarily constituted by these individual issues and addressed by separate and mostly technical and scientific communities. Reproductive health at ICPD, in part, grew out of and in response to the issue of rapid population growth and country experience with family planning programs. During the 1970s and 1980s, population and population policy were an integral and highly visible part of the international development agenda. Neo-Malthusian arguments about the impact of overpopulation on efforts to reduce poverty and sustain the environment were compelling for many at the time and evident in the outcomes of two high-level United Nations conferences on population—Bucharest in 1974 and Mexico City in 1984 (Finkle and Crane 1985, 1975). The Bucharest conference became widely associated with the slogan, "development is the best contraceptive," while the

Mexico City conference was well known for the U.S. role in politicizing the issue of abortion. While the processes and outcomes of these conferences were different in their policy implications, they both placed population and family planning squarely on the global agenda.

The resources allocated by the international community to population activities also reflect the importance of population on the global policy agenda. Figure 1 is a reproduction of Schindlmayr's (2004) analysis of donor trends in population assistance and shows an increasing but inconsistent flow of international financial resources allocated to population activities from the 1960s to 1995. As Schindlmayr points out, funding for population assistance increased rapidly by 1970 and continued to increase throughout the 1970s. After falling off in the early 1980s it began to spike prior to both the Mexico City and Cairo conferences and was then followed by a visible decline. This pattern may reflect the increased advocacy leading up to these conferences. Schindlmayr's analysis describes variation in the share of overseas development assistance (ODA) going to population activities over this time period, with a large increase in the 1960s and 1970s when population was roughly 2 percent of ODA. During the 1980s, population as a share of ODA declined to an average of 1.2 percent.

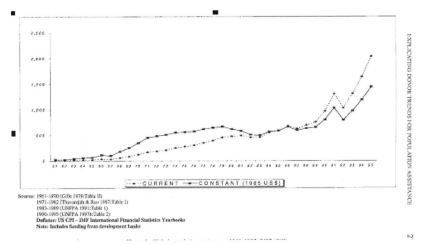

Figure 1. Global population assistance, 1961–1995. Reproduced from Schindlmayr (2004: 27, Fig. 1).

During this period, the issue of population growth became closely linked by demographers, government officials, and policy makers with its solution—the need to decrease fertility and halt rapid population growth in underdeveloped countries perceived as a threat to global environmental and political stability. The intervention proposed by demographers and population scientists to achieve this was widespread use of family planning. Demographers and population scientists took ownership of the population issue; many of them worked closely with and advised policy makers, ensuring family planning and population's visible status on the development policy agenda.

Reproductive Health and the Global Policy Agenda During the Preparatory Committee Process and at ICPD

During the preparatory committee process, which included several years leading up to and during ICPD itself, reproductive health (defined beyond provision of family planning) actively engaged with a broader set of development issues (e.g., gender equality and equity, women's empowerment, education, environmental sustainability, and improved health outcomes). This is evident in the expanded base of institutions involved in the ICPD preparatory process, which included NGOs and activists working on environmental, poverty, population, and reproductive health and rights issues. Reproductive health was portrayed as integral to realizing a range of development objectives based on arguments beyond fertility reduction and environmental sustainability. The preparatory process was marked by well-organized regional and international meetings of women's health and rights activists. These meetings resulted in a series of dialogues and debates that provided the foundation for the concepts and language that came out of ICPD. A number of articles in the academic and lay press and high profile political speeches related to reproductive health were published during this time. The women's health advocates who spearheaded this work were extremely savvy about ensuring opportunities for media and other coverage of their concerns. As a result, reproductive health became more entrenched and visible on the global policy agenda.

As part of the ICPD preparatory process, economists, demographers, and other experts prepared resource estimates for implementing aspects of the Programme of Action. Referred to as the "costed package," paragraph 13.15 states that these resource estimates are for implementing "programmes in the area of reproductive health, including those related to family planning, maternal health and the prevention of sexually transmitted diseases, as well as other basic actions for collecting and analyzing population data, [and] will cost: $17 billion in 2000, $18.5 billion in 2005, $20.5 billion in 2010, and $21.7 billion in 2015" (para. 13.15). The Programme of Action designated that donors pay one-third of these estimated costs while national governments cover the remaining two-thirds. ICPD was the first UN conference to prepare such resource estimates and they were intended to serve as an advocacy tool for both donor countries and governments of developing countries. Prior to and just after ICPD there was an increase in funds for population and reproductive health (see Figure 1).

Unlike rapid population growth, reproductive health as defined at Cairo did not have a single solution or technological intervention associated with it. ICPD resulted in a paradigm shift in thinking about how to improve women's lives by proposing a rights-based approach to the provision of reproductive health services, to achieve broader development goals of gender equality, equity, and women's empowerment. While several of the Programme of Action's individual components (e.g., family planning or maternal mortality reduction) continued to be associated with particular solutions, the reproductive health agenda in its holistic form was not characterized by a specific intervention. The lack of specific interventions at the time of ICPD has had implications for its operationalization post-ICPD.

Reproductive Health and the Global Policy Agenda After ICPD

Immediately following ICPD and until the late 1990s, reproductive health continued to be an integral part of the broader development agenda. This is documented in the deliberate adoption of Cairo in a series of high level international conferences. The specific language and/or underlying principles of Cairo were reaffirmed in several global conferences including the Fourth World Conference on Women in Beijing in 1995, the World Summit for Social Development in Copenhagen in 1995, the five-year review of ICPD in New York, and various sessions of the UN Commission on Population and Development (see Girard, this volume). Attention to ICPD was also reinforced in the large number of country case studies and academic articles assessing the implementation (Haberland and Measham 2002; Hardee et al. 1999). Discussions about how to implement ICPD were common among donors, academics, and international and national policy makers during the 1990s.

However, since 2000, many implementers and practitioners have maintained that reproductive health is less visible on the global policy agenda (Langer 2006; Glasier and Gulmezoglu 2006). As evidence, they point to the decision not to hold a high-profile ten-year review of the ICPD conference and, perhaps most glaring, the exclusion of reproductive health as a Millennium Development Goal (Sinding 2005a; Crossette 2005). The implications for reproductive health of its omission as a separate MDG are debated by academics, advocates, and practitioners alike.[3]

Some academics and activists feel exclusion from the MDG list is not necessarily a disaster (Basu 2005), while some policy makers put it bluntly, "If
you're not an MDG, you're not on the agenda. If you're not a line item,
you're out of the game" (Steve Sinding, in Crossette 2005: 77). Some
women's health advocates and practitioners (Langer 2006) have been assuaged by the inclusion of reproductive health as an MDG target at the
2005 World Summit (UN 2005a, para. 57(g)). Regardless of the implications, most agree that reproductive health was not a specific MDG because of its political nature[4] and the hesitancy to put it front and center
on the global agenda at a time of conservative politics.

At the risk of unfairly generalizing, women's health advocates, many
of whom were pivotal to the Cairo process, tend to project a more positive attitude about the current status of reproductive health. Some, like
Adrienne Germain, argue that ICPD is a "living document" with its fundamental principles and intent adapted and reflected in evolving policies and statements (Germain and Kidwell 2005). Sonia Correa cautions
that ten years in the ICPD process is not a long time and that a more
realistic longer term view must be taken when assessing the fate of reproductive health and rights (Correa et al. 2005).

Other evidence offered for the demise of reproductive health is a
decline in resources for reproductive health and rights since ICPD
(Merrick 2005; Speidel 2005). The resource targets for the "costed package" in the Programme of Action have not been met. As Table 1 shows,
neither donors nor developing countries met their targets for the year
2000. Since then, donor funding has increased, but it is still below what
is thought necessary to implement the costed package. In 2002 and
2003, donors met only 40 percent of their ICPD commitments (in real
terms) (Ethelston and Leahy 2006). (See Merrick, this volume for analysis and explanation of donor assistance trends post-Cairo.)

There are several explanations why the resource targets set at Cairo
have not been met. These include a sense that population and reproductive health are no longer salient as a development issue because of
the fertility decline that has occurred in many parts of the world
(Gillespie 2004; Blanc and Tsui 2005); that donor priorities have shifted
to other issues; and that the resource estimates no longer reflect the reality of programming reproductive health. For example, the original
ICPD cost estimates significantly underestimated the HIV/AIDS epidemic. In the Programme of Action the $18.5 billion estimated for re-
productive health in 2005 included $1.4 billion for "sexually transmitted
infections, including HIV/AIDS. Ten years later, HIV/AIDS alone needs
more than $10 billion for 2005" (Ethelston and Leahy 2006: 39).

Although the Programme of Action cost estimates have not been met,
the trend in donor resources for population and reproductive health

TABLE 1. Programme of Action Resources for Costed Package: Estimated and Actual

	2000	2001	2002	2003	2004	2005	2010	2015
Targets for costed package	$17 billion $5.7 billion (donors) $11.3 billion (domestic)	n.a.	n.a.	n.a.	n.a.	$18.5 billion $6.1 billion (donors) $12.4 billion (domestic)	$20.5 billion $6.8 billion (donors) $13.5 billion (domestic)	$21.7 billion $7.2 billion (donors) $14.3 billion (domestic)
Actual resources by source	Donors $1.975 billion Domestic $3.5 billion	Donors $2.06 billion Domestic $1.5 billion	Donors $2.878 billion Domestic (data not collected)	Donors $4.189 billion Domestic $11.7 billion	Donors $5.2 billion Domestic $14.5 billion	Donors $5.8 billion Domestic $14.9 billion	n.a.	n.a.

Sources: UNFPA, NIDI (various years).

has increased since 2000. Estimates of donor spending on population, reproductive health, and HIV/AIDS show an increase from $4.7 billion in 2003 to $5.3 billion in 2004. "Estimates for 2005 show that donor funding increased to $6.1 billion" (statement by A. Pawliczko, New York, 3 April 2006). Population as a percentage of ODA reached a high of 5.12 percent, up from 3.65 percent in 2002 (UNFPA 2005a). In 2003, population assistance was 11.45 percent of U.S. total overseas development assistance (UNFPA 2005b). Figure 2 shows primary population assistance funds from the decade beginning in 2003.

While overall amounts of international assistance for population and reproductive health have increased, the reproductive health community has expressed concern that the distribution of those resources has been shifted from family planning and reproductive health to HIV/AIDS. Figure 3 shows quite clearly that during the period 1995-2003 resources for family planning declined while resources for HIV/AIDS increased sharply. Donor spending on reproductive health in 2002 and 2003 was close to $3 billion. Shiffman's (2008) analysis of donor spending shows that donor spending on HIV/AIDS in 1992 was 7.7 percent of health and population assistance and this figure had risen to 23.5 percent of donor health and population assistance by 2005. During the same time period, aid for population decreased from 32.1 percent to 8.0 percent of health and population aid. A recent meeting of the UN Commission on

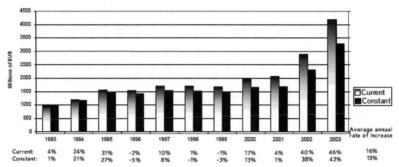

FIGURE 2. PRIMARY FUNDS FOR POPULATION ASSISTANCE, IN CURRENT AND CONSTANT DOLLARS, WITH PERCENTAGE CHANGE, 1993-2003

Figure 2. Primary funds for population assistance, current and constant dollars, with percentage change, 1993–2003. UNFPA 2005a.

Population and Development reported that ICPD estimates are not being met. While ICPD estimated 8 percent of total population assistance for STDs/HIV/AIDS, actual spending in 2005 was 72 percent. Absolute dollar amounts for family planning "are lower than they were in 1995" with family planning as a percentage of all population assistance decreasing from 55 percent in 1995 to 7 percent in 2005; funding for reproductive health services declined to 17 percent (Deen 2008: np).

There is evidence that funding for HIV/AIDS has increased dramatically, and possibly at a cost to family planning and reproductive health (Shiffman 2008). "During the last 10 years, spending on HIV/AIDS has increased by 300 percent" (Sinding 2005b: 5). Of the $6 billion in population assistance projected for 2005, "donors are deploying close to 60 percent to address the HIV/AIDS pandemic, while reproductive health and family planning activities are benefiting from less than 25 percent and 10 percent of total funds, respectively" (Ethelston and Leahy 2006: 1). During this period there was also the creation of funding mechanisms that specifically targeted HIV/AIDS. For example, the creation in 2003 in the United States of the President's Emergency Plan for AIDS Relief (PEPFAR) called for $15 billion to be spent in 16 countries over five years. Reproductive health areas beyond HIV/AIDS also show a dilution of funds. A recent estimate of donor spending on maternal, newborn, and child health found that $2.935 and $3.481 billion of ODA went to maternal, neonatal, and child health activities in 2005 and 2006; however, child health accounted for more than two-thirds of ODA in these areas (Powell-Jackson et al. 2006; Greco et al. 2008).

The interventions for achieving the Programme of Action after ICPD were not clear-cut, and evidence did not point to a clear or easily imple-

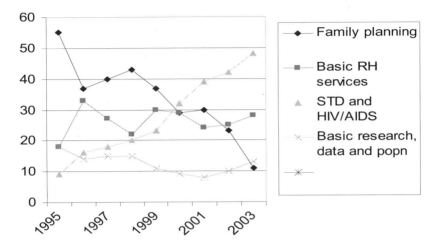

Figure 3. Donor expenditure for population assistance by category. UNFPA 2005b.

mented solution. Different approaches to operationalizing reproductive health were offered; calls for rights-based approaches (Jacobson 2000) and interventions that addressed health sector reforms were made (Ravindran and de Pinho 2005). These different approaches were not always clearly articulated among all stakeholders and resulted in discussion and debate as to how to address reproductive health. This made it difficult to advocate a solution for reproductive health on the agenda. Furthermore, national examples and case studies produced during this time showed variation in models and approaches to implementing reproductive health thus moving the evidence base away from a single easily replicable approach.[5]

Based on this brief analysis of measures of policy attention, financial resources, and advocacy of solutions or interventions, there does appear to have been a decline in the status of reproductive health on the global policy agenda since 2000. What explains this decline, and what are its implications for the future of reproductive health?

Explaining the Decline in Reproductive Health on the Global Policy Agenda

Several explanations have been offered for the decline in attention to reproductive health, including lack of financial resources to effectively implement the ICPD agenda (Speidel 2005; UNFPA 2005b); insufficient political will to address reproductive health and rights (Jahan and Germain 2004); the effect of successful fertility decline in much of the developing world (Gillespie 2004a; Blanc and Tsui 2005); and an agenda thought to be too diffuse to be easily implemented (Sinding 2006). Three reasons for the decline in attention will be examined below: the current political and policy environment in which reproductive health operates; the changing development policy agenda; and the increased focus on global health.

The Global Political and Policy Environment and the Reproductive Health Agenda

An important factor in the declining status of reproductive health on the global agenda is the political context in which reproductive health and rights must operate. The current conservative political environment in the United States has had a particularly significant impact. The U.S. influence is evident in the highly visible role the U.S. played at earlier UN conferences on population (see Finkle and MacIntosh 2002; Finkle and Crane 1985). It is also apparent in its long history of financial support for global population and reproductive health activities: "Since 1965, USAID has obligated over $6.6 billion in assistance for international population planning" (Nowels 2003: CRS-11). The United States remains the leading donor in terms of global share of development assistance for HIV/AIDS and population; it provided 11 percent of donor assistance in 2003 (Speidel 2005). A recent study comparing the average share of funding for population activities for the 21 OECD donor countries found the United States to be the major donor over the period 1996-2002, providing more than 75 percent of donor support for family planning activities and 60 percent for HIV/AIDS (Van Dalen and Reuser 2006).

While not the only donor—continued financial support for reproductive health and rights by European and especially Scandinavian countries is considerable—the United States remains an important influence on the reproductive health agenda at both global and national levels. U.S. influence at the national level is manifest in its provision of technical assistance to countries around the world as well. In 2003 67 percent of U.S. funding for population and reproductive health was provided through cooperating agencies that provide funds and technical assistance at the country level (Speidel 2005). The U.S. can put political pressure on recipients of U.S. foreign assistance for population and reproductive health. The threat of withholding assistance when the recipient organization or government does not abide by certain expectations (such as adhering to the Global Gag Rule[6]) is a powerful influence on the content of the reproductive health agenda at the national level.

The conservative politics and policy decisions of the George W. Bush administration have also imposed significant political barriers to reproductive health. A detailed recounting of this has been done elsewhere in this book (Girard and Kissling, both in this volume). Bush's reinstatement of the Mexico City Policy, the increasing role of the religious right in public health policies, and the lack of political support for reproductive health from the U.S. delegation at regional conferences in preparation for ICPD+10 represent attempts to "turn back the clock" in the language and scope of reproductive health and rights. A change in U.S. administration might alter this conservative agenda, depending on the composition of the government. However, in the current political climate, the reach of U.S. influence on reproductive health and rights has broadened beyond the issue of abortion to include issues related to sexuality, contraception, and women's rights. It may take sustained effort to redirect the effects of eight years of Bush administration policies, especially since they are but one of the factors which have constrained ICPD.

The Influence of Broader Development Policy

The status of reproductive health has also been affected by changes in the broader health and development policy environment since ICPD. The growing HIV/AIDS epidemics, increased attention to poverty reduction, and new funding mechanisms have had important effects.

The increasing HIV/AIDS epidemic has affected funding, political attention, and human resources for reproductive health (see Gruskin, this volume). As already discussed, spending for HIV/AIDS has increased at the expense of reproductive health and family planning, and further increases in HIV/AIDS spending are expected, based on revised estimates of the costs of addressing the epidemic. "The 2006 UN General Assembly high level meeting on AIDS called for annual HIV expenditure in low and middle income countries to rise from $8.3 billion in 2005 to around $23 billion by 2010" (England 2007: 344). There is debate as to whether current spending on HIV/AIDS is justified given the burden of HIV in the context of other diseases (see DeLay, Greener, and Izazola 2007; England 2007).

The rapid growth and sheer size of funding for HIV/AIDS has affected the structure of health spending and systems. Some argue that HIV "has produced the biggest vertical programme in history, with its own staff, systems, and structure" (England 2007: 344). The impact is the potential underfunding of other diseases and the creation of separate health structures and delivery systems that hinder other health services. Others see HIV funding as an opportunity to strengthen the health system: HIV "should provide an opportunity and entry point for strengthening health and social service systems if it is used appropriately" (DeLay, Greener, and Izazola 2007: 345). While potential exists for reproductive health to be integrated into HIV service provision, some may view the proposition in zero-sum terms (see Gruskin, this volume).

Poverty Reduction and the MDGs

Poverty reduction has become the focus of the larger development agenda as witness the huge focus on achieving the MDGs. Reproductive health is overshadowed by the MDGs not just by exclusion (as discussed earlier) but because of the need to justify reproductive health interventions and ICPD in terms of achievement of the MDG goals, particularly the first MDG on poverty reduction. The reproductive health field is under pressure to document the relationship between reproductive health and poverty. As Greene and Merrick (2005) find in their review of the literature on reproductive health and poverty, there is a dearth of evidence on this relationship; what does exist has not been used in a compelling way, and the pathways are not clear. There is a need for more research and evidence collection to convince Ministries of Finance and Planning that investments in reproductive health contribute to poverty reduction.

New Funding Mechanisms

The increased attention to poverty reduction has created new funding strategies in development assistance that present challenges for reproductive health. Donors have moved to broader mechanisms such as general budget support or the Poverty Reduction Strategy (PRS) process, which devolves allocation of specific funds to the country level. The number of countries participating in the PRSP approach has more than doubled since 2002 to over 50 (Vogel 2006). The PRSP process makes it easier for specific health issues to become lost and more difficult to track funds allocated to a particular issue (Merrick, this volume).

At the other end of the funding spectrum are highly visible disease-specific funding campaigns. One high profile example is the Global Fund to Fight AIDS, Tuberculosis, and Malaria created in 2002. "Since its birth, it has approved $6.6 billion in proposals and dispersed $2.9 billion toward them. . . . The fund estimates that it now provides 20 percent of all global support for HIV/AIDS programs and 66 percent of the funding for efforts to combat TB and malaria" (Garrett 2007: 4, online version). Countries spend time and resources submitting proposals to the Global Fund through a unique process involving country coordinating mechanisms. Beyond the obvious attention to HIV/AIDS, reproductive health writ large is usually not part of these proposals. Perhaps in response to this exclusion, a global fund for maternal and child health has been suggested as a mechanism to ensure that funds are made available and donors are held accountable for the achievement of MDG-4 (Reduction of child mortality) and MDG-5 (Improve maternal health) (Costello and Osrin 2005).

Because of their predominance on the global health agenda, HIV/AIDS and the MDGs are seen by some as carts that reproductive health should hitch itself to in order to remain on the policy agenda and ensure continued funding. The reproductive health community has been left scrambling to respond to calls for how reproductive health relates both to HIV/AIDS and poverty reduction. ICPD could not have predicted these new forces on the global agenda. As a result, the groundwork in terms of evidence collection was not laid at ICPD and is now being done so hurriedly, perhaps adding to the sense by practitioners of reproductive health being left behind.

The Increased Importance of Global Health

As mentioned in the introduction to this volume, the increased importance of global health, which adopts a particular approach to funding, accountability, and measurement, has troubled the status of reproductive health on the policy agenda.[7] Global health is driving the increase in U.S. and European overseas development assistance, as well as that of the World Bank and private foundations (Garrett 2007; Ethelston 2004a). Despite this increase in funds for global health, recent estimates suggest that more money is needed. Jeffrey Sachs in 2001 argued that $20 billion a year was needed to address global health (Sachs 2001). "Estimates of the additional donor assistance required every year to achieve the MDGs by 2015 range from U.S.$50 billion to $100 billion" (Ethelston 2004a: 39). Whether accurate or not, these global estimates have been useful for advocacy for global health issues. While more money is available for global health, reproductive health still must compete for financial and other resources among an agenda of a larger set of issues.

The way these funds are programmed also impacts reproductive health. Popular interpretations of global health are marked by a vertical approach to programming with a preference for disease-specific large-scale interventions that often take the form of high profile global initiatives (e.g., WHO 3 x 5 Initiative). Reproductive health is unique in the breadth of issues that define it; it encompasses an array of health issues and interventions—some, such as improving women's empowerment, which requires multisectoral approaches. Reproductive health is a complex concept as opposed to a specific health strategy to be addressed through a well-financed and highly publicized international initiatives such as Roll Back Malaria or Stop TB Initiative (Shiffman et al. 2002). There is no "magic bullet" approach for reproductive health that easily fits the focus on vertical programs so popular in global health today.

The increasingly dominant funding and agenda setting role of a few large U.S.-based private foundations in today's global health environment cannot be overlooked. "As of August 2006, in its six years of existence, the Bill and Melinda Gates Foundation had given away $6.6 billion for global health programs. Of that total, nearly $2 billion had been spent on programs aimed at TB and HIV/AIDS and other sexually transmitted diseases" (Garrett 2007: 3, online version). While this increase in funding for global health is laudable, the grant making of large private foundations may "influence the decisions of other funding agencies" and not necessarily be reflective of needs at the national level (Okie 2006: 1087).

The Programme of Action stated that the original resource estimates for ICPD were to be revised and officially reviewed. Official revisions have not been done, however one well accepted estimate suggests that $35 billion to $45 billion annually is required over the next few years (Ethelston and Leahy 2006). The UN Millennium Project estimated total costs for family planning, maternal and newborn health, treatment of selected sexually transmitted infections, and prevention of HIV/AIDS in 2005 at $18.2 billion, in 2010 $29.8 billion, and in 2015 $35.8 billion.[8] Estimates for the resources to achieve MDG-4 and MDG-5 are a minimum of $7 billion per year (Powell-Jackson et al. 2006).

Measurement and Priority Setting in Global Health

Another impact of global health on reproductive health is the increasing reliance on evidence-based priority setting and application of summary measures of population health to set health priorities (Van Der Maas 2003; Murray et al. 2002; Murray and Lopez 1996a; World Bank 1993). One widespread measure is burden of disease (BOD) analysis.[9] Its appeal to policy makers and donors is understandable. It calculates the burden of ill health for a wide range of conditions using the same measure, the disability-adjusted life year (DALY), purportedly allowing for comparison among a range of health issues. It also ranks a set of health interventions based on their cost-effectiveness measured in DALYs, giving policy makers the sense that they are prioritizing the health intervention that provides the biggest return for each dollar spent.

Efforts to measure the burden of disease due to reproductive health conditions have been useful yet flawed. The first global burden of disease (GBD) exercise in 1990 estimated that reproductive ill health contributed 5-15 percent of the burden, with the main contributing factors being death and disability due to pregnancy and childbirth, sexually transmitted infection (including HIV/AIDS), and reproductive tract cancer (Murray and Lopez 1996b). Furthermore, the 1990 GBD analyses found that reproductive ill health accounted for a greater global burden of disease for women than men (22 versus 3 percent). These early calculations of the DALYs associated with reproductive ill health served a constructive role in getting reproductive health on the global health policy agenda (Petchesky 2003; Allotey and Reidpath 2002; AbouZahr 1999; Murray and Lopez 1998). The quantification of disability associated with reproductive health conditions complemented the efforts at ICPD to generate policy attention to reproductive health. An update in 2001 reported that the burden of disease related to sex and reproductive health accounted for 18 percent of GBD among women aged 15–44 and 32 percent among women aged 15–44 (Lopez et al. 2002).

While DALYs represent an important technical advance in the field of global health, there are technical limitations in the assessment of the burden of sexual and reproductive ill health (AbouZahr and Vaughn 2000) that affect where reproductive health fits on the global agenda.[10] One critique is that the basis for calculating DALYs, the International Classification of Diseases (ICD), which allows for DALYs to be classified as diseases, injuries, and their sequelae, is problematic when measuring reproductive morbidities that go beyond anatomical diagnoses (see AbouZahr and Vaughn 2000). A second critique considers the valuation of health states. Reproductive ill health is underreported because symptoms are often unrecognized, undiagnosed, or asymptomatic; shame and stigma associated with sexually transmitted infections or infertility create strong social and cultural reasons for under reporting them (AbouZahr 1999). The valuation of health states, a critical component in BOD calculations, is therefore especially challenging for reproductive health issues. Finally, a lack of reproductive health data creates a tendency to underreport some reproductive health conditions, thus skewing incidence estimates essential to the DALY calculation. This is exacerbated by the fact that the reproductive health field has struggled to agree on indicators to measure progress, show results, and make linkages and associations with other development issues. The challenge of finding indicators for reproductive health that are both measurable and manageable remains (Kaufman, this volume).

The limitations of summary measures such as DALYs for reproductive health are significant. They shape policy makers' perceptions of the relative importance of reproductive health in the overall global health agenda. This translates into a large portion of the reproductive health agenda, as defined by ICPD, being left out. These measurement limitations directly affect the resources allocated for reproductive health. As described earlier in this chapter, resources for reproductive health have been declining over the past decade. While the mismeasurement of reproductive health issues is not the only explanation for diminishing resources, it could be argued that more accurate measurement of the burden of reproductive health may lead to increased attention and allocation of resources.

Conclusion: Moving the Reproductive Health Agenda Forward

The analysis in this chapter suggests that reproductive health has slipped in its status on the global policy agenda since ICPD. This conclusion, based on evidence of declining policy attention, diminishing resources, and lack of a clear intervention that all stakeholders agree on, is made with several caveats. First, this judgment is based on interpretation of an incomplete set of evidence. Second, the analysis focused only on the global reproductive health agenda; the results may be more encouraging at the national level, depending on the country context. While beyond the scope of the analysis here, evidence at the national level seems less pessimistic, and it is important for the field to continue to document success at the national level. Bangladesh is one such example (Jahan and Germain 2004). This ownership at the national level was an overall goal of ICPD and should therefore be considered as successful implementation of ICPD.

Third, the conclusion depends on the definition of reproductive health one adopts. A more holistic definition of reproductive health views ICPD as a "living document" with the major principles and underlying concepts of its agenda being adopted and adapted into other documents and settings since ICPD. Some women's health advocates have argued that "Cairo provided the foundation for the MDGs" (Germain and Kidwell 2005) and that the UN Millennium Project moves the ICPD agenda forward (Glasier and Gulmezoglu 2006). If reproductive health is defined as the set of individual components, one may be less optimistic. As for funding, the evidence is pretty clear that there is diminishing attention to reproductive health in the global donor community, particularly when HIV/AIDS is separated from reproductive health activities.

How then do we think about the reproductive health and rights agenda in the future? What are some strategies for maintaining and increasing its status on the global agenda? It is important to consider the reproductive health and rights agenda in the current policy context it operates in, and in particular, the unique factors that the current interest in global health bring to bear. The impact of global health should not be considered just in how reproductive health relates to other health and development issues (e.g., HIV/AIDS or MDGs) but in how it interacts with and responds to the changing global health and development environment itself. Such a view suggests that maintaining and increasing reproductive health's visibility on the global agenda will require a multipronged approach that addresses new funding mechanisms, improvements in measurement of progress, and expanding advocacy. On today's global policy agenda, reproductive health is more recognizable in terms of the underlying concepts of ICPD that have been explicitly or implicitly adopted in a range of new policy agendas. This provides the opportunity for the ICPD agenda to be adopted and adapted into a larger network comprised of new relationships. This should be seen not as a weakening of reproductive health but as a testament to the inherent and enduring strengths of ICPD and its Programme of Action.

Chapter 3
The Conundrum of Population and Reproductive Health Programs in the Early Twenty-First Century

George Zeidenstein

The title of this volume does not include the word population. Yet reproductive health programming originated in the international development field of population policies and programs, as I explain. But, for reasons discussed below, reproductive health programs are now largely severed from their original base in population policies and programs. The unfilled gap presents the conundrum referred to in the title of this chapter. The chapter is intended to explain the conundrum and advance some suggestions about resolving it.

The concept of reproductive health programs was first articulated at the 1994 ICPD conference in Cairo. The programs were conceived and articulated as population activities: they were described as absorbing and integrating what had formerly been vertical family planning programs within a broader array of reproductive health services that would be more responsive and broadly useful to clients.

But since the 1994 conference international concerns about population policy have waned, along with diminished fertility in most countries. What, then, about the creatures of those population policy concerns, reproductive health programs? Somehow or other, without discussion of where things came from and how they are affected by their antecedents, reproductive health programs seem to me to be understood nowadays by most professionals as having become pure public health activities, planned, operated, and evaluated as if they have nothing to do with population dynamics. Well, one may ask, is there anything wrong with that? Are not public health activities worthy in and of themselves? Is not achievement of improved public health goals justification enough? These are fair questions, and I believe the answers to them are all affirmative. Public health programming needs no further justification, no props from other sectors. It has its own validity and worth.

The problem in this case, however, arises because reproductive health programs, bereft of their former population policy support (and beset with political obstacles originating in their connection with sexual behavior) are doing poorly in the competition for public health attention and funds. International support seems wavering and uncertain at best. International and national financial support for reproductive health programs has consistently fallen below the Cairo funding recommendations every year since 1994. And when effort was finally exerted in 2000 by the global community of nations to produce the Millennium Development Goals (the overriding standard, it was thought then, for international development objectives to be achieved by 2015), all reference to reproductive health program achievement was omitted. The words "reproductive health" with or without modification by the word "programs," are totally absent from the MDGs, even though it is plain now that several of the stated goals cannot be realized without underlying progress in reproductive health programs (Freedman et al. 2005a).

In my view, both the waning interest in population policy and the inadequate financial support for and constructive attention to reproductive health programs are unjustified and counterproductive for achieving the sorts of human well-being goals so often articulated internationally, but so seldom achieved.

Historical Perspective

The history of what became known everywhere as the global population problem is well known (e.g., Ehrlich 1968). From the beginning, there were pessimists and optimists confronting the same facts. Malthus late in the eighteenth century, and a sturdy line of scholars and activists during the years and centuries after him, feared that rapid population growth would outstrip resources, causing huge human misery (Malthus 1986; Meadows, Meadows, Randers, and Behrens 1972). Condorcet and a thinner line of scholars and activists during those same centuries disagreed; in their view, humanity was not endangered by rapid population growth and could even benefit from it (Condorcet 1976; Boserup 1978). To this day, the fundamentals of that divide have not been bridged (Sinding 2000).

Notwithstanding that endless debate, the prevailing modern view has been concern that rapid population growth, especially in poor countries, would outstrip resources, or prevent or slow economic development and poverty alleviation, or cause or add to environment degradation, or foster ill health especially in mothers and children, or cause or exacerbate social instabilities, all or some of these (and more) to one degree or another (Demeny 2003; Seltzer 2002; Birdsall and Sinding 1999; Harkavy 1995).

This concern was expressed in an array of population policies seeking reduction in total fertility, a term used by population professionals to mean the average number of children born to women during their fecund years (NCHS 2004). Papers and books about programs and projects undertaken to implement those policies are plentiful; descriptions, assessments, appreciations, and criticisms of actions address what was seen as the global population problem, and its national manifestations abound (e.g., Demeny 2003; Ashford 2001; Tsui 2001; Jain 1998).

National efforts began slowly and haltingly in the 1950s and rose to a peak in the 1970s and 1980s, as did international financial and technical support for them (Donaldson and Tsui 1994). Indeed, national efforts depended heavily on international donor support, and that trended downward toward the end of the twentieth century and seems to be in question (or less) in this early part of the twenty-first century (PAI 2004b; Merrick, this volume).

The whole complex of policies, programs, and projects, their conceptualization, articulation, and implementation, was led by international donor country interest, especially in the United States and Scandinavia, and following its establishment in 1969, by the United Nations Population Fund (UNFPA). This was followed after various lags and often without notable enthusiasm by developing (i.e., poor) countries where the actual problems of rapid population growth were occurring. Generally, national interest in identifying and addressing rapid population growth arose first in South and East Asia, later and with less conviction in Central and South America, and more recently, but even now without uniform enthusiasm, in some Middle Eastern and African countries (Seltzer 2002; Tsui 2001). The first national family planning program was established in India in 1952 (Bose 1995).

Family planning program, one may ask? What is that? National family planning programs were the early and nearly exclusive poor country actions (devised largely by rich donor countries) to reduce high rates of fertility, thus addressing the global problem at the national, poor country level. The hope in fielding them was that fertility rates would be reduced by couples avoiding pregnancies through use of modern contraceptives during sexual intercourse (Seltzer 2002; Tsui 2001; Freedman 1997).

The daily contraceptive pill was approved by the U.S. Food and Drug Administration in 1960. Its availability and characteristics suggested something that had never before been possible. For the first time, the pill made it possible to think of sexual intercourse with hardly any chance for pregnancy and no contraceptive action to be taken at the time of intimacy. The timing of ingestion of pills and intercourse need not be related in any particular way, and the contraceptive required no manipulation of genitals. Effectiveness in pregnancy prevention was said to be in the hugely impressive high 90th percentile, indeed above 95 percent (Hatcher et al. 1998). The availability of such a seemingly ideal contraceptive made the family planning program idea seem more feasible than ever.

To program professionals, the contraceptive pill seemed to offer a near perfect line of action to address the population problem they had identified. There had, of course, been other means of preventing pregnancy, both traditional and industrial, and efforts had been made to include some of them in the first family planning programs. But none were thought by the professionals to be as convenient, or easily deliverable as the pill. Indeed, the professionals regarded the pre-pill contraceptives more or less cumbersome, unaesthetic, unreliable, ineffective, or combinations of these.

The pill was joined a bit later by the copper-T intrauterine devices (IUDs), which professionals believed would certainly solve the problem of high fertility in India. IUDs have the characteristic (attractive to those early professionals) that removal is ordinarily not possible without professional assistance. A further advantage over the pill was thought to be that once inserted, no further contraceptive action was necessary by the user.

Both contraceptives are still important means of pregnancy prevention, but neither proved to be the perfect instrument for which professionals had hoped. There was a huge revulsion in India about the IUD, and serious health risks associated with the original pill required fundamental reformulations (Grimes 1998). There was the further hope that through what is usually called IEC (information, education, and communication), family planning programs might also induce couples to desire smaller families and so to avoid, limit, or space pregnancies by using contraceptives. Thus, in the first, broader instance, family planning programs were thought to provide the contraceptive *supplies* that couples were assumed to desire to limit pregnancies. There was the further hope that family planning programs might induce that desire (create demand) where it did not already exist (Seltzer 2002; Freedman 1997).

Family planning programs quickly became the core, worldwide, of all action intended to control, moderate, reduce, stabilize, harmonize, limit, or restrain population growth through fertility reduction; all these terms and more were used at one time and context or another (Demeny 2003; Bulatao 1998). So much was this the case that the labels became mostly conflated. That is, "family planning programs" equaled "population programs" and vice versa (Jain 1998). This nearly exclusive reliance on family planning programs (and related IEC efforts) for population policy implementation occurred in the face of a robust line of understanding that fertility behavior is causally and consequentially related to economic and social development. That is, programs to affect economic and social outcomes, underway in the very same poor countries during the very same time periods as family planning programs, affect and are affected by people's desires about family size (Demeny 2003; McNicoll 2003; Bongaarts et al. 1990). The economic and social quality of people's lives affects their desires for children, and vice versa. Put another way, the demand of couples, or women, or men, for fertility regulation (contraception) depends heavily on the economic and social quality of their lives (Bruce 1994). Consequently, to the extent family planning programs themselves do not create that demand (and ordinarily, demand creation is not in their mandates), they hope to satisfy a demand that development efforts (among other things) have created.

In some cases population programs, that is, family planning programs, were actually combined with other sorts of development initiatives intended to improve economic and social well-being of their clients. The Grameen Bank and its programs of microcredit for small business entrepreneurship by poor women was an encouraging example in Bangladesh (Engelman 1998). There was even a well-known slogan first articulated at the International Conference on Population in Bucharest in 1974 (noted later in this chapter) by Dr. Karan Singh, minister of health of India, and taken up by developing country officials and others quite seriously. It stated, "Development is the best contraceptive," deploring the international development funds going into family planning programs at the expense of more obviously positive development programs of, say, education (especially of girls), gender equity or equality, health care, community development, poverty alleviation, and the like (Bose 1995; Finkle and Crane 1975). Obviously, the statement itself had (and has) legs. But even if one understood that economic and social development had *lots* to do with family size desires, and family planning programs *fairly little*, the hard fact was (and remains) that people at work in population policies and activities had (and have) little or no influence, let alone control, over development programs in other sectors. Family planning programs were the only actions in their hands for implementing policies of reducing rates of population growth in poor countries.

It was natural then, one might say, that throughout the rising levels of international and then national interest to moderate high fertility from the 1950s to 1960s, 1970s, and 1980s (with exceptions and amid considerable, even furious, internal debate and name calling) actual program activities in the population field focused narrowly and vertically on family planning programs (contraceptive delivery), even though most people understood and accepted that family planning programs had the serious limitations noted earlier. They addressed only the supply-side of a complex equation with hugely important and poorly understood demand-side elements. These, in turn, seemed to be affected substantially by events in other sectors of economic and social development. Population policies and activities were only one sector among numerous others in the larger, older, wider, more comprehensive, continuing, and, many believed, more positive work of international economic and social development. But administrative, professional, personnel, and budgetary separations preserved verticality. For all the talk of integration (which continues to seem never ending), ministries, disciplines, and professions operated within their prescribed remits and budgets (compare, for example, great universities where, most power is in discipline-defined departments and outsiders are usually not welcome).

Origins of ICPD

Perhaps because of the limited nature of what could be reasonably expected of truly voluntary family planning programs to create demand for contraception, excesses and worse occurred (Hartmann 1995; Bose 1995). Material incentives for contraceptive use were offered to people so poor they could not refuse, and burdensome disincentives (read, penalties) were imposed on people who failed or refused to use contraceptives (Isaacs 1995). Social pressure was applied through traditional channels of authority to monitor and control the fertility of one's neighbors. Women were hounded by local officials to abort pregnancies beyond prescribed fertility limits (Boland, Rao, and Zeidenstein 1994; Bok 1994). These are not exhaustive examples. Excesses of these and additional kinds in family planning programs were becoming widely unacceptable, and it was not only the increasingly well organized and cogent international groups of feminists who were saying so (Garcia-Moreno and Claro 1994).

It was with this background and in this environment that planning began at the opening of the 1990s for what became in September 1994 the ICPD, after which, as the cliché goes, nothing would ever be the same. Earlier UN-sponsored international population conferences had been held in 1954 in Rome, 1965 in Belgrade, 1974 in Bucharest, and 1984 in Mexico City. Rome was for experts in their individual capacities and was undertaken in collaboration with the International Union for Scientific Study of Population. Belgrade, too, was mostly for experts but also recognized for the first time that fertility was a policy variable in the context of development planning (Mertens 1994). Bucharest and Mexico City were for country representatives, so political positions and concerns became important, if not central (Finkle and Crane 1975, 1985).

Overall, one may say that at Bucharest the bureaucrats and politicians pulled the rug from under the experts (heavily represented by Americans and Scandinavians). The latter hoped to focus on population program details (principally family planning programs), including development of new contraceptives, but the former wanted central attention to the need for increased investment in economic and social development activities (Finkle and Crane 1975). At Mexico City, with the Reagan administration in Washington, formerly reluctant (if not truculent) poor countries supported population programs (again mostly family planning), but the United States turned equivocal to doubtful about the pressing need for them (Finkle and Crane 1985). Here too, what has become known, and continued under the Bush administration, as the Global Gag Rule, was announced for the first time (Finkle and Crane 1985). In 1968, at Teheran, the International Conference on Human Rights proclaimed in paragraph 16 that

Parents have a basic human right to determine freely and responsibly the number and the spacing of their children. (UN 1968)

This language or some close variant has been included in the final document of all the UN-sponsored international population conferences that came afterward. In the Cairo Programme of Action, it appears this way in Principle 8:

All couples and individuals have the basic right to decide freely and responsibly the number and spacing of their children and to have the information, education and means to do so.

It seems to me that the main thing about what finally emerged from ICPD in 1994 is that it opened space between family planning programs and population policies, and filled it with concerns, articulated as elements of population policy, for economic and social development outcomes and individual well-being. We should note that, of the three quantitative goals agreed to be achieved by 2015 among the 179 states represented at ICPD, only one relates directly to reproductive health care, including family planning services. The others are reduction of infant, child, and maternal mortality and universal education, particularly for girls.

Similarly, of the 16 chapters in the ICPD Programme of Action, only one, Chapter 7, addresses reproductive rights and reproductive health, including family planning. Other chapters take up interactions of population change with several economic and social development sectors: sustained economic growth and sustainable development; environment; poverty; gender equality, equity, and empowerment of women; health, morbidity, and mortality; and education. In fact, ICPD is the first of the UN-sponsored international population conferences to have the word Development in its title. Paragraph 1.5 of the Programme of Action states:

The 1994 Conference was explicitly given a broader mandate on development issues than previous population conferences, reflecting the growing awareness that population, poverty, patterns of production and consumption and the environment are so closely interconnected that none of them can be considered in isolation.

After ICPD no longer would family planning and population programs be conflated, synonymous. No longer would family planning programs be the almost exclusive action available for implementing policies to reduce or moderate fertility. The delegates and perhaps even more so the impressively well prepared, organized, and transnationally effective nongovernmental organizations in attendance (especially feminists and others concerned about the well-being of women in a largely man's world) successfully refocused population policy from programs to people. Before ICPD, population policy had been mostly about contraceptive service delivery programs; ICPD directed that it be mostly about the well-being of individuals, with special attention to women, not because their well-being is more important than that of men, but because it is more neglected (Sen, Germain, and Chen 1994).

The Conundrum

Under ICPD, family planning programs became elements of a new, more comprehensive something called reproductive health programs, but only one of their several important elements. In turn, reproductive health programs were seen as only one of the economic and social development sectors enumerated in the Programme of Action as interacting causally and consequentially with population behavior. What *were* the reproductive health programs referred to in ICPD? Where had *they* come from? The world had little program implementation experience with reproductive health programs before ICPD. They were born whole at the ICPD to address needs that had been identified over years of contentious experience with vertical family planning programs. Therefore, an effort was made in paragraph 7.6 of the Programme of Action to list the elements to be included in reproductive health programs. Summarizing, they should include family planning (contraceptive services); prenatal care, safe delivery, and postnatal care; infertility prevention and care; abortion but not illegally or "as a method of family planning"; treatment of reproductive tract infections and sexually transmitted diseases (including HIV/AIDS); and information, education, and counseling on human sexuality, reproductive health, and responsible parenthood.

Although the Programme of Action directs considerably more space and attention to various population and development interactions than it does to reproductive rights and health, nothing in the Programme of Action suggests that policy or program action in these other economic and social sectors should or would, after ICPD, come somehow into the hands of practitioners in the population sector. In the past, family planning programs had been their nearly exclusive population policy instrument. After ICPD, what? Were reproductive health programs simply to replace family planning programs as the nearly exclusive instrument of post-Cairo population activities? Indeed, we may ask what seems currently to be an open question—were they thought to have anything at all to do with population policy? Did anybody believe that reproductive health programs (beyond their family planning components) might in some way affect fertility behavior? Did anyone care whether that was so or not? All this was left ambiguous. Purposely?

This strikes me as a groping moment for those of us who continue to believe that population is an important sector among the economic and social development processes that are transforming the world. Population behavior—understood as family formation decision-making and behavior, mortality, and migration—whether fertility is high or low, remains causally and consequentially connected to those changing economic and social processes; it is affected by them and affects them. As I read it, the Programme of Action says so, too. Perhaps this should have been stated more explicitly. If it had been, perhaps there would be less doubt today than there seems to be about the importance of reproductive health programs, including their family planning components.

Rethinking the Links Between Population Policy and Reproductive Health Programs

Reproductive health programs are not doing well on their own (that is, divorced from population policy considerations) in health sector resource competition. HIV/AIDS work has been mostly extracted into vertical programs. Other health sector initiatives seem consistently to be given higher priority in resource allocation. These include programs for safe motherhood, maternal and child health, primary health care, and health sector reform. Burden of disease theory and practice seem to cast doubt on the priority to be accorded to reproductive health programs (WHO 1998, 2005; Aitken 1999; Merrick and Reichenbach, both in this volume).

Neither reproductive health programs nor their family planning components were seen in the Programme of Action as creating demand for contraceptive services. Rather, the underlying sense was that already in 1994 substantial unsatisfied demand existed for these services, estimated at around 350 million couples and 120 million more women (para. 7.13). The presumption seems also to have been that more demand would certainly arise through advancing cohorts and in response to life transformations from continuing economic and social development improvements, including, of course and especially, the expected greater gender equity and equality.

So then, I ask, what is the current situation? Are reproductive health programs abandoned by the international style setters to twist in the wind of changing fashions in development activities? Might it be different if they were understood to be vital elements of population policy, and population policy—no longer focused solely on fertility reduction—were widely acknowledged as important? Is anybody besides me prepared to argue the case for population policy and for reproductive health programs as important elements of its implementation?

If we *were* to want to draw attention once more, in this early twenty-first century, to the relevance of population policy for international development undertakings, what might we be looking at? We ask this question with reference to policy rather than demography. That is to say, we hope for first rate demographic research to inform us, but our objective would be to affect international development policies rather than the social science of demography. We would want to affect those policies in ways responsive to demographic realities and possibilities.

Of course, fertility would always concern us and we would seek to ensure its front and center presence in the forums considering all sorts of international development issues. In some parts of the world, perhaps especially in sub-Saharan Africa and the Middle East, high fertility still seems to be a pressing human and development problem, notwithstanding the devastations of AIDS. In others, differential fertility among different ethnic groups might be the element drawing most (political) attention. In still others, low fertility might be the paramount focus of policy attention.

But there would be additional population concerns that might be introduced into twenty-first-century population policy discussions. Migration and possible fertility pressures upon it, including brain drain questions; population aging and mortality; and issues of gender equality and equity, have large-scale importance in contemporary development policy. Often they are of professional interest to demographers; most likely they are also appropriate for policy attention in the population sector. How that might differ from the attention they are currently receiving is worth vigorous consideration.

And, if reproductive health programs, including family planning activities, *were* accepted as closely related to operations under population policy, how might they be affected? The close connections between demographic desires and behavior and health, education, and gender equality and equity, for example, might be attended to more actively and effectively. And the natural locus of attention in reproductive health programs to some of the pressing issues with respect to HIV/AIDS might be more readily supported and encouraged, creating a more horizontally integrated supplement to the existing largely vertical programs. This would certainly produce a wider spread of health benefits, especially in places where the epidemic is generalized in the population. That is to say, vulnerable groups of people confronting the pandemic may not be reached easily by regular reproductive health programs and therefore may require specialized vertical programs to reach them, but where the pandemic has spread into general population, it is likely that reproductive health programs are already in the most effective position to reach them. It seems to me that engaging and potentially fruitful possibilities for development policy emerge if we could turn our attention to the many ways in which population policies and programs plus related reproductive health programs continue to be vital and relevant in the twenty-first century.

Chapter 4
Population, Poverty Reduction, and the Cairo Agenda

David E. Bloom and David Canning

Decisive evidence is emerging that reproductive health and the age structure of a population matter considerably to the achievement of the Millennium Development Goals (MDGs). This statement is a major departure from academic thinking over the past two decades. Until recently, the dominant view has been "population neutralism," a view that emerged from a lack of evidence that population numbers or growth rates affect economic development. This absence was said to imply that population neither impedes nor promotes development and that on average the positive and negative effects tend to cancel out. "Population neutralism" was the dominant view in the 1986 report of the U.S. National Research Council (NRC 1986); most significantly, it contributed to population and reproductive health sliding off of the radar screen of many influential international donor agencies.

Research done over the past several years has revealed a major defect in the academy's conclusion and the research on which it was based, which, in its preoccupation with population numbers and growth rates, missed the consequences of changes in population age structure. The population neutralist view, therefore, must be replaced by a more nuanced position. Although the overall rate of population growth may not affect economic growth, the changing age structure of the population can have a sizable effect on economic well-being. Reproductive health and fertility decline are at the heart of this mechanism.

We argue here that new evidence on the connection between fertility reduction and economic growth suggests that the link between population policies and poverty reduction is stronger than previously believed. The 1994 ICPD conference enunciated a progressive, feminist agenda that sought to bring development actions to the local level and to

promote grassroots involvement in defining and implementing reproductive health programs. The importance of this agenda to economic
development is strengthened by recent findings in demography and
economics about the relationships among fertility rates, demographic
change, and economic development.

The Demographic Transition and Poverty Reduction

World population doubled from 1960 to 2000, from 3 to 6 billion, and
is projected to increase by another 3 billion by 2050. These increases,
which are concentrated in developing countries, are associated with a
phenomenon known as the demographic transition. This term refers to
the transition from high fertility and high mortality to low fertility and
low mortality. Mortality declines first, and in high-mortality populations
this decline is mainly concentrated among infants and children (due
typically to the spread of vaccines, antibiotics, safe water, and other public health measures). A baby boom ensues because more babies survive
to adulthood than in previous generations. The high-survival-rate baby
boom ends when fertility subsequently declines, as couples realize that
fewer births are needed to reach their targets for surviving children, as
desired fertility abates, and as women are empowered to realize their fertility desires.

This baby boom cohort initially lowers income per capita because the
output of the working-age population must be divided among more people. More young people need to be fed, clothed, housed, and provided
with medical care and schooling, which limits the resources available for
other uses such as building up a country's infrastructure. The diversion
of resources from investment tends to slow the process of economic
growth in absolute terms, as conventionally measured.

In 15 to 25 years, when the baby boom cohort reaches working ages,
the productive capacity of the economy expands on a per capita basis
due to the expansion of labor supply. The large, working-age baby boom
generation is in sharp distinction to the small number of elderly and the
reduced number of children. At this time in the transition, a country's
potential output also grows because the working ages are the prime
years for savings, a key to capital accumulation and technological innovation. Savings get a further boost as longevity increases in the latter
phases of the demographic transition. People save more in anticipation
of longer periods of retirement, promoting further capital accumulation
and economic growth.

Poverty reduction—the first and most important MDG—follows
from this process because economic growth is to some extent a rising
tide that lifts all boats. The poverty rate can be thought of as a function

of the average level of income and the distribution of this income across members of society. There is evidence that, on average, the poor enjoy a similar rate of growth of income as the population in general. Rising average incomes lift substantial numbers of people out of poverty. It should be noted, however, that this average relationship does not hold true in every country, and there are examples of economic growth in which the poor have gained little and of poverty decline with little economic growth taking place.

Considerable evidence has now been accumulated that the mechanism described above—known as the demographic dividend—has had a huge, positive effect in some developing (and some developed) countries. The demographic dividend in part explains the exceptionally good performance of the East Asian "Tiger" economies, particularly in comparison to the poor performance of sub-Saharan Africa. The huge differences between sub-Saharan Africa and East Asia—geography, governance, educational attainment, and economic policies—help explain their disparate macroeconomic performances, but cannot account for it entirely (Bloom, Canning, and Malaney 2000; Bloom, Canning, and Sevilla 2003).

Recent research has demonstrated that the demographic dividend can account for about one-third of East Asia's phenomenal economic growth during 1965-90. Health improvements and subsequent rapid declines in fertility in East Asia generated a baby boom cohort whose entry into the labor market coincided with the start of economic booms. In contrast, poor health and high fertility in sub-Saharan Africa have generated high levels of youth dependency and low income growth. In accounting for economic growth, there are no significant unexplained differences between the two regions once demographic change is taken into account.

High fertility in sub-Saharan Africa is usually due not to unmet need for family planning services but to high desired fertility. Evidence suggests that desired fertility will only fall when infant mortality rates fall, female educational attainment increases, opportunities for female employment outside the home are created, opportunities to educate children increase, and mechanisms to acquire financial assets to save for old age are in place. When these conditions are met, as is now the case in South Asia and particularly India, desired fertility can fall dramatically, leading to rapid reductions in actual fertility if family planning services are available. When this happens, the effects of the demographic transition can act as an accelerator, turning slow economic development into a sustained economic boom.[1]

Mason and Lee (2004) summarize research on the effect of the demographic dividend on poverty reduction and conclude that it had a significant effect in Latin America and Asia between 1960 and 2000. Moreover, they say that, as a result of the dividend, the developing world could see a 14 percent reduction in the share of the population living in poverty between 2000 and 2015, and they predict that Africa will for the first time share in these benefits. They also estimate, using Indonesian data, that a 10 percent reduction in the fertility rate would lead to an 11 percent reduction in the poverty rate.

Demographic change, along with changes in economic policy, is occurring in most countries. The pace and timing vary, but the trend is unmistakable. Dollar and Kraay (2002) point out that, primarily because of the rapid income growth in China and India, economic inequality in the world is decreasing and global poverty is declining. Even if countries do not change their economic policies, the first MDG will likely be substantially met by 2015. Projected economic growth, based to a large extent on the beneficial effects of demographic change, will lift hundreds of millions out of poverty by that date (Bloom et al. forthcoming).

The facts summarized above have significant policy implications. Because family planning programs have led to lower birth rates, and because the demographic transition has had large positive economic benefits, reproductive health issues matter not only to families, communities, and health ministries, but also to finance ministries. Improving the reproductive health of women and expanding the choices available to them can lead to fewer, healthier, and better-educated children. A baby boom generation, when it reaches working age, can work more productively, save more, and, especially if there are continued reductions in fertility, have fewer dependents to support. Economic growth can follow quickly, as it did in East Asia. But none of this is guaranteed. Sustained investment in education and in opportunities for youth to enter the workforce are essential (Jimenez and Murthi 2006).

A comparison of the experience of China and India provides some telling lessons about the importance of policies in bringing about the economic fruits of the demographic transition. China's early commitment to basic education, in combination with a rapidly falling fertility rate (which fell precipitously even before full implementation of the one-child policy and continued to fall afterward) helped propel economic growth and poverty reduction. China also managed to lower the infant mortality rate very rapidly when India's was falling steadily but slowly. India, much more recently experiencing economic growth (and at a less dazzling pace than China), did not educate nearly so broadly, and its fertility rate fell much later. There are, of course, numerous other very significant factors that may explain the difference between China's sustained and rapid economic growth (and concomitant reduction of poverty) and India's slower progress, but a successful focus on education meant that China's relatively large generation of working-age people had the skills they needed to interact productively with an increasingly globalized economy. When China made the decision to export labor-intensive goods to the world economy, it did so with a well-prepared workforce.

Although the first MDG may be met on a "business as usual" program, high poverty rates in sub-Saharan Africa and Latin America will remain. Because any program or policy intervention that reduces the unmet need for contraception will promote fertility decline, reproductive health programs have a potentially vital role to play in the achievement of the MDGs. Reducing the unmet need for contraception is beneficial whether or not it promotes economic growth and poverty reduction. But it is even more beneficial if it also promotes achievement of the MDGs, though this also depends on public policies that extend beyond the realm of population and reproductive health.

ICPD and the MDGs

The foregoing arguments point to the relevance of reproductive health concerns and to demographic change as highly relevant to the first MDG. A crucial issue to be addressed is how the ICPD Programme of Action contributes to the achievement of development goals, including the MDGs.

One key point is that the evidence base for the linkage between population issues and poverty has changed. In particular, the Programme's Chapter 3, on Interrelationships Between Population, Sustained Economic Growth, and Sustainable Development, although it discusses the effects of population age structure on the economy, could be rewritten to emphasize the strong connection that has been found between demographic change and economic growth.

Chapter 6, on Population Growth and Structure, describes actions that will contribute to the alleviation of poverty in a number of ways, many of which are related to the processes described above. For example, paragraph 6.4 calls for countries that have not completed their demographic transition to take effective steps in this regard. This requires development and strengthening of family planning programs. Although the effectiveness of such programs in reducing fertility has been debated extensively, recent research by Miller (2005) provides a careful and compelling analysis of the positive effects of ProFamilia, Colombia's long-standing family planning program. The program has led to women having fewer children and at a later age, getting more education, and working more. Girls (and boys even more) benefited by delaying the start of their working lives.

Paragraph 6.5 appropriately highlights the importance of under-standing the interaction between fertility and mortality levels and the need "to reduce high levels of infant, child and maternal mortality so as to lessen the need for high fertility and reduce the occurrence of high-risk births." To the extent that high desired fertility is a consequence of high infant mortality rates, an emphasis on reducing infant mortality can have multiple benefits, as described above. Furthermore, in para-graph 6.6 the primacy of making family planning services available to all who want them is clearly laid out. When desired fertility is lower than ac-tual fertility, family planning services have been instrumental in reduc-ing fertility levels.

The issue of early marriage is highlighted in paragraph 6.11, which draws attention to the fact that in areas of the world where the practice is common, women's potential to contribute to economic development is severely constrained by the need to take care of and spend meager family assets on young children. In addition, of course, these mothers are able to earn much less in the paid workforce, making it much more difficult to emerge from poverty.

Paragraph 6.15 calls for reproductive health services, sex education, prevention of early pregnancies, and education about HIV/AIDS pre-vention. As explained above, lowered birth rates are the key to the de-mographic transition. HIV infection tends to target the poor and uneducated and to further immiserate them by impeding their produc-tivity and depleting their savings. It follows that the further spread of HIV/AIDS will create great difficulty for many already poor or near-poor families and communities, who will have great difficulty emerging from poverty (Bloom et al. 2004).

Additional statements on the relationship between reproductive health and economic growth are found in Chapter 7, Reproductive Rights and Reproductive Health. The key statements are in paragraphs 7.12 ("The aim of family-planning programmes must be to enable cou-ples and individuals to decide freely and responsibly the number and spacing of their children") in paragraph 7.14, on preventing unwanted pregnancies. Carrying out these parts of the ICPD will not only in-crease the welfare of families directly by allowing them to achieve their family planning goals but also help promote economic growth and poverty alleviation by the effects of this fertility reduction on age struc-ture, and on the immediate ability of parents to better provide for their children.

Although evidence suggests that lower levels of fertility will promote economic growth, this does not imply that governments should act coer-cively to lower fertility. The ICPD argues that family planning policies should aim to meet the desires of families, not be based on coercive polices by governments: "The principle of informed free choice is essential to the long-term success of family-planning programmes. Any form of coercion has no part to play" (para. 7.12).

Indeed, there is no economically or morally defensible argument or evidence that can rationalize a return to coercive family planning policies. Even if those policies were to promote achievement of the MDGs, they are economically unjustified if they diminish the well-being of women. And even if the overall benefits of fertility control are positive, when they are achieved by coercion some women will have had their will and rights violated with no redress. To be crystal clear about this, population and reproductive health programs that reduce unmet need *and* promote the MDGs are win-win and therefore incontrovertibly good. Furthermore, programs that reduce unmet need are incontrovertibly good even if they do not promote the MDGs. Finally, programs that coerce fertility outcomes are bad policies, whether or not they promote the MDGs.

Family planning policies should allow women to achieve their desired levels of fertility without coercion, yet there may be some scope for policies that affect this desired level. Population policies that attempt to change fertility levels by incentives that affect desired fertility rather than coercion of actual fertility or fixed family size targets allow families to still achieve their goal by forgoing the incentive.

The rights-based approach evident throughout the ICPD and the instrumental argument that strengthens that approach are complementary. The principles agreed on at Cairo speak effectively to both the value in itself of reproductive health and the indirect but significant effects of reproductive and population health programs in alleviating poverty. New evidence on the connection between fertility reduction and economic growth suggests that the link between population policies and poverty reduction is even stronger than the ICPD set out. Indeed, the existence of the demographic dividend can be used as a political lever to argue for increased attention to reproductive health, since such a focus can have huge economic benefits.

Five points sum up the relationship between the ICPD and the MDGs, keeping in mind that "welfare" involves far more than just income. First, population and reproductive health programs and policies that reduce the unmet need for family planning as set out in the ICPD promote welfare directly *and* will help promote the achievement of the MDG of reducing poverty in developing countries. As families have fewer children, they are better able to make sure that those children are educated and healthy. As adults, these children will be more likely to escape poverty since both education and health improve earnings. In addition, as an earlier, large generation of children reach working age, the extra production they can generate can lead to an increased rate of economic growth and higher incomes. These outcomes, although not sufficient for poverty reduction, are generally necessary if it is to be achieved.

Second, the main effects will be felt only after a level of development is achieved at which desired fertility falls. Until then, individual workers are inevitably forced to devote much of their earnings to care of their young dependents. More broadly, society as a whole (via workers' earnings) must provide housing, food, education, and health care for children. This need places limits on the resources that can be invested, thus limiting future economic growth.

Third, the beneficial effects on poverty reduction require appropriate policies that promote employment and savings and that channel savings into productive investments. Even when fertility falls and the share of the working-age population rises, economic benefits may not be realized. A large set of factors, some of them at least partially under government control, affect whether the economic boom made possible by the demographic transition actually comes into being. If young people are not educated and do not have sufficient opportunity to find productive employment, the potentially positive effects of the demographic transition will be squandered. If a large working-age cohort suffers from significant unemployment, the overall level of income is unlikely to rise, aggregate savings may not increase, investment will be constrained, and poverty may not be alleviated at all.

Fourth, population and reproductive health programs that reduce unmet need are also directly beneficial by enlarging the choices of women, even if they do not promote the MDGs. It is important to remember the central goal of such programs: improving the lives of women (and families as a whole) and empowering them to control and better their own lives in ways that are often not possible when they have no option but to have more children. Programs that respond successfully to the unmet need for family planning are crucial in and of themselves, totally apart from their effects on economic well-being and poverty reduction.

Finally, population and reproductive health programs that coerce fertility outcomes cause large direct welfare losses by limiting choice. Freedom to make reproductive choices is the antithesis of coercion; unrelated to economic status or outcomes; that freedom is itself a central element of welfare. Moreover, there is no evidence that coercive policies increase welfare, whether conceived in terms of overall well-being or in narrower economic terms.

This chapter has, in effect, made the case that greatly increased access to reproductive health services should have been its own MDG. First, good reproductive health is central to human well-being and is distinct from, though closely entwined with, the other health-related MDGs. Second, greater access to reproductive health services can be a crucial element allowing families to escape poverty. And third, widespread access to such services can speed the demographic transition, allow greater public and private investments in health and education, and lift major sectors of society out of poverty.

Chapter 5
Mobilizing Resources for Reproductive Health

Thomas W. Merrick

What Happened to the Money for ICPD, and Why?

The 1994 ICPD Conference moved the rationale and content of "population" activities beyond the macrolevel concerns about the effects of population growth and structure on economic growth that were the predominant themes of earlier conferences. ICPD was the culmination of efforts by many reproductive health and rights advocates to ensure that programs were responsive to the reproductive rights and health needs of women, men, and their children, especially the poor.

ICPD was also a first in that it attempted to estimate the costs of the broader program of action agreed upon at the conference. There was a general expectation that funding for population programs would be expanded to support the new approach. But after an initial increase during the years immediately after the conference, funding levels stagnated. Several factors contributed to this, including a shift in donor funding modalities from "project" to broader budgetary support for poverty reduction and for achievement of the Millennium Development Goals (MDGs) at the end of the 1990s. At that time, the ICPD goal of universal access to reproductive health services was excluded from the MDG list due to political pressures.

Figure 1 summarizes available information on development assistance for population and reproductive health activities over the past several years.[1] Overall donor assistance for health has favored infectious diseases, particularly HIV/AIDS, malaria, and TB, and health systems development. HIV/AIDS accounts for most of the increase in overall donor aid shown in the chart. Family planning assistance increased slightly after ICPD, but has declined recently. Funding for research and policy and for

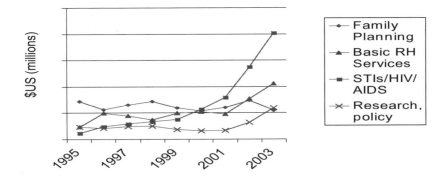

Figure 1. Donor assistance for population, reproductive health, and HIV/ AIDS/STDs, 1995–2003. UNFPA 2002; UN Commission on Population and Development 2005b. Ethelston and Leahy 2006 estimated that overall population assistance rose to $5.3 billion in 2004 and projected $6 billion for 2006. They noted again that the bulk of this increase went to HIV/AIDS; reproductive health and family planning assistance remained about 25 and 10 percent of the total respectively.

other reproductive health has increased since 2000, but not as much as funding for HIV/AIDS. Detailed information on patterns of donor assistance can be found elsewhere (UNFPA 2002; Ethelston 2004; Speidel 2005; UN Commission on Population and Development 2005).

Tracking donor assistance for population and reproductive health has never been easy despite strong efforts by UNFPA and others to compile this information. While bilateral donors and foundations report "population" program activities, other donors and lending institutions like the World Bank do not always track the specific programmatic focus, particularly when reporting line items like salaries, buildings and equipment, medicines, and supplies rather than program areas. Recent shift from project to program or sectorwide funding has further complicated the reporting problem, so that comparisons of information for earlier and later years may misrepresent actual spending trends.

Some donors, the United States in particular, channel funding through nongovernmental organizations (NGOs), while others support governments or channel resources through multilateral organizations like UNFPA, WHO, and the World Bank. Private foundations have been an important source of financial support for population and reproductive health and account for about one-sixth of overall funding, with a few large foundations accounting for most of the funding at the international level. Foundations support a range of population and reproductive health activities, including advocacy and provision of controversial services like abortion. Some foundations have been rethinking their grant-making priorities, raising concerns about how long they will continue support in this arena (Speidel 2005).

Several authors (Gillespie 2004a; Blanc and Tsui 2005; Kantner and Kantner 2006) have discussed reasons for the stagnation in family planning funding. These include (a) the perception that because population growth rates have declined there is no longer a need for family planning assistance, (b) loss of interest in population growth in the face of the HIV/AIDS epidemic, (c) opposition to family planning by social conservatives, and (d) the ICPD shift from population to reproductive health and undermining the sense of urgency that once motivated funders' interest in solving population problems. The future of family planning funding appears to be problematic, particularly in view of perennially proposed cuts in the U.S. foreign aid budget.

Another factor in the apparent stagnation in family planning funding, one that has made tracking of funding even more difficult, is that many donors have shifted from funding vertical projects for specific services (maternal health, family planning, etc.) to financing an entire health sector program, or to a combination of sectoral support and targeted funding to address high priority problems (HIV/AIDS, infectious diseases). These donors, and the legislative bodies that approve their budgets, have grown impatient with funding inputs that appear to get few results. They now favor reforms and results-oriented assistance that address underlying systems and structural problems. The MDGs and their focused objectives dovetail nicely with this results orientation, and sector-wide or multisector program funding has been used to support both reforms and health system development initiatives.

Overall patterns of development assistance have been affected by the growing recognition that traditional approaches to aid have benefited the rich more than the poor. In response, poverty reduction has moved to center stage in setting of priorities for program funding. Countries seeking debt relief are required to prepare Poverty Reduction Strategy Papers (PRSPs) to guide the reallocation of funds previously used for debt service to social services that will help the poor to escape poverty. Poverty analyses are also guiding priority-setting for program funding in countries that are not seeking debt relief. Though disease-specific projects are not completely gone, current health funding is more likely to be embedded in broader sectoral or multisectoral grants and loans and aimed at priority goals like those embodied in the MDGs, the first of which is the elimination of extreme poverty and hunger.

This shift has given special importance to having a strong evidence base to demonstrate that population and reproductive health outcomes affect poverty and that investment in such outcomes helps poor households escape poverty. Part of the problem is that with the shift from the old "population" paradigm to the broader reproductive health approach we are dealing with a much broader range of outcomes and factors affecting those outcomes in addition to fertility, for example, early childbearing, maternal mortality and morbidity, sexually transmitted diseases, and sexual violence.

In this context, HIV and infectious disease advocates have done a better job demonstrating the impact of those adverse health outcomes on poverty than have the champions of reproductive health. New funding mechanisms like Global Fund for HIV/AIDS, TB and Malaria, the U.S. President's Emergency Fund for HIV/AIDS Relief, and the World Bank Multi-Country HIV/AIDS Program have played a major role in the increase in HIV/AIDS funding noted above. Further increases in HIV/AIDS funding are projected, though actual spending will depend on whether governments live up to their pledges for these initiatives.

While maternal health and HIV figure in the MDG list, other dimensions of reproductive health, including unintended pregnancy and early childbearing, which disproportionately affect poorer women, are not mentioned. Even maternal mortality tends to get short shrift in the allocation of resources for MDGs. There have been calls to restore the ICPD goal of universal access to reproductive health services (or indicators or progress toward that goal) to the MDG list, and for a global funding channel similar to the one for HIV/AIDS, TB, and malaria, but political support for these initiatives remains problematic.

Large amounts of money are being channeled to poverty reduction initiatives through budget support mechanisms. The case can and should be made for funding the full range of reproductive health services, including family planning, for poor women and men both as a right and as a means of helping them escape poverty. A stronger evidence base is needed to demonstrate that poor reproductive health outcomes do, in fact, undermine the chances of the poor to escape poverty. While common sense suggests that such outcomes—early pregnancy, unintended pregnancy, excess fertility (when actual births exceed desired fertility), poorly managed obstetric complications—adversely affect the chances of poor women and their children and families to escape poverty, the evidence base to support this argument is thin and the evidence that does exist could be more effectively marshaled.

Who Decides Where the Money Goes?

A key consequence of the move to program/budgetary support is that decisions about the allocation of donor funds are made by finance ministries and their macroeconomist counterparts in development banks and donor agencies, rather than by sectoral ministries and their counterparts. Finance ministries evaluate a broad range of competing investment possibilities (infrastructure, institutional development, health, education, etc.) against a range of criteria, including poverty reduction, economic growth and stability, good governance, and aid effectiveness. The MDG targets have been adopted as performance measures, and progress toward country level MDG goals has become part of the ongoing policy dialogues among donors and countries receiving development assistance.

For the poorest countries, poverty reduction (the first MDG) is a high priority in these dialogues. Countries seeking debt relief are required to prepare Poverty Reduction Strategies (PRSs) that map the extent of the country's poverty problem and the factors that perpetuate poverty, identify investments that will help to reduce poverty, develop an expenditure plan for these investments, and provide mechanisms for tracking expenditures and their impact on poverty reduction (Klugman 2002). Once a PRS is agreed on, countries may receive a Poverty Reduction Credit (PRC). PRCs are generally program/budget funds that are allocated among the various investments called for in the PRS. The PRS/PRC process is also dominated by finance ministries and donor economists. The ground rules for preparation and monitoring of the process call for participation by civil society institutions, but their involvement has generally proved to be marginal at best.

Sectoral ministries such as health and education are confronted with two tasks: making the case that investments in their sector have an impact on poverty reduction, so that they receive an adequate allocation in the intersectoral resource allocation process, and demonstrating the specific investments within their sector are cost-effective. These economic criteria reflect economists' concerns about ensuring that when resources are scarce (as they almost always are), specific spending decisions will bring the largest improvements in outcomes the amount of money available can buy. Macroeconomic policy often "trumps" sectoral agendas. For example, budgetary ceilings are often imposed as part of the macroeconomic stability "package," so that when donors offer targeted funding for a specific priority area, the sectoral ministry may lose part of its share of the overall program budget to the extent that the added targeted funding puts its annual spending above the agreed expenditure plan ceiling (Ooms and Schrecker 2005).

In the case of health, the effort to achieve cost-effectiveness has employed burden of disease (BOD) analysis to identify "best buys" among competing health investment opportunities. BOD was developed and has been promoted by health economists in institutions such as the World Bank and WHO as a metric for measuring health outcomes (reductions in death and disability attributable to specific disease conditions) that permits comparisons among outcomes that are not themselves comparable. In translating these outcomes into the number of years of healthy life lost to a range of health conditions, BOD analysis has enabled decision makers to rank-order investments in terms of years of healthy life gained (MacKellar 2005).

While economic criteria have come to play a central role, they are not the only criteria used in the priority setting process. Consumer preferences, human rights, and political processes (for example, the Millennium Summit that brought the MDGs) continue to play important roles. What gives the economic arguments an edge in the process is the struggle for resources and who controls that process-when there are many competing needs for resources and not enough money to meet all needs, decision makers are pushed by parliaments and donor agencies to prioritize, and the broad economic criteria above (poverty reduction, economic growth and stability, good governance) tend to take center stage.

Recent funding trends suggest that reproductive health and rights have not done well in the resource allocation process. While poor reproductive health outcomes (for example, high maternal mortality and morbidity rates) are reflected in country-level burden of disease reports, the BOD associated with them is typically lower than that for infectious diseases. Inclusion of maternal mortality reduction in the MDG list has helped ensure that it remains a priority even when its contribution to the BOD is lower. While pregnancy involves health risks, it is not a disease, and the social and economic impacts of early or unintended pregnancies do not get counted in the BOD. Furthermore, the health consequences of unintended pregnancy tend to be poorly measured or not measured at all, so exclusion of fertility regulation from the MDG list has further eroded its position in the priority-setting process (AbouZahr and Vaughn 2000).

Another limitation of the BOD approach is that it fails to address distributional issues, a reflection of the utilitarian ("greatest good for the greatest numbers") value system on which it is based. The recognition in many quarters that raising overall average income levels or reducing overall mortality rates may do little to improve the lives of the poorest groups in society has prompted new thinking about the meaning of poverty and approaches to poverty reduction (Gwatkin 2000).

What About Rights?

An important shift brought by ICPD was its emphasis on reproductive rights, including the right to decide whether and when to engage in sexual activity, bear children, and marry; freedom from sexual violence; and the right to adequate reproductive health services as embodied in the ICPD goal of "universal access to reproductive health services." While economists may agree with the rights approach, particularly the broadly stated right to adequate health care, they typically counter with the question "How do you decide which health care services to fund when resources are limited?" Their inclination, as noted above, is to employ economic approaches such as BOD analysis to decide. Rights advocates counter that certain groups, particularly poor women and children, have special claims, and the inclusion of maternal and child health in the list of MDGs can be viewed as recognition of this. But what about the dimensions of reproductive health and rights that were excluded from the MDGs?

Reproductive rights advocates may be able to gain traction in the dialogue with economists by getting them to recognize that reproductive ill health is one of the multiple dimensions of poverty the World Bank 2000/2001 *World Development Report* defined as "pronounced deprivation in well-being" (World Bank 2000: 15). According to that report, poverty encompasses not only material deprivation (income and consumption poverty) but also low levels of education and health when they accompany material deprivation. Additional dimensions of poverty include vulnerability and exposure to risk as well as voicelessness and powerlessness. Where income and health are concerned, vulnerability means that in addition to falling into income or health poverty, there is exposure to other risks, including "violence, crime, natural disasters and being pulled out of school." The report cites Amartya Sen's (1999) characterization of these forms of deprivation as restricting the "capabilities that a person has, that is, the substantive freedoms he or she enjoys to lead the kind of life he or she values."

The capabilities approach recognizes the connections between income/consumption poverty and capabilities, but views that former as "instrumental" in achieving the latter. In this approach, health and education are viewed as important ends (or rights, though Sen does not use that language) in themselves as well as means to reducing poverty measured in terms of income and/or consumption. Health and education are also core assets in the economists' calculations of human capital. Other aspects of well-being include adequate nutrition, social inclusion, and opportunity to earn. There is debate whether and how to measure how these capabilities add up to "well-being," which leads many economists to prefer poverty metrics based on income/consumption. On the other hand, if health and education indicators are poverty reduction ends in themselves as well as being instrumental to the reduction of income-consumption poverty, it may ease possible tensions between rights and economic rationales for including reproductive health and rights in setting priorities if, indeed, it can be shown that failure to help poor women achieve them undermines their chances to escape poverty.

There is much survey evidence to show that poor women have worse reproductive health outcomes and make less use of health services (for example, delivery attendance by a medically trained person) than the non-poor. For example, tabulations by wealth quintiles of Demographic and Health Surveys data carried out during the late 1990s for 56 countries show that an average of one-third of women in the poorest quintiles had attended deliveries compared to over four-fifths for women in the richest quintiles (Gwatkin et al. 2004). These tabulations rely on a measure of household assets (ownership of a bicycle or radio) and housing characteristics (numbers of rooms, toilet facilities) that has been shown to work as a good proxy for household income/consumption levels, which DHS surveys do not measure.

Does Poor Reproductive Health Undermine Poverty Reduction?

If the answer to this question is "yes," then there is a strong case for donors and countries to support a range of reproductive health services for poor women. Available research is less helpful than one would hope. Economists are quick to point out that the association between poverty and poor reproductive health outcomes does not prove that these outcomes cause poverty. Some of the main findings from a review of available research on the effects of selected reproductive health outcomes (early childbearing, complications of delivery, and unintended pregnancy) on household level variables relating to health, education, and well-being, and of gaps in the evidence base about them are highlighted below (Greene and Merrick 2005). Generally speaking, the evidence base on health effects is strongest, household well-being weakest, and education between the other two.

Looking at early childbearing, there is strong evidence that very early pregnancy adversely affects the health of children and mothers, including lifelong morbidities (for example, obstetric fistulae). With regard to educational outcomes, there is some evidence of links between early childbearing and dropping out of school, but reasons other than pregnancy (poor performance, cost) are often more important than pregnancy. In the realm of well-being (earnings/consumption), there is more evidence that early childbearing adversely affects household economic conditions in Latin America (where marriage age is later) than in Africa and Asia (where early marriage and childbearing are more closely linked).

Turning to complications of delivery, a number of studies point to lower survival chances and poorer health outcomes for children of mothers who died as a result of delivery complications; women who survive often have lifelong morbidities, but these are poorly documented. There is limited evidence that children of mothers who die get less education, but this is mediated by fosterage and other contextual factors; much more evidence is being compiled on the condition of AIDS orphans. Finally, there is little or no evidence of impacts of pregnancy-related mortality and morbidity on the well-being of households.

Considering the outcomes of unintended pregnancy, there is substantial evidence that short birth intervals affect child survival; for mothers, the number of births has more impact than birth intervals; unsafe abortion is a widely documented health risk associated with unwanted pregnancy. In some contexts, large family size reduces investment in children's education, and there is some evidence that large family size creates competition in household spending on children, with adverse effects on girls in some settings.

Several caveats emerged from the review. There was general agreement that more household level analysis was needed, and that the relationships of interest are more complex at this level than at the macroeconomic level. Causal relationships are difficult to establish because reproductive health outcomes and other household level explanatory variables are themselves influenced by each other. One of the themes that occurred repeatedly was that relationships tend to be context specific and that one cannot look at individual characteristics without taking account of the context in which they are observed.

One of these contextual variables is the level of economic development. When there are no schools and health clinics, parents have few options for improving their children's health and schooling. The consequences of early marriage and childbearing depend in part on the structure and cost of schooling. Increasing returns to educational investments may motivate parents to subsidize the cost of younger children by relying on the labor and inputs of older children, particularly daughters.

As countries move through the transition from high to low fertility, they experience changes in age structure at both the societal and household levels, moving from high child dependency through periods of rapid growth in the young adult and mature adult populations and eventually to rising old-age dependency (see Bloom and Canning 2003). Much of the recent discussion of macrolevel economic-demographic linkages has focused on the temporary windows of opportunity afforded by these age shifts for the accumulation of physical and human capital (see World Bank 2007). There may be parallels at the household level. Groups in society at the leading edges of such change may be able to take advantage of them by educating their children and finding good jobs that bring higher income and asset accumulation. Those at the trailing edge may lose out because of the adverse impacts of poor reproductive health outcomes.

Intrahousehold decisions are affected by local labor market conditions. For example, Hausmann and Székely (2001) investigated the premise that child rearing requires resources that have opportunity costs related to the mother's earnings potential in the labor market. They found that the number of children a mother has, her husband's earnings, her own earnings potential, and labor market conditions are key determinants of where she will work—at home, in the informal economy, or in the formal labor market, and that these relationships, in turn, affect the educational attainment of the next generation. Adult and child market wage rates help determine the extent to which work competes with schooling for children's time (poverty makes child labor more attractive, so children do not attend school).

Cultural and institutional factors also affect the process in a variety of ways. While mothers may be more child-oriented in their expenditures than fathers, their capacity to act on this will depend on their access to resources and their autonomy in using household resources. In cultures where responsibilities for child support extend beyond children's own parents to grandparents, aunts and uncles, and others, the number of siblings may be a less important determinant. Where child fostering is common, the impact of additional children is spread across a wider kin network. Another aspect of variation in household dynamics relates to gender roles, and the child-rearing responsibilities assumed or not assumed by men and women.

All this underscores the importance of marshaling country-level evidence on relationships between poor reproductive health outcomes and poverty reduction and of ensuring that this evidence gets to the attention of those who are preparing Poverty Reduction Strategies and other documents that guide resource allocation. While care is required when contextual factors may be influencing the impact of poor reproductive health outcomes in specific settings, policy decisions do not need to wait for replication of "gold-standard" causal analysis in every case. When available country-level data are consistent with more robust findings that do meet such standards, policy makers should not ignore them, though they should recognize that the strength of the relationships may not be estimated with complete accuracy. This has been the practice in other realms, for example, the recent emphasis on the importance of good governance, where the evidence base is still being developed but common sense argues for addressing the issue. Nor should we have to wait for a full and complete understanding of these relationships to make the kinds of investments that will ensure that poor women have the information and access to services that will enable them to achieve the better reproductive health outcomes that their better-off sisters already enjoy.

Who Is at the Table When Priorities Are Set?

It is critically important that all stakeholders be effectively involved in setting priorities and guiding financing decisions, and that they follow up to ensure that money is actually spent on improving reproductive health outcomes. To ensure that the resource allocation process does not shortchange reproductive health and rights, its champions need to understand the process, assess the risks to reproductive health associated with the methods and approaches used, and act strategically to mitigate those risks. Rather than stand on the sidelines and lament what is going wrong, reproductive health advocates need to engage in the process through a variety of mechanisms. A key step is to establish clear goals and agreed-on measurable indicators of progress toward these goals—one of the main shifts in approach under reform is that progress in implementing programs focuses on results rather than inputs. It is also critical to involve the user community in program design, management, and oversight. New approaches in donor assistance and the reproductive health approach share a concern that the needs/demands of users of health services inform the design and management of those services. There are encouraging examples of effective community involvement in this area (Jahan and Germain 2004).

Supporters of reproductive health programs must ensure that there is adequate financial and technical support for priority program areas. The budget process is an entry point for this, but should be complemented by expenditure tracking to determine whether funds that are allocated are actually spent on provision of information and services for poor women and children. A number of countries have developed reproductive health and HIV/AIDS sub-accounts for national health accounts. Public expenditure reviews are another tool that reproductive health advocates can employ.

Last, champions of reproductive health and rights should take part in change management to ensure an effective transition process. Many countries have established change management units to guide the change process and to bring in experts in such areas as management and organizational capacity building, personnel systems, and financial management. Reproductive health interests need to be represented in such units.

Health resource allocation and efforts to improve and expand reproductive health services can and should be mutually reinforcing, but this is not guaranteed. Both require changes in the way of doing business. It is not enough to leave the design and implementation of expenditure plans to health economists. Champions of reproductive health must be "at the table" when plans are being discussed. They need to employ the language and analytical tools of expenditure planning to track the ways in which specific investments are affecting reproductive health outcomes. They must also demonstrate to financiers that investments in reproductive health will help countries to improve the well-being of poor women and their families, goals that economists and reproductive health advocates share.

Chapter 6
Measuring Reproductive Health: From Contraceptive Prevalence to Human Development Indicators

Joan Kaufman

The reproductive health field burst upon the scene in the years leading up to the historic ICPD in 1994 and the Fourth World Conference on Women in Beijing the following year. With its roots in population and family planning, the new world of reproductive health reached out to bring in important new perspectives on human sexuality, women's health, women's rights, sexual rights, and women's empowerment. Reproductive health spurred a major rethinking about human reproduction and its biological, social, economic, cultural, and political determinants and outcomes. Separate from other primary health care services, a new paradigm was launched, but one connected to a broader vision of factors, especially those related to development. Distinct from and yet part of the health and development sectors, reproductive health after Cairo immediately faced the complication of developing measures of its own success. The separation of the field from a basis in primary health care and its "balkanization" within the larger development agenda has ended up marginalizing reproductive health in more contentious current political environment. Without consensus on evidence-based indicators, the place of sexual and reproductive health and rights risks becoming sidelined, as evidenced by its omission from the Millennium Development Goals (MDGs) in 2000 (Crossette 2005). All this is taking place in a world increasingly challenged by an expanding sexually transmitted AIDS epidemic, making links to reproductive health programs even more urgent. Moreover, breakdowns in access to needed health services for the world's poor intensify the implications of sidelining crucial lifesaving sexual and reproductive health interventions.

This chapter reviews the history of measurement in the reproductive health field, and examines current methodological and political challenges associated with measuring reproductive health. It then offers a broader framework for evaluating sexual and reproductive health and rights as a central component of human development. It provides a historical overview on measurement and evaluation in reproductive health, highlighting the choice and appropriateness of indicators used, and links measurement approaches to the evolution of the concepts and debates about sexual and reproductive health and rights in the last twenty years. It argues that the balkanization of the reproductive health agenda within primary health care and the development field is and has been counterproductive beyond the standard political debates. Reintegrating the health and rights constituents into other development areas and a poverty reduction framework, as has been done by several Millennium Project task forces, may be a first step in recentralizing these essential issues for human development. The chapter concludes with suggestions for institutionalizing measures of reproductive health and rights into assessments of development determinants and impacts.

Measurement of Reproductive Health Before ICPD: Demographic Outcomes

The international population and family planning movement emerged in the 1960s as a central part of the global development agenda. Following the earlier work of Margaret Sanger and birth control advocacy groups in the United States (Chesler 1992; Harkavy 1995), the U.S. government launched a concerted international development assistance effort to promote contraception through family planning programs. It was based primarily on a neo-Malthusian rationale linking population control and reduced fertility to economic development and environmental sustainability. Evaluation indicators in the family planning field focused almost exclusively on measures of contraceptive use, that is, births averted and fertility decline. The "proximate determinants of fertility" framework developed by Bongaarts (1978) was the accepted effects model, and most measurement approaches were derived from it. Within family planning programs, measures of progress included Couple Years of Protection (CYP, a measure of supplies distributed), Contraceptive Prevalence Rate (CPR, a point in time measure of all women using contraceptive methods), Contraceptive Acceptance Rate, and in some cases, Contraceptive Continuation Rate. Social and economic determinants were important for driving fertility decline. However, organized family planning programs were shown to be essential to achieve population decline in less developed countries in the short term (Lapham and Mauldin 1985; Simmons and Lapham 1987) and became the accepted dogma.

The World Fertility Surveys (1972–84), Contraceptive Prevalence Surveys (1977–85), and their successor Demographic and Health Surveys (DHS, 1984–present), were then designed and launched to provide data on family planning use, contraceptive prevalence, and fertility. These measures remain a central focus to this day. The surveys have been conducted in over 75 countries for 30 years. Many important new indicators have been added in recent years to measure new challenges such as HIV/AIDS, gender-based violence, and service use issues for both family planning and maternal and child health services. The DHS and the frameworks that drive them, despite shortcomings, have been incorporated into mainstream development discussions. While providing evidence about the natural course of the demographic transition, these surveys have documented the role that family planning programs have had in expediting reduced fertility and improving child and maternal survival. They have also shown the effects of smaller, spaced families on women and girls' education and increased labor force participation. With a widely agreed upon outcome (fertility reduction) and a large evidence base provided by the DHS and their predecessors, family planning access became a central strategy for development, especially women's development, in the developing world.

Reproductive Health as Redefined by ICPD: Sexual and Reproductive Health and Rights

The ICPD revised the paradigm for understanding fertility and human reproduction. Whereas the dominant rationale for family planning programs was based on the consequences of fertility, the ICPD articulated a set of health, rights, and development determinants that drove fertility as well as other health outcomes related to sexual behavior. The ICPD agenda shifted the focus of the population control movement from fertility control measured on a population basis to the social, political, and economic circumstances of the individuals whose behaviors result in aggregate outcomes. ICPD broadened the need for programs beyond family planning provision alone to more comprehensive approaches that incorporated services provided by other parts of the health system, such as safe pregnancy and delivery services and gynecological care including screening and treatment of sexually transmitted infections and reproductive tract infections (STIs/RTIs), nutrition, and HIV/AIDS care. It also broadened its scope to address important determinants affecting reproduction and health, including a stronger focus on women's social status and rights protection across the life span. Within the realm of family planning programs, service quality was reoriented to focus more on client needs, presuming that attention to such matters would result in more effective contraceptive use and continuation. The WHO definition of reproductive health outlined a set of required health services and outcomes. This definition formed the basis for developing new indicators for reproductive health in the post-ICPD period (WHO 1994). An influential volume published by the National Research Council in the U.S. in 1997 identified key areas of services required for achieving reproductive health acknowledging the cultural context for healthy sexuality and taking as its framework that sex acts should be free of coercion and infection, pregnancies should be intended, and each birth should be healthy (National Research Council 1997).

While this broader definition of what constituted reproductive health was based on strong evidence, the expansion and myriad nature of these factors have made it more challenging to measure, especially when some of these factors lie outside the medical or health services realm. As a result, there is a lack of consensus about what to measure, particularly about which factors outside the health system should be included in indices of reproductive health. Most agencies have tried to devise a short core set of indicators that can be feasibly collected in diverse settings, rather than a comprehensive list of harder to measure indicators (e.g., power in sexual decision making). As a result, most of the measurement effort has focused on specific health problems related to pregnancy, STIs/RTIs, contraceptive use, and abortion, albeit including a defined set of proxy measures for social and economic status and enabling factors, such as the legal status of abortion. Major development agencies (e.g., United Nations Population Fund, USAID, WHO) that provided financial and technical support to reproductive health programs in the years following ICPD have developed indicators and evaluation approaches for measuring reproductive health determinants, service provision, and outcomes (UNFPA 1998; Bertrand, Magnani, and Knowles 1994; Bertrand and Tsui 1995; Bertrand and Escudero 2002; WHO 2006a). These efforts involved numerous experts and practitioners working together to specify the pathways to better reproductive health.[1] Large compendia of indicators and boiled down shorter lists have resulted from these efforts. In particular, the framework and indicators published by the USAID Evaluation Project (Bertrand, Magnani, and Knowles 1994; Bertrand and Tsui 1995) and Measure Evaluation Project (Bertrand and Escudero 2002) (framework attached as Figure 4 below) have provided the most commonly used framework for understanding the determinants of reproductive health and their measurement. One glance at the framework reveals the complexity, if not daunting nature of the undertaking. Crosscutting issues like women's status, the policy environment, management, training, and logistics systems are detailed, and male involvement is often included as well. However, the main indicators are within programs and services, and measured outcomes are mainly related to individual behaviors, contraceptive use, use of pregnancy and delivery services, and RTI/STD/HIV outcomes. The relationship of enabling factors like women's agency and autonomy, health infrastructure and access to services, and the presence of civil strife are rarely incorporated into determinants, even though all would agree that the "supply environment" of reproductive health services cannot be really understood without considering such factors.

Moreover, development changes take time. Focusing on point in time process and outcome indicators belies the reality that women's agency, poverty reduction, and other determinants like nutrition and education are longer-term processes. On the flip side, the relationship between these outcomes and broader development objectives has received insufficient attention (until the Millennium Project forcefully made the connections) (Bernstein and Juul Hansen 2006), unlike in the pre-ICPD era when aggregate demographic trends were closely linked to social and economic outcomes.[2] The post-ICPD reproductive health field has been less focused on providing the evidence base for the development benefits of reproductive health, partly because it has been preoccupied with defending core turf on issues like sexual rights, access to abortion, and safe sex programs for youth (see Merrick, this volume for another perspective). Rights issues have dominated the discussions, while the public health and development benefits have received less attention.

A Broader Approach to Measurement and Evaluation

The Fourth World Conference on Women in Beijing the year after ICPD reaffirmed the new paradigm of reproductive health and rights espoused at Cairo and further articulated the social, economic, and political determinants required to insure women's right to health. The Beijing Conference emphasized the important links between women's poverty and social inequity, especially gender inequity, for the achievement of reproductive health and population goals (UN Department of Economic and Social Affairs 1995). The larger mandate of these and other UN Conferences in the 1990s as well as the regular UN Human Development Reports has been to highlight the critical importance of not only social investments in health and education by governments but also the protection of rights and promotion of freedoms and agency for achieving basic social and economic advancement.

U.S.-based private foundations such as the Ford Foundation had been heavily investing in advocating for and implementing the ICPD

Programme of Action. Ford's Asset Building and Community Development Program Reproductive Health team established a working group[3] in 1998 to develop a broader framework for understanding and measuring the determinants of and progress toward achieving sexual and reproductive health and rights, drawing on the work of Amartya Sen[4] and the human development assessments of the United Nations. The work of the group was driven by the perception that indicators and measurement approaches available at the time were insufficient. Nor were the research or evaluation frameworks capable of demonstrating the centrality of reproductive health and rights for the achievement of other development goals. The Ford Foundation team and other like-minded colleagues saw a need for a new conceptual framework to lay out the role of reproductive health and rights in social and economic development, from an intergenerational as well as a gender perspective.

The working group began by drafting its own framework for thinking about reproductive health and rights and its broad and difficult to define determinants, such as social development and women's empowerment. The group then commissioned an inventory of available indicators that might be deployed to measure the different components of that framework and the specific reproductive health services required to achieve reproductive health and rights goals (Ford Foundation and IPPF 2002). The following areas were included: family planning, safe motherhood, abortion and post abortion care, RTIs and STDs, HIV/AIDS, youth sexual and reproductive health, male involvement in sexual and reproductive health, and sexuality. Women's empowerment categories included gender equity, rights, education, and prevention of violence against women. Social and economic development categories included social context and culture, migration, and health sector reform.

With the help of a group of external experts,[5] a conceptual framework was developed (see Figures 1–3). Despite the complexity of those frameworks, two clear key goals were developed: (1) healthy sexuality free from violence and discrimination and (2) the highest possible standard of sexual and reproductive health and rights. A combined framework that graphically shows the relationship of these two goals to the ultimate goal of overall well-being and maximized human potential (human capability in Sen's term) also developed, highlighting its importance for an enabling context for reproductive health and rights as well as critical prerequisite conditions. Some of these enabling environment factors include political security and freedom from conflict, investment in human capital, cultural, secular, and religious legitimacy for positive sexuality, democratic governance and strong civil society, economic security, and respect for human rights. The prerequisite conditions in-

GOAL #1: Pleasurable (Healthy) Sexuality
Freedom from Violence & Discrimination

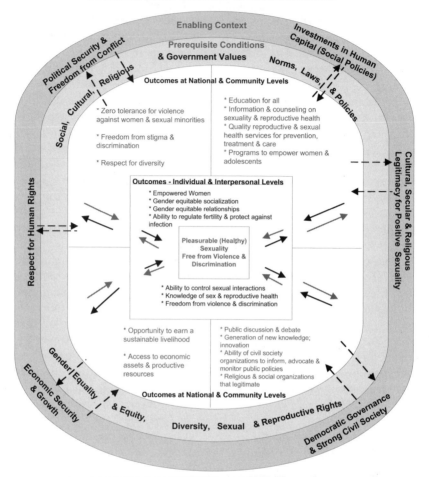

Figure 1. Goal 1: Pleasurable (healthy) sexuality; freedom from violence and discrimination. Ford Foundation Reproductive Health Indicators Working Group 2001.

clude supportive government values and norms, policies and laws, gender equality and equity, sexual and reproductive rights protection, and health equity. These enabling and prerequisite conditions lead to many other positive outcomes at the national and community level, such as economic opportunity, education, and open public debate. They also have a direct impact on individual and personal circumstances that are necessary for achieving reproductive health and rights goals, such as

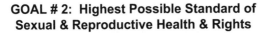

GOAL # 2: Highest Possible Standard of Sexual & Reproductive Health & Rights

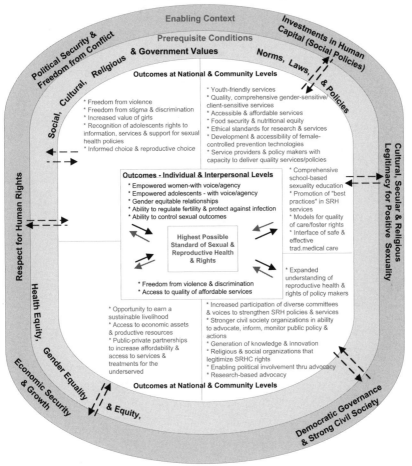

Figure 2. Goal 2: Highest possible standards of sexual and reproductive health and rights. Ford Foundation Reproductive Health Indicators Working Group 2001.

women's empowerment, gender equitable relationships, knowledge of sex and reproductive health, and freedom from violence.

The framework illustrates the complex set of factors that ideally must be measured to adequately represent the conditions for achieving reproductive health and rights. Furthermore, the framework places these outcomes within a larger development model, since all enabling and prerequisite factors are central components of social and economic and

Relationship Between Two Goals - Overlapping & Synergistic

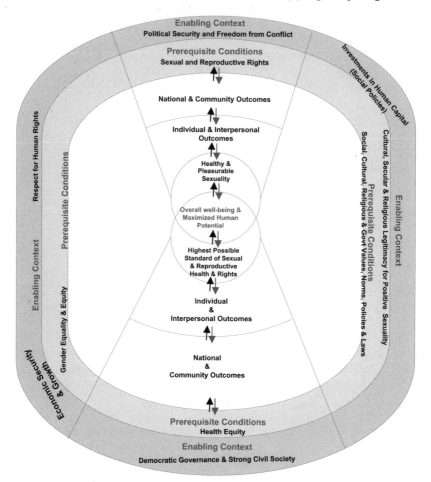

Figure 3. Relationship between two goals—overlapping and synergistic. Ford Foundation Reproductive Health Indicators Working Group 2001.

political development. Seen this way, achievement of reproductive health and rights becomes a key component of development and an outcome necessary for overall well-being and maximized human potential.

Issues of sexuality and reproductive health are inseparable as outlined above. However, it is precisely the connection to sexuality and sexual rights that has become a stumbling block in advancing the field to its rightful place as a central component of development. These topics have become highly contested in recent years, and as a result are often not measured in current reproductive health programs. When the components of reproductive health become contested politically, measurement of the factors contributing to key reproductive health outcomes becomes more difficult, contributing to a vicious cycle in which both the evidence base and the political support for reproductive health programs are undermined.

Challenges in Developing Frameworks for Measurement

A main factor driving the sidelining of reproductive health in development policy is the attack on sexual rights and abortion from the conservative and religious right both in the U.S. and abroad. The Catholic Church has long opposed abortion and contraception (Mumford 1986), including condom use for HIV prevention. Along with social conservatives in the U.S. and abroad, the religious right has changed the terms into a defense of the nuclear family and family values; in their terms reproductive health presumably threatens a woman's primary role as mother and homemaker. "Reproductive rights" have been construed by opponents to mean abortion rights and the right to have same sex partnerships, and thus many groups have avoided discussion of rights so as not to threaten their work on and funding for other issues. The repercussions for the reproductive health field have been enormous (see Girard, Berer, and Kissling, all in this volume). As funding has decreased, measurement efforts have retrenched to specific service areas (WHO Department of Reproductive Health Rights 2006c). In an effort to avoid losing ground and minimize the risk of further antagonizing hostile actors, many policy makers have chosen to invest in a more limited set of interventions. Little mainstream effort is underway to tie in the important and inseparable evidence related to the impact of access to legal abortion, youth sexual behavior, or women's agency and empowerment. All this may change under a different political climate, but politics are not the only factor.

The second major challenge to reproductive health has come from the new priority setting approaches to health. Even as WHO estimated in 2001 that sexual and reproductive health problems accounted for 18 percent of the global burden of disease (BOD) among women ages 15–44 (Singh et al. 2003), reproductive health services are receiving decreasing attention for investment and focus in health care. In part this is because of the preeminence of the BOD methodology that measures ill health caused by disease or life style and behavior, known as disability adjusted life years (DALYs), for priority setting (Murray and Lopez 1996). Allotey and Reidpath (2002) provide an overview of the problems of using DALYs in the reproductive health field. The deficit to a healthy life that the DALY is supposed to capture is thought to be underestimated in the area of reproductive health morbidity (AbouZhar 1999). This underestimation is likely due to several problems involved with measuring reproductive health burden. Women often underutilize the health system for many of their main reproductive problems, despite the potentially dire sequelae for morbidity. Moreover, both culture and context affect the experience and subsequent reporting of morbidity (e.g., infertility; see van Balen and Inhorn 2002). Because the BOD methodology is based on the International Classification of Disease, which is organ- and pathology-based, it tends to miss the real experience of morbidity and its consequences in developing countries, such as social exclusion, divorce, and resulting depression due to infertility. In addition, the linkages regarding risks for maternal morbidity are not adequately captured, such as the impact of malaria in pregnancy or the consequences of unsafe abortion on future fertility. The implications of intergenerational impacts, such as the role of maternal nutritional deficiencies on subsequent birth outcomes, are hardly captured in the BOD framework (Stillwaggon 2006; Inhorn 2004).

A fundamental limitation of applying BOD analysis to reproductive health is that reproductive health services are most often preventive in nature, and measuring non-health determinants that influence health-seeking for women, like empowerment and self-efficacy, is not part of the BOD approach. Essentially, measuring problems averted is more difficult than measuring years of working life lost to a disease or event. For example, measuring obstetric fistulae averted by attended deliveries and reduced numbers of births would be more difficult than measuring the occurrence of fistulae. Carla AbouZahr (1999) raises similar concerns but links them to the challenges of quantifying health gains due to the provision of key reproductive health interventions, such as family planning. The value of these preventive interventions is not well captured in the BOD approach, although these interventions are a major acknowledged contributor to health and development. She notes that to the degree that the BOD method does capture maternal conditions and their impacts, it is heavily biased toward pregnancy and pregnancy-related issues and biased against other less visible conditions that lead to measurable ill health for women, such as uterine prolapse or reproductive tract infections.

Efforts to measure reproductive health face several other hurdles. Together with the burden of disease methodology, donors are increasingly partitioning development issues and focusing funds in new neovertical funding mechanisms, like the Global Fund for AIDS, TB, and Malaria or the Global Alliance for Vaccines and Immunizations. As key health and development issues become more separated for both funding and global attention, the trend is away from complex systems analysis and comprehensive paradigms. Moreover, the capacity of the health system to deliver reproductive health interventions, especially preventive ones, is rarely calculated. One study in rural China clearly showed that health service utilization for key reproductive health services like prenatal care, safe delivery, and screening and treatment of RTIs was adversely affected by women's inability to pay for those services. The study also showed that the breakdown in health education about the importance of seeking preventive services for these conditions undermined health seeking and health outcomes further (Kaufman and Jing 2002). In other words, weakened health systems intersect with poverty and gender inequity to erode women's right to basic health services. Therefore it is important to include measurement of systemic processes such as the impact of health sector reform and human resource shortages when evaluating reproductive health service availability and outcomes.

At the same time, identifying measures of persistent gender inequalities in health access and utilization are important. Structural gender inequity intersects with weakened health systems to affect not only what services are provided but the ability of women to shape and use them. Lack of women's participation in health planning and gender insensitivity at the local level often undermine the appropriateness of services offered. Germain explored the "Culture of Silence" (International Women's Health Coalition 1994) that prevents women from seeking medical assistance for embarrassing reproductive tract infections from male doctors; similarly the Gender and Health Equity Initiative studies in China, India, and Mozambique are currently exploring how women's lack of participation in health planning within weakened health services impedes availability of appropriate services to meet their real needs (Sen, George, and Ostlin 2002; Gender and Health Equity Network nd). Efforts have been undertaken to incorporate gender perspectives into measurement such as the International Planned Parenthood Federation *Manual to Evaluate Quality of Care from a Gender Perspective* (IPPF/WHR 2002 with Latin American Women's Health Network) but these efforts have not been scaled up and incorporated into any global measurement approaches.

New Challenges to the Measurement of Reproductive Health: MDGs

Current global measurement approaches for development are now focused on achievement of the Millennium Development Goals (MDGs). Of the eight MDGs, three have substantial health and gender equity components that will be hard to meet without achieving full access to reproductive health services and protection of reproductive rights: Combat AIDS, malaria and other diseases (Goal 6); Promote gender equality and empower women (Goal 3); and Improve maternal health (Goal 5). Political factors resulted in the lack of mention of reproductive health and rights in the formulation of the MDGs, and substantial effort has been underway to integrate them. Much of that work has been concentrated in the actions and analysis of two Millennium Project task forces: Gender Equality and Safe Motherhood. The work of these two task forces resonates with the pathways to development outlined in the conceptual frameworks presented earlier.

The background to the establishment of these task forces is an important part of the measurement story. Reproductive health, as a number of chapters in this volume note, was left out of the Millennium Development Goals, a UN-led effort, despite international endorsement of the ICPD Programme of Action, an earlier UN-led effort. Haslegrave and Bernstein (2005) note that the two MDG goals on maternal health and HIV/AIDS have explicit reproductive health content, but there is no reference anywhere to access to contraceptive services provision—a key aspect of international development efforts over several decades. After the Millennium Summit established the MDGs in 2000, there was considerable outcry and advocacy about the omission of the ICPD goals; therefore, when the Millennium Project was established to work out specific measurable targets and indicators for each MDG, task forces were composed to include academic and program representatives working on women's empowerment and reproductive health and rights. The task force working on MDG 5 (Improve Maternal Health) added a new target on universal access to sexual and reproductive health, endorsed by the UN General Assembly in October 2006, and added language on equitable access for the poor and marginalized (Freedman et al. 2005a).[6] The task force specified goals related to achieving levels of contraceptive prevalence, reducing HIV prevalence among 15–24-year-old women, increasing the proportion of births attended by a skilled birth attendant, measuring the proportion of demand for family planning satisfied, reducing adolescent fertility rates, and increasing the availability of emergency obstetric care. These are all goals also specified in the ICPD Programme of Action in 1994.

The task force working on MDG 3 (Promote Gender Equality and Empower Women) outlined seven strategic priorities which include both guaranteeing sexual and reproductive health and rights and combating violence against girls and women (Grown et al. 2005). Most important, the task force also developed and adopted an operational framework of gender equality in three dimensions that are critical to achievement of MDG 3: capabilities, access to resources and opportunities, and security domains. This framework echoes the determinants outlined in the frameworks presented earlier, particularly Sen's capabilities framework. The task force also noted the need to ensure reproductive health services within often constrained national public health systems. Despite the rigorous efforts of these task forces to develop goals and indicators, there is still no consensus on what needs to be measured to monitor reproductive health service provision to achieve these MDGs. Dixon-Mueller and Germain (2006) examined sets of indicators proposed for use by the MDG task forces—contraceptive prevalence rate, total fertility rate, unmet need for contraception and unplanned births, unsafe abortion, and abortion mortality. They concluded that no measure of contraceptive use or total fertility will be sufficient without measuring unplanned pregnancies and births as well as the ability to terminate pregnancies safely. Furthermore, Crossette's (2005) review of the political process surrounding the MDGs concludes with skepticism about whether the Millennium Project task force reports will succeed in reintegrating attention to reproductive health given its original omission from the Millennium Report and Declaration.

Unresolved Debates

The work of the MDG Task Forces has successfully made the case for measuring reproductive health and rights within the now commonly accepted development goals of the MDGs. Still, debates continue about the inclusion of other core aspects of the ICPD agenda that have implications for measurement; furthermore, lack of measurability has implications for their inclusion in policies and programs such as the place of sexuality and sexual rights on the overall agenda, the comprehensiveness of the service packages promoted (i.e., women's health or reproductive health), whether reproductive health should continue to be problem-defined or should focus instead on healthy sexuality, and how to include measurement of enabling factors for achieving and pursuing a healthy sexual and reproductive life.

In 1994, the ICPD stated that reproductive health included having a safe and satisfying sex life. However, WHO recently defined sexual health as "broader and more encompassing than reproductive health" (WHO 2004). WHO argues that in order to have good reproductive health, women need to be in control of their sexual lives and have access to health services.[7] However sexual rights, other than sexual satisfaction, are omitted from this definition. These rights include freedom to choose one's sexual partner, including sexual orientation, freedom from coerced sex within and outside marriage, and the rights to sexual health information and services, particularly for adolescents. These are the precise areas of political debate that have contributed to marginalizing the reproductive health agenda and remain largely off the screen for measurement. This creates a vicious cycle—when these issues are not included, there are few attempts to measure them, but without effective measurement it is more difficult to make the case for their inclusion. One symptom of this is that WHO's Department of Reproductive Health Research guidelines on reproductive health indicators (published in 2006) revert to a short list of medical, problem-defined factors related to fertility and contraceptive use, safe pregnancy and delivery, and sexually transmitted diseases and HIV/AIDS. They omit any enabling factors now commonly agreed upon as the important determinants of individual behavior and service utilization. Moreover, most international agencies, including the MDG task forces, have defined reproductive health around a set of focused services related to contraception and abortion access, prevention and treatment of STIs, including HIV, and safe pregnancy and delivery; some propose that women's reproductive health over the lifespan, from menarche to menopause, be addressed. Many bemoan the exclusive focus on women, noting that by ignoring half the world's population (men) and not focusing on couples and sexual networks, key driving factors are ignored (Sonfeld 2002; Becker 1999). Measurement continues to focus on problems, not healthy mental and physical outcomes associated with quality of life resulting from one's sexual and reproductive life. Insufficient attention has been paid to measurement of the enabling environment to achieve individual reproductive goals, such as access to adequately trained health providers within weakened health systems and the development of laws and policies about such critical issues as child marriage, same sex unions, abortion access, and women's inheritance.

The Way Forward

While the ICPD paradigm broadened the understanding of factors that must be examined to address and improve reproductive health outcomes, efforts at implementation have resulted in an unfortunate separation of the reproductive health and rights field from the rest of primary health care and from the overall development field. While the family planning and maternal and child health fields of earlier times may have had limited visions, they were firmly incorporated into development planning and their contributions to social and economic development were not contested. That is not the case with reproductive health. While the reason for this may be largely political, nevertheless there is also a need for a better focus and marshaling of the evidence to

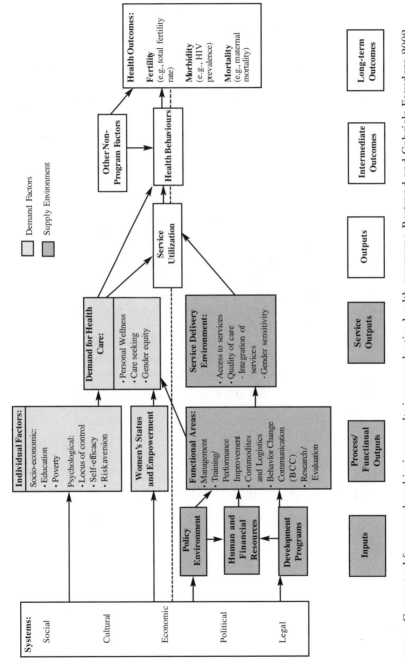

Figure 4. Conceptual framework: achieving results in reproductive health programs. Bertrand and Gabriela Escudero 2002.

support the importance of reproductive health and rights for achieving development. On the other hand, it is important to deliberately devise measures of the context and enabling environment affecting reproductive health and related development outcomes, such as gender equity and state of the health sector. A multilevel evaluation approach—as is mapped out in the frameworks provided in this chapter—is needed that measures the enabling environment and social, economic, and political determinants of reproductive health as well as incorporating core primary health care assessments such as access to clinical and prevention services. This evaluation framework also ought to measure not only reproductive health outcomes for individuals but intergenerational impacts as well.[8] This is not easy. It will take creativity to devise indicators that are feasible, easily available, and validated for such categories. However, this challenge must be addressed because reliance on individual and service measures and point of time assessments alone are insufficient. Provision and measurement of reproductive health and rights needs to resume a central place in the development agenda and the evidence must be marshaled to demonstrate its rightful place therein. Reproductive health services should be core constituents of primary health care service packages promoted by health agencies and donors in resource poor settings. Using a broader framework, as outlined in this chapter, to capture the key determinants and examine the outcomes for individuals and then connect the dots back to development impacts will help to restore reproductive health services and reproductive and sexual rights protection to its rightful place as an essential investment for achieving social justice in the world.

Part II
Human Rights Realizations

Chapter 7
Bearing Human Rights: Maternal Health and the Promise of ICPD

Mindy Jane Roseman

Women continue to suffer and die due to childbirth at the same stagger-ing levels they did at the time the Programme of Action of the 1994 ICPD Conference was adopted (Ronsmans and Graham 2006).[1] Is this surprising? In terms of policy direction, ICPD contains several refer-ences to maternal health services and includes an entire chapter de-voted to "safe motherhood." The Programme of Action (UN 1995) moreover benefited from the confluence of the international maternal health movement—a movement that predated, and coexisted with, ICPD's reproductive health and human rights advocacy movement. The persistence of maternal mortality and morbidity is a disappointment for both the reproductive rights movement and its allied safe motherhood movement.

Despite the consensus of ICPD, there continue to be diverging views on the best approach to reduce maternal mortality and morbidity. An emerging school of thought would, in effect, replace the human rights and empowerment approach of ICPD with the sole focus of achieving Millennium Development Goal (MDG) 5 of improving maternal health, with or without regard to rights. This approach advocates better data collection, improved financing, and the wholesale repair of the mater-nal health care system (Borghi, Ensor, Somanthian, et al. 2006; Ronsmans and Graham 2006). Conversely, there are those who believe that if MDG 5 is to be realized, the commitment to ICPD and reproduc-tive rights and health needs to be intensified, not jettisoned (Freedman et al. 2005a). This school of thought believes that ICPD does and will continue to provide an efficacious program for improving all aspects of reproductive health (Germain and Kidwell 2005). Finally, there is a third response that falls in between and advocates community health solutions as well as recognizes the importance of human rights (Costello, Azad, and Barnett 2006).

In light of these revisionist attitudes toward ICPD, this chapter examines the current state of global maternal health policy in terms of what is considered the unique contribution of ICPD to achieving health—its connection to human rights. While some work has tried to describe the impact of human rights on reproductive health (Cook, Dickens, and Fathalla 2003; Sundari 1992; Cook 1989), only a small portion has been concerned with its effects on maternal health (Sen, Govender, and Cottingham 2006; Cook and Bevilacqua 2004; Cook and Dickens 2001). The objective of this chapter is to identify the difference human rights has made for maternal health, particularly in light of ICPD. Human rights, the chapter argues, was the vehicle that uncoupled women's health during and after pregnancy from the health of the children they bore. Maternal health became a component of reproductive health, as reflected in ICPD. Moreover, human rights have been used in various ways to improve maternal health outcomes. The chapter examines some of the ways the human rights norms expressed in ICPD (and likeminded documents) have been relevant to maternal health. It concludes by assessing whether the human rights approach to reproductive and maternal health in ICPD has added any value, despite the lack of progress in reducing maternal mortality.

One of the challenges in assessing "value added" is agreeing on how human rights is being defined and measured. It is a slippery term that is used differently by different actors. When activists and scholars refer to human rights, they sometimes mean a system of formal accountability, sometimes advocacy, and sometimes an approach to programming. These different elements are related to each other, as will be discussed below; however, it is important to keep the categories distinct in order to assess the "value added" of human rights.[2] This chapter finds that human rights as advocacy has generated important norms that should guide national government and international agencies in their efforts to address maternal health; the formal international human rights system has issued such normative guidance, largely as a result of advocacy. Finally, human rights approaches, relatively recent developments that are inspired by human rights principles such as participation and nondiscrimination, may well help move the rhetoric closer toward implementation. While the value added of human rights to maternal health has been fundamental, it has also not been fully made manifest.

Maternal Health Before ICPD

International efforts to improve maternal health that predated ICPD for the most part conflated women with the children they bore. Maternal mortality was thought to be inevitable if tragic, until technological advances such as anesthesia and aseptic/antiseptic practices were developed in the late nineteenth and early twentieth centuries in the industrialized West and used to save women's lives (Loudon 1992). Preserving the life of a mother was often measured instrumentally, as important for, if not entirely conflated with, the health and well-being of her infant. No doubt this reflected a genuine concern for children who were nearly universally assumed to need the care of their mothers (Roseman 1999).[3] It is a telling point of departure that for much of the twentieth century the field was termed "Maternal and Child Health" (MCH).

In the mid-1980s, some voices in international public health drew attention to the persistence of maternal morbidity and mortality despite improvements in child health. A 1985 article with the provocative subtitle, "Where Is the M in MCH?" starkly presented an inherent bias in maternal and child health approaches; maternal and child health programs neglected women while laudably focusing on infants and children (Rosenfield and Maine 1985). Prevention and treatment of diarrhea, promotion of breastfeeding and growth monitoring of infants, and provision of immunizations were able to reduce the rates of infant and child death and disease. These interventions had no impact on women suffering injury or dying in childbirth or from pregnancy related causes. The authors noted, "not only are the causes of maternal death quite different from those of child death, but so are the potential remedies" (83). The recognition that the etiology and epidemiology of maternal morbidity and mortality diverged from those of children created some space to consider how to intervene to improve maternal health outcomes, as well as how women's individuality had been effaced in MCH programs.

Equally important were the contemporaneous social movements outside public health—especially feminism—around rights and health in particular countries and globally. The women's health and rights movements viewed women as human agents and not instruments to achieve governmental objectives stated in population policies (Correa and Petchesky 1994). The lack of autonomy women possessed to make decisions surrounding their health, and in particular related to motherhood, became the basis for conceptualizing "reproductive rights." State population control policies that coercively sterilized women and were driven by achieving targets were denounced; women's rights and health activists advocated for legal and policy measures to ensure voluntary access to quality family planning and safe termination of pregnancy services and information. A combination of good public health research and feminist political activism thus helped pave a new way forward for maternal health.

This recognition of the separation of women from their children is reflected in the International Conference on Safe Motherhood, held in Nairobi, Kenya, in February 1987. At this conference, international agencies, governments, and a few international nongovernmental organizations created the Safe Motherhood Initiative (SMI).[4] SMI asserted that maternal mortality persisted because of discrimination against women: in a keynote speech Dr. Halfdan Mahler, director general of WHO, stated that maternal morality

is a neglected tragedy, and it has been neglected because those who suffer it are neglected people, with the least power and influence over how national resources shall be spent; they are the poor, the rural peasants, and above all, women. (Starrs 1987: 4)[5]

Human rights did not yet figure in addressing this neglect. The 1987 SMI program of activities embraced intuitive solutions that seemed well tailored and sustainable, such as risk screening during prenatal care or training traditional birth attendants. These interventions, it was hoped, would make a difference for maternal health outcomes. They did not entail any significant change in gender relations. In other words, while maternal health researchers and advocates were converging on an analysis somewhat similar to human rights discourse about the causes of maternal mortality and morbidity (e.g., discrimination), their actual approaches did not contribute to women's empowerment.

ICPD: MCH Becomes Part of Reproductive Health

ICPD, as many of the chapters in this volume point out, brought human rights into matters of reproduction and sexuality (see Berer and Shepard, both in this volume). The basic definition of reproductive health is predicated on reproductive rights, and ICPD emphatically asserts that good health outcomes require the promotion and protection of human rights (Chapter 7). This emphasis reflected ICPD's central thesis: persistent inequality and discrimination against women fueled (over)population and (under)development. Rights guarantees, therefore, and not demographic targets would lift populations out of poverty. Furthermore, by emphasizing reproductive rights, ICPD focused attention principally on women as individuals, with due deference to the reality that for many women motherhood is a central aspect of their reality. It captured the momentum building through the Safe Motherhood

Initiative and assimilated it into the Programme of Action as "Women's Health and Safe Motherhood" (Chapter 8). ICPD also integrated maternity related health care services, such as those proposed by SMI, into the broader mosaic of services bundled and labeled as "reproductive health." This was a significant if not mini-paradigm shift within the overall ICPD paradigm shift: ICPD severed the ideological tie between maternal and child health. As if to highlight maternal health, ICPD proposed a clear goal: to cut the number of maternal deaths by half by the year 2000, and in half again by 2015—one of the few elements of ICPD directly translated into an MDG. To reach that goal, governments promised, in ICPD and subsequent agreements, to develop comprehensive strategies to ensure universal access to reproductive health services, with particular attention to maternal and emergency obstetric care, especially in underserved areas.[6]

Safe Motherhood as a "Human Right"

The effect of ICPD's reconceptualization of maternal health as part of reproductive health can be seen in the ten-year review of the Safe Motherhood Initiative in 1997. It turned out that ten years of effort promoting prenatal care and training birth attendants did relatively little to stop maternal death. Rather, research revealed that women were dying from hemorrhage, toxemia, obstructed labor, and the consequences of unsafe abortion. These conclusions led to a collective sense of disappointment over a previous decade's efforts and a strong difference of opinion as to which interventions should be prioritized,[7] as well as a certain degree of soul searching. Women, whose lives were each independently valued, deserved better; ICPD underscored this. Given that many individuals who were active in SMI were involved at ICPD, reproductive rights was considered a readily available concept to reenergize, if not reorganize future SMI efforts. James Wolfensohn, president of the World Bank and keynote speaker, put the fine point on the SMI malaise in his address to the conference: "Safe motherhood is a human right . . . if the system lets a woman die, then the system has failed" (quoted in Tinker, Finn, and Epp 2000). He focused on the systemic failures of the health sector in relation to women. His naming these deaths a human rights failure was a rallying point that resonated deeply with ICPD's reproductive rights framework.

While the SMI platform launched a salvo in the direction of governments, intergovernmental agencies, and NGOs to approach maternal mortality as a human rights violation, what exactly would that mean? Wolfensohn's speech raised as many questions as it answered for scholars and activists. Scholars recognized that "safe motherhood," like reproductive rights, was arguably a composite right—cobbled together from interpretations of existing rights, including those relating to life, health, and security of the person. It therefore might have potential to be the one-stop organizing principle for health interventions that would refocus attention on neglect of women and redirect efforts to strengthen maternal health systems.

To advocates and other actors, different questions were raised. Would ministers of health be liable for a woman's death? Could the poor staffing, training, or provision of a maternal health facility be a violation of a woman's right to life (Chapman 1996)? These questions produced anxiety, not only among governmental officials responsible for health and other sectors, but for the human rights movement itself.[8] Traditional human rights methodology focused on individual fact finding and reporting and had little familiarity with aggregate public health data. It was not altogether clear how to attribute systemic failure to the wrongdoing of an individual actor. Therefore to address the range of human rights issues raised by maternal mortality, a credible analysis toward accountability would have to be developed, as well as appropriate methodologies to connect practices, outcomes, and remedies.

By the late 1990s, thankfully, a significant body of scholarly literature discussing theories and methodology of accountability concerning the human rights dimensions of maternal mortality had developed. Some of this work has been foundational. Rebecca Cook's efforts defined how existing human rights have been interpreted so as to address maternal mortality (Cook 1999, 1998). Deborah Maine and Alicia Ely Yamin (1999) wrote more instrumentally, on using international health systems indicators as a standard to monitor governments and holding them to account for actions (or inactions) related to maternal health.[9] Lynn Freedman (2002, 2001) has also investigated the rhetorical force human rights bring to questions of motherhood and health and how that might be translated into programming. These articles have helped to frame and assess the value added of applying human rights to maternal health. The next logical progression is implementation: putting the ideas of human rights toward maternal mortality reduction into practice.

Maternal Mortality and Human Rights

Advocates, scholars, activists, and policy makers set out to do just that, and it is worth the effort to map out just what has been done in the name of human rights for maternal health. Human rights as a term has a certain mercurial quality. Its meaning often depends on the objectives of those who use it. What it must mean in the context of ICPD, however, is that women are valued as human agents in and of themselves, and not instrumentally as a function of their children's, families, communities, or state's needs. In other words women, at a minimum, must be able to exercise their agency—be free from violence and coercion and have the information and means to make decisions regarding their own reproduction and health. Governments would have an obligation to protect, respect, and fulfill these rights: for example, to provide a functional reproductive health system (including maternal health care) and ensure that third parties (such as husbands or mothers-in-law) do not interfere with a woman's right to access reproductive health services (including maternal health care). There are concrete examples of human rights influencing maternal health research, policy, and programming interventions. The next section of the chapter describes the ways in which human rights have been used within a formal system of accountability, as advocacy and as an approach to programming. The chapter then assesses their value, if any added, and concludes with a discussion of potential challenges and successes.

Maternal Health Policy: Human Rights as Accountability

Human rights, insofar as they are state obligations, can also be thought of as a formal system of international "legal" accountability, established through the UN institutional mechanisms. The treaties that contain rights related to maternal health (such as the rights to life, health, or information) require governments to ensure that their laws, policies, budgets, and other activities promote and protect these rights. Governments must regularly submit progress reports to treaty monitoring bodies. These bodies review the reports, hold discussions with the governments, and issue advisory statements called concluding observations or comments. These statements are a good measure by which to evaluate activity related to maternal health and the influence of the rights discourse.[10] While they are not binding law, they are evidence of emerging norms in state behavior and can help create the corpus of international customary law. At a minimum, they support standard setting for international policy making and the concrete work of local NGOs.

It is beyond the scope of this chapter to undertake a systematic, scientific review of all reports (governmental and nongovernmental) submitted, issues presented, and concluding observations issued by all the treaty bodies before and after ICPD.[11] (Nor, for that matter, does this chapter examine the incorporation of ICPD and reproductive rights into the national and transnational jurisprudence, legislation, and policies.[12]) However, a brief survey of the concluding observations issued by the major treaty bodies shows that prior to 1994, consideration of pregnancy and maternal mortality in human rights terms was rare.[13] By 1995 and thereafter, it was commonplace that maternal mortality rates give rise to some comment. For example, the Human Rights Committee (HRC),[14] which monitors the International Covenant on Civil and Political Rights, provided a detailed observation with regard to Mali:

While noting the considerable efforts made by the State party, the Committee remains concerned at the high maternal and infant mortality rate in Mali, due in particular to the relative inaccessibility of health and family planning services, the poor quality of health care provided, the low educational level and the practice of clandestine abortions. (UN Human Rights Committee 2003, para. 81(14); UN 1966a, Article 6)

The committee continued that in order to guarantee the right to life, Mali should ensure "the accessibility of health services, including emergency obstetric care. . . . It should help women avoid unwanted pregnancies . . . and ensure that they are not forced to undergo clandestine abortions, which endanger their lives. In particular, attention should be given to the effect on women's health of the restrictive abortion law" (para. 81(14)).

Linking Article 6 (the right to life) to measures the government of Mali should take to reduce maternal mortality is a direct reflection of the human rights analysis. Similarly, many of the treaty monitoring bodies have issued comments on abortion, noting that its criminalization violates human rights principles (UN Human Rights Committee 2005; Committee Against Torture 2004). It is also significant to note that Committee on the Elimination of Discrimination Against Women employs the ICPD to normatively evaluate a government's compliance with the right to health (UN CEDAW 1995).

Beyond the treaty bodies, there are other UN institutions that are responsible for human rights promotion and protection. The recently created Human Rights Council (replacing the Commission on Human Rights) has retained the mechanism of appointing Special Rapporteurs on thematic issues. The reports of the Special Rapporteurs arguably can help establish international norms concerning human rights and their interpretation. The Special Rapporteur on the Right to Health has investigated and issued reports that consider maternal (and reproductive health) as an indispensable aspect of the right to health and has presented cogent and forceful guidance to states on the measures they should enact to improve maternal health outcomes—especially as they relate to abortion. Importantly (and boldly given the highly politicized context of the UN (see Larson and Reich, this volume), the Special Rapporteur, Paul Hunt, in the 2004 report to the General Assembly notes that 68,000 women die annually from unsafe abortion, raising "a right to life and right to health issue of enormous proportions" (UN

2004). He directs states to offer (or allow to be offered) to women facing an unwanted pregnancy "reliable information and compassionate counseling, including information on where and when a pregnancy may be terminated legally" (2004a: 30). Given the attempts to weaken international agreements such as ICPD, restatements in other international forums are important.

Maternal Health Research: Human Rights as Advocacy

Perhaps the most intuitive way in which human rights have been used in regard to maternal health is to advocate for the issue or make it visible by identifying it as a human rights violation and mobilizing public sentiment to address the problem and hold those responsible accountable for the harm. Typically, human rights advocacy relies on research—fact finding, documentation, and report writing—to accomplish its ends. Two notable contributions to advocacy around maternal mortality come from the Center for Reproductive Rights and Physicians for Human Rights.[15]

The Center for Reproductive Rights (CRR), in partnership with a local NGO in Mali, documented the ways women lack access to affordable, quality health services, as well as facing pervasive discrimination. The report presents vivid examples of the hardships all Malians face due to an inadequate health care system, but with particularly tragic consequences for pregnancy. For example, the report presents the experience of Kadja, a young woman, married at 14, dead at 19. The story of her pregnancy and maternal death is contextualized to illustrate how social expectations, economic constraints, and pervasive gender discrimination undermine the exercise of human rights. Kadja lived with her husband's family, typical in many societies; atypically, however, her husband took over her task of collecting firewood when Kadja was pregnant. While gathering wood, he was bitten by a snake and died, and his family blamed Kadja. When her water broke, she did not realize this meant that she would soon be in labor, and she delayed telling anyone until a few days later when she was in pain. The family chose not to take her to the hospital due to distance and cost. She and the baby died unattended.

Kadja's lack of information about her own condition, her lack of direct access to health care, and her subordination within her family were a matter not of individual fault, but of systemic governmental failure, and the CRR report places Kadja's and a number of such stories in that broader context. It finds that inadequate health care facilities, women's low social status, and cultural practices that harm women's health conspire to make pregnancy unsafe. These conditions violated the human rights of women, and CRR recommended concrete actions that government civil society and the international community should take to ameliorate the situation: law and policy reform to change the perceptions of women's worth and social roles as well as technical and financial support to Mali (CRR and Association des Juristes Maliennes 2003). CRR launched this report in Mali and used the information to submit an alternative report to the UN Committee on the Rights of the Child (CRLP 1999). The Committee issued a concluding comment which did address, in part, maternal mortality (UN CRC 1999). The committee recommended that Mali, among other things, "strengthen reproductive health education and counseling services. In this regard, the Committee encourages the introduction of training programmes on reproductive health" (UN CRC 1999, para 27).

Similarly, Physicians for Human Rights (PHR) in 2002 examined maternal mortality in Afghanistan and found that women were dying at an extraordinarily high rate (PHR 2002).[16] In addition to employing methods of traditional fact finding, the PHR study was population based and used data-driven, epidemiologic methodology to estimate the maternal mortality ratio in Afghanistan. The report identified factors that likely were leading to maternal deaths in the region: inadequate health facilities to care for normal and complicated deliveries; insufficient supplies of medication and equipment for complicated pregnancies and births; a strong cultural norm for women to deliver at home; and lack of transportation to hospitals in urban centers and poor roads in rural areas. These conditions are the expected consequences of years of war and poverty. In addition the PHR report focused on the denial of individual freedoms such as freely entering into marriage and access to birth control. Unlike most human rights reports, the target of criticism was not the state of Afghanistan, but rather the international community, which at the time was rebuilding the state and its infrastructure. PHR used the report to induce donor nations to infuse funds into the Afghan health sector to stem the number of fatalities in childbirth. It is difficult to attribute causation; however this report received widespread attention and reducing maternal mortality in Afghanistan has become a stated objective of the Canadian and U.S. governments, as well as UNICEF (see, e.g., USAID 2007; CIDA 2007; Sahil 2007). Physicians for Human Rights has continued its work investigating maternal mortality with an innovative report and advocacy strategy in Peru (Physicians for Human Rights 2007).[17] This report focuses on the lives and deaths of seven women in representative parts of Peru (supplemented by 32 key informant interviews), narrating the circumstances along the "three delays" model (Thaddeus and Maine 1994)—delay in seeking care, delay in reaching care, delay in receiving appropriate care once there—and analyzing the corresponding human rights obligations of state (and non-state), using, where appropriate, internationally agreed upon health indicators. The report contains unprecedented recommendations for improving access to emergency obstetrical facilities by examining Peru's resources, and speculating how it could maximize their availability to be justly and equitably invested in the health system, for example, by increasing the overall revenue base by raising taxes.

Maternal Health Programming and Interventions: Human Rights as an Approach

Human rights advocacy and accountability strategies often position the state and its agents as perpetrators of violations and seek redress legally, politically, and morally. A different strategy is to constructively engage with the state to achieve its obligations through human rights-based approaches to issues—such as programming. Although there is no set definition of what "rights-based approaches" (RBAs) are or must be, they generally attempt to integrate the human rights principles of nondiscrimination, participation, and accountability into governmental (or nongovernmental) activity. A number of international NGOs and intergovernmental agencies have adopted RBAs in an effort to unravel what seem to be intractable knots in supporting governments in their provision of services, to promote human rights (Hawkins et al. 2005).

Two programming attempts by UN, governmental, and nongovernmental agencies, in conjunction with university-based health and human rights programs, have been undertaken in the area of maternal health; they are worthy of review. The first is the Columbia University Averting Maternal Death and Disability program (AMDD), built on the previous work of Columbia's Prevention of Maternal Mortality Program (1987-97). AMDD was inspired by the analysis that "most of the obstetric complications that lead to maternal death can neither be predicted nor prevented, but the vast majority of women can be saved through prompt treatment" (AMDD 2007). Strictly speaking, AMDD did not concern itself with the formal system of human rights and focused on ensuring the availability of emergency obstetrical services. Still, because its analysis was inspired by rights claims—providing adequate facilities for emergency obstetrical care as a fundamental obligation of governments—for the purposes of this chapter it will be considered a rights-based approach to intervention.

As just mentioned, AMDD's primary objective was to upgrade health facilities to address the causes of maternal death and disability, including missing or poor equipment, lack of emergency drugs, insufficient blood supplies, inadequate or nonexistent life-saving and other skills, and poor provider attitudes. These health facility/systems interventions were based on an analysis of national and local medical, social, and policy obstacles to providing emergency obstetrical care and engagement with communities in improving and extending health care services. Supported by a $50 million Bill & Melinda Gates Foundation grant, AMDD established, refurbished, trained, staffed, and provisioned emergency obstetric facilities. In order to connect this work to the formal system of human rights accountability, the health professions were to "use the UN process indicators," so that eventually when the government would "report on progress in implementing international conventions," the treaty bodies would be equipped to evaluate the progress made in understandable and accepted terms. However, these process indicators related to health systems, so reporting on them (e.g., for every 500,000 population, one comprehensive emergency obstetrical care facility) would not reveal much about whether women were unable to use the facility because of the fees charged or other barriers to access.

AMDD was evaluated in 2004 pursuant to its Gates grant (Caro, Murray, and Putney 2004). The review noted that AMDD contributed to an increase in the availability and use of maternal health services. The natural inference, therefore, is that more pregnant women received life saving care. There was also some evidence that governments changed their policies and revised their budgets to provide emergency care, which may have been motivated by use of UN indicators described above (Caro, Murray, and Putney 2004). In its own report of its activities in 1999-2005, AMDD identifies human rights as one of its three conceptual areas of action (AMDD 2006: 2). It mentions a finding of the 2004 Gates evaluation that "AMDD was also responsible for framing access to emergency obstetric care as a human rights issue. Although the program struggled with articulating how to operationalize the perspective, it resonated with policy makers, donors, and civil society groups. . . . This was the most experimental aspect of the program, but it has had a large impact on how the issue is framed in international and national discussions" (AMDD 2006: 15). Most intriguing is its synopsis of an external evaluation of its joint activities with CARE-Peru, which used an explicitly rights-based approach; the evaluation compared the AMDD/CARE health care facility in Ayacucho, Peru, with a similarly situated one. It found significantly greater use of the AMDD/CARE facility for emergency obstetrical care (59).

A different rights-based approach originated with WHO in conjunction with the Program on International Health and Human Rights at the Harvard School of Public Health, entitled "Using Human Rights for Maternal and Neonatal Health: A Tool for Strengthening Law, Policies and Standards of Care" (the "tool") (WHO and Program on International Health and Human Rights 2001).[18] The objective of the tool is to assist governments in meeting their human rights obligations related to maternal (and newborn) health. It defines a rights-based approach as identifying and addressing legal, policy, and regulatory barriers related to maternal and newborn health and facilitating governments to overcome those barriers. Governments are the principal recipients of this policy intervention, although civil society and other "stakeholders" are participants in the assessment process as well. The tool has two parts: a data collection instrument and an accompanying process that incorporates human rights principles and analysis. The data collection component uses human rights and internationally agreed upon conference targets, laid out by the ICPD, to frame the collection of information—the national (and other appropriate levels) legal, policy, regulatory, and practice situation—and connect it to health indicator data (e.g., Caesarian section rates, proportion of women exposed to domestic violence, or female literacy rates). This permits the identification and assessment of the laws, policies, strategies and plans—in sum, the government's efforts and practices—that present barriers to or opportunities for the reduction of maternal and neonatal mortality and morbidity. This assessment is linked to a facilitated, multisectoral, participatory process in which governments, civil society, and other stakeholders can establish and shape priorities, recommendations, and interventions to promote accountability and assist in fulfilling governmental human rights obligations, as well as achieve international political commitments for maternal health, such as MDG-5.

Insofar as the assessment and analysis are based on human rights (and human rights principles), the WHO-Harvard project requires translation into "lay" understanding, adaptation to local conditions, and ongoing training by WHO and Harvard staff. The tool was pilot tested in Mozambique, Brazil, and Indonesia between 2003 and 2006. The preliminary results from the Mozambique and Brazil tests are at the time of the writing of this chapter in the process of being analyzed. The Indonesia field test yielded evidence that using the tool does help to make visible gaps in government efforts and human rights promotion. For example, through application of the tools, researchers were able to show that discrimination on the basis of marital status kept adolescents and single women away from information and care. The tool mapped poor reproductive health indicators in those populations to this discriminatory regulation, which in turn has led to proposed legal and policy reform to remove married status as a prerequisite for reproductive health services (Gruskin et al. 2006).

Discussion

What might be said, therefore, of the value added overall by these efforts to improve maternal health by using human rights?

The acknowledgment of maternal mortality as a human rights concern by the UN human rights machinery cannot be overstated. These normative statements are a necessary, although insufficient, step toward changing governmental priorities and improving maternal health outcomes. That concluding observations remains abstract and do not offer implementation guidance is an all too common, but serious shortcoming. Advocates and scholars are working to improve the quality of the recommendations that the treaty bodies and other mechanisms issue. Using the normative language to change governmental, donor, and local practices remains the challenge for advocates and those who wish to eliminate maternal death, as well as discrimination against women.

The value of the normative human rights standards generated by these accountability mechanisms is reflected in their use in advocacy. Both of the human rights reports examined addressed maternal mortality and therefore were unusual in their subject matter and conceptualizations. However, they approached the genre of human rights advocacy in a conventional fashion—document facts, publish a report, and engage in advocacy. Typically, this form of advocacy has been labeled "name and shame." However because the harms associated with the denial of rights relating to maternal health are systemic, blame can be diffuse. This approach is unlikely to be able to point a finger at one actor or ministry, when many factors contribute to a nonfunctional health care system and discrimination against women. It is hard to mobilize the conscience of the community and media when there is no clear perpetrator and a number of suspect practices. It is even harder to measure success. Nonetheless, merely making these deaths visible and framing maternal morbidity and mortality in human rights terms are an important contribution to human rights (as a discipline) and to reproductive health for the creation of a more enabled legal and policy environment for pregnant women. To date, most mainstream international human rights organizations have not reported on maternal mortality as a human rights violation, although this is likely to change in the future. With organizations including Amnesty International and Human Rights Watch campaigning and investigating economic and social rights such as health, additional leverage may well be brought to bear. Even greater leverage could be exerted by the International Initiative on Maternal Mortality and Human Rights[19]—a newly launched coalition of organizations—the mission of which is to focus attention and activities on the human rights dimensions of maternal mortality and morbidity.

Insofar as enhancing public health approaches to maternal mortality, the human face that fact finding reports put on population-based data might well lead to changes in policies and practices. Even with the issuance of an international recommendation such as in the Mali case, the unavoidable question regarding advocacy reports is has anything changed (or will anything change) for women? Will, for example, Mali revise its priorities and solicit international financial and technical assistance to fulfill their human rights obligations related to maternal health? This would be incontrovertible evidence that using human rights advocacy can make a difference. Short of such proof (and such proof is short), human rights advocacy can be said to raise the visibility of maternal death—certainly an accomplishment, but not the change in practice that advocates (and others) wish to achieve. While at this point there is scant evidence that such advocacy results in identifiable changes, there is every reason to believe that over time human rights advocacy will be shown to be effective. In other settings, laws and practices change after the uncovering of abusive, unjust, and appalling practices. For example, after the imprisonment of women for obtaining abortions in Nepal was exposed, the king released some of these women and a law legalizing abortion was passed (CRLP 2002). Understanding broad social issues in rights terms—such as was done in addressing primary education—has been shown to alter government practices. A good example is Kenya, which made primary education completely free in 2003 and then had to direct resources and new revenues to that sector. Over the longer term, human rights advocacy—especially when it can be used to move formal international and national accountability mechanisms—should prove to be an effective avenue for improving maternal health systems.

Finally, advocacy and accountability can help create a demand for governments and other maternal health implementers to use human rights-based approaches in their programming efforts. Rights-based approaches are the newest consequences of ICPD; the two examples provide the basis for a provisional assessment, as these approaches are too new to show anything but promise. Both AMDD and the WHO-Harvard initiatives have potential inherent weaknesses—with sustainability and government buy-in being the greatest challenges. As far as sustainability is concerned, there are several challenges. For example, the executive branch may well want to improve maternal health and introduce legislation to legalize abortion while the legislature or certain sectors of civil society may be differently inclined; or one government can easily give way to a different government with a different set of priorities. However, as models for using human rights in programming to improve maternal health outcomes, both projects hold merit, especially when human rights is explicitly part of the health system analysis or intervention.

These types of approaches inherently set aside the adversarial aspects of human rights and seek instead to involve the government as a partner. They stress that cooperation with civil society is essential in listening to what communities want and in improving the acceptability and use of maternal health services.

The chapter has argued that human rights has made an enormous, fundamental difference in the conceptualization of maternal health and in efforts to implement maternal health policies and programs. Women still die and suffer due to pregnancy and childbirth. Initially, the conflation of women with the children they bore led to a poor analysis of the causes of maternal mortality and poorly targeted interventions to address it. The women's rights and health movement did much to clarify the situation. ICPD and other international efforts such as SMI called for the integration and use of human rights to end death and injury due to pregnancy. Human rights, whether as advocacy, formal norm generation, or programming, has attempted to operationalize ICPD. It is reassuring that human rights NGOs have shown their willingness to investigate the deaths and illness of pregnant women on par with other deprivations of human rights.

The attention the various UN human rights mechanisms pay to maternal mortality (particularly in the context of unsafe or illegal abortion) holds much potential, particularly as a corpus of international human rights standards gets incorporated into national law and jurisprudence. A notable example is the 2006 Colombian Constitutional Court decision legalizing abortion in certain cases; the Court based its ruling on international human rights law (Women's Link Worldwide 2007). Rights-based approaches to programs that seek to improve maternal health have also been launched. Although too early to tell, their advocates believe that if supported at a reasonable level and duration, they could well demonstrate that human rights, in fact, has a role in this field. Most promising is the study, carried out by Peru's Ministry of Health, of human rights approaches to emergency obstetrical care mentioned in the AMDD report; it suggests measurable added value of human rights regarding the use of services. Human rights, especially when combined with advocacy leading to enhanced articulation of norms, and as a way to harness government effort, is therefore a promising way forward, even if it appears not to have yielded much to date in terms of tangible results.

ICPD cemented the foundation of human rights to achieve, among other things, health. This has permitted the construction of a framework for advocacy, accountability, and programming, one that makes visible the legal and policy environment in which the health system operates, internationally, nationally, and locally; it permits an analysis of government action and inaction in terms of conduct and results. The most fundamental gain that human rights has brought to maternal health is in securing woman's individual agency, as apart from her pregnancy. Already, the language and programming around maternal health has changed. Maternal mortality, which entails both maternal morbidity and discrimination against women, evolved from "maternal and child health" (sometimes called maternal and newborn health) to "maternal health," "Safe Motherhood," and, most recently, "Safe Pregnancy." Presumably the evolution in terminology reflects an evolving view of the individuality of the woman.

However, there are some countervailing trends regarding the efficacy of human rights in relation to maternal health. First, on the level of terminology, the Safe Motherhood Initiative has transformed itself into the Partnership for Maternal, Newborn, and Child Health and is reported to be the vehicle for administering a Global Fund (WHO 2007). Perhaps this reorganization has very laudable ends, but the rearticulation of M with CH (as opposed to reproductive health) may be a harbinger of concern for viewing women as worthy of attention on their own merits. It also portends the creation of yet another "vertical" fund for maternal (and newborn and child) health (Costello and Osrin 2005). This may splinter off yet one more of the components of reproductive health, diminishing the comprehensive breadth of ICPD.

Second, since 2002, the United States administration and its allies, such as the Holy See, have tried to amend and retract the understanding of the Cairo consensus. The ostensible sticking point has been abortion. As a significant percentage of maternal mortality is caused by unsafe abortion, women will continue to die until opposition can be overcome. As long as a conservative configuration of the U.S. government and the Vatican endures (the latter more intransigent than the former), human rights is not likely to be a winning argument. For example, Amnesty International recently took a position on sexual and reproductive rights that incorporated access to abortion for women in certain limited circumstances (Amnesty International 2007); the Vatican announced it would stop its donations to Amnesty International and called on all Catholics to do so (McFeely 2007). However, the Vatican's menace has had little impact on Amnesty International.

Furthermore, there are recent decisions in the Inter-American Commission and the Human Rights Committee that hold the governments of Mexico and Peru (respectively) accountable for human rights violations by denying women access to abortion to which they were legally entitled under law (Inter-American Commission on Human Rights 2007; Human Rights Committee 2005). Similarly, the European Court of Human Rights upheld its decision against Poland, awarding

39,000 Euros to a woman who was refused an abortion although she qualified for one under the "health" exception under Polish law (European Court of Human Rights 2007). These are important statements that overcome some of the ambivalence toward pregnant women's individual rights and may in time be considered something of a trend. These victories on the national level underscore the observations made in other chapters of this book that international efforts to advance the Cairo consensus might not be the most fruitful at this point in time (see Girard, this volume). Bilateral action may be the way forward, as the United Kingdom and Sweden embrace ICPD and sexual and reproductive rights as the basis for their overseas maternal health assistance (SIDA 2006; DFID 2004). Given the power the United States exerts internationally, it may be time to rethink international strategies and use human rights on the national level to mobilize communities, engage with governments, and improve health services for women—on their own, eventually without dependence on foreign assistance.

Third, there may have been some wishful thinking at work among women's rights and health activists that by identifying maternal mortality as a human rights violation, the struggle to reduce the number of women dying from pregnancy-related causes could be magically surmounted. Human rights, it was the hope, could somehow trump utilitarian considerations of costs and benefits. But human rights is not a "trump card" that can automatically shift resources and long-held policy approaches. It is a discourse and a claim, and while it may have moral and legal force, it operates in an environment of competing claims that must be taken into consideration and progressively realized over time.

Nonetheless, bringing the claims of human rights to the issue of maternal mortality offers a blueprint for future action. And here the connection between human rights and health outcomes forged at ICPD remains vital, resilient, and indispensable. It will initially take much advocacy to move public lamentations into public action; there may at times be resistance and budgetary impasses, particularly as those wanting better health systems for women argue with advocates for better education systems for children. One way to overcome the competing demands against each other is through coalition politics at the local, national, and international levels. Through coalition building, a constituency can be created to direct resources to support a functional health system as a matter of human rights. The case can be made that just as the leading medical causes of maternal mortality and morbidity—hemorrhage, septicemia, pre-eclampsia, and obstructed labor—can be ameliorated though functioning high quality emergency care, many other lives beyond those of pregnant women will be saved.[20] An unintended consequence of the proliferation of neovertical health programming as well may be the building of a new coalition of advocates—say, among maternal health and traffic safety. A gender- and human rights-responsive health care system may also improve services for HIV/AIDS, malaria, and water-borne illness, to name a few. The sum of these constituencies is larger than each individual part, able to leverage more resources and create a better integrated health system that functions for all. Maternal health, like reproductive health, is not a discrete outcome. It requires that women have access to a range of interrelated services and have the ability to act. Reproductive health requires functioning and accountable health, education, judicial, and other state systems. This, in fact, is an enduring legacy of ICPD.

Chapter 8
Advocacy Strategies for Young People's Sexual and Reproductive Health: Using UN Processes

Bonnie Shepard

The ICPD Programme of Action and ICPD+5 made important commitments to adolescent sexual and reproductive health. The section on adolescent reproductive health in the Programme of Action (UN 1995, paras. 7.41-7.48) recognizes adolescents' vulnerability and their need for reproductive health education and services. It urges governments to provide family planning information and services to sexually active adolescents and recognizes an obligation by governments to ensure access to reproductive health programs and services that are private and confidential, "including on sexually transmitted diseases and sexual abuse."

This is particularly important, as the current generation of young people aged 10-24[1] is the largest in human history, approximately 1.7 billion in 2005 (World Bank 2005).[2] This chapter reviews the health and development risks faced by young people internationally, focusing on the sexual and reproductive health risks of the most vulnerable young people in developing countries. It argues that advocacy on behalf of young people is crucial to promoting their reproductive rights. This advocacy requires strategic use of internationally agreed upon norms and goals articulated in United Nations conference consensus documents and human rights treaties. This chapter analyzes the strengths and weaknesses of these agreements, in terms of both their language on young people's sexual and reproductive health and the mechanisms for implementation and enforcement of these agreements.

Gender discrimination and related social norms defining appropriate masculine and feminine behavior have a determining influence on young people's health and development. Discrimination, in particular, increases the risks faced by adolescent girls and young women.

Addressing discriminatory gender norms is essential to all efforts to promote the sexual and reproductive health of young people.[3] Gender discrimination within families in access to food leads to stunting, anemia, and heightened maternal risks for young women, as do harmful traditional practices such as female genital mutilation/cutting. For girls and young women worldwide, maternal mortality is one of the leading causes of death among female adolescents aged 15–19. For females under age 15, maternal mortality risks are five times higher than for those in their twenties (UNICEF 2002). Social norms governing sexuality differ for young men and young women and strongly influence constraints, behaviors, and risks, especially for girls after they reach puberty. Girls face greater sociocultural barriers to access to sexual and reproductive health services than do boys, since social disapproval of girls' sexual activity outside marriage is often extremely intense. Gender-based violence and economic dependency on spouses leave women of all ages powerless to protect themselves against HIV and unwanted pregnancies within marital relationships. Young girls may face sexual harassment in schools from teachers or male peers or in workplaces from employers.[4] Early marriage leads to too early childbearing with risks to both mother and infant and increases the risk of contracting HIV for young girls married to older, more sexually experienced men.

Gender norms also increase health risks for young men, but in different ways. Traditional social norms about masculinity encourage risk-taking behavior, multiple sexual partners, and violence. Young men who have sex with men face stigma, discrimination, and often violence, leading to increased physical, mental, and sexual health risks.

An estimated 10.3 million youth ages 15–24 are living with HIV/AIDS, and half of all new infections—over 7,000 daily—occur among this age group (WHO 2004). Young women in the highest prevalence countries are especially vulnerable; in sub-Saharan Africa, young women 15–24 are at least three times as likely to be HIV-positive than young men (UNAIDS/WHO 2005). Of the 333 million new cases of curable sexually transmitted infections (STIs) occurring worldwide each year, the highest rates are among 20–24-year-olds, followed by 15–19-year-olds (Dehne and Riedner 2005). Young women's vulnerability to STIs, including HIV infection, is exacerbated by sexual coercion within marital and sexual relationships and by rape in war. Studies in Asia, Africa, and the Caribbean have demonstrated that prevalence rates for sexual abuse were between 19 and 48 percent among young women and 5 and 32 percent among young men (Blum 2005). Recent studies have shown that in several countries, as many as 23 percent of women have experienced forced sex within their marriage, usually initiated early in the marriages of young women (Population Council 2004).

In spite of widespread knowledge about the severity of these risks at both global and country levels, policies that protect young people's sexual and reproductive health (YPSRH) are weakly implemented and enforced, and they are not translated into needed programs and financial resources. Even the most basic interventions for young people, such as provision of information on modes of HIV transmission and means of protection against infection, reach only half or fewer of adolescents in the higher prevalence countries. In recent studies in 24 sub-Saharan countries, two-thirds or more of young women (15–24) lacked comprehensive knowledge of HIV transmission (UNAIDS/WHO 2005). Although the 2001 UN Declaration of Commitment on HIV/AIDS aimed for 90 percent of young people to be knowledgeable about HIV by 2005, the latest surveys indicate that fewer than 50 percent have achieved comprehensive knowledge levels (UNAIDS 2006a).

This worldwide failure to protect young people's health calls for advocacy at all levels. The rest of this chapter focuses on the global political context for advocacy to protect young people's sexual and reproductive health and discusses the strengths and limitations of UN consensus agreements and international human rights law as advocacy tools. First, the chapter briefly discusses trends leading up to the transition in "framing" young people's sexual and reproductive health that the ICPD officially inaugurated. Then the protections provided by these agreements and human rights conventions are analyzed using two illustrative examples of policy goals—young people's access to sexual and reproductive health education and services and elimination of child/early marriage. These issues are chosen because they are essential to protecting young people's sexual and reproductive health, especially for young women and girls.

The advances and gaps in UN consensus agreements will be compared with those in international human rights law, and use of these tools in global and national policy advocacy will be discussed. Although several consensus agreements have made important advances in the protection of YPSRH, at this point in history strategies involving the international human rights system are a necessary complement to use of the ICPD and Beijing agreements and indeed might provide a more solid basis for advocacy for the most contested sexual and reproductive health issues affecting young people.

Historic Trends in Young People's Sexual and Reproductive Health Programs

Consideration of young people's sexual and reproductive behavior predates the health- and rights-based framework of ICPD. Since the 1970s, large-scale, effective programs in most countries in Europe have combined almost universal access to comprehensive sex education and contraception for unmarried young people with universal access to high quality secondary education, resulting in the lowest adolescent pregnancy and abortion rates in the world. However, conservative pressure groups in the United States and developing countries view this "European model" as too dependent on government funding and too accepting of adolescent sexuality. As a result, fruitless and even harmful attempts to find another way to protect young people's sexual and reproductive health continue to receive millions of dollars in donor funding. However, the European policy framework, based on political and social acceptance of young people's human right to sexual and reproductive health information, education, and services helped lay the groundwork for the commitments in the ICPD Programme of Action.

Spurred by the unprecedented involvement of women's organizations and civil society groups, concern at ICPD for overpopulation gave way to concern for the health and rights of individuals—especially women. This new focus led to the three major emphases in the ICPD framework: comprehensive approaches to sexual and reproductive health, empowerment of women, and fulfillment of human rights, specifically reproductive rights. Applying this focus to adolescents, ICPD affirmed that adolescents' right to health, development, and survival—as stipulated in the Convention on the Rights of the Child—gives them the right to access to sexual and reproductive health information, education, and services (paras. 7.41–7.48).

ICPD's comprehensive and rights-based framework both sprang from and subsequently reinforced three shifts beginning in the 1980s that led to a transformation in the underlying goals and approaches of YPSRH programs. First, throughout the 1980s evidence mounted that narrowly focused family planning or sex education programs for young people often stimulated community and political resistance, such that programs either fell apart once external donors halted support or remained but on a small scale with low coverage. Furthermore, many were successful in changing knowledge and attitudes but without the expected changes in behavior. Beginning in the 1990s, programs began to apply findings from research on the mutually reinforcing strategies needed to promote behavior change among young people and to systematically involve adult gatekeepers.

Second, the human rights system and the youth development field experienced parallel shifts beginning in the 1980s. The human rights system has recognized that governments have both negative obligations (avoiding violations of rights) and positive ones (protecting and fulfilling rights). Likewise, the youth development field has recognized that a negative focus on problems is insufficient, that effective programs have a positive focus on building strengths and assets—often called positive youth development, or the assets-building approach. One expert noted:

It is clear from research that focusing on risk reduction alone is not sufficient to reduce risks and that most such strategies have proven ineffective. Rather, successful interventions build on the strengths and confidence of young people, creating meaningful roles and opportunities to contribute. . . . A caring adult, opportunities to contribute, school and community activities, and a safe place for young people all appear to be part of a critical formula for improved health and social outcomes. (Blum 2005, paras. 25–26)

Third, the urgent need to address the HIV/AIDS epidemic and the high proportion of young people among those infected each year has pushed governments and reproductive health programs to expand their focus and push past cultural and political resistance to provide young people with comprehensive sex education and access to condoms. In the late 1990s, HIV programs paid more attention to the cultural factors influencing sexuality and to how gender and human rights issues affected young people's vulnerability to infection and access to HIV prevention, voluntary counseling and testing, care, and treatment.

However, in spite of the increased political will stimulated by ICPD and the spread of the HIV/AIDS pandemic among youth, the information, education, counseling, and services needed to prevent these sexual and reproductive health risks for young people are still sadly lacking, especially for young married girls and for unmarried young people of both sexes. The political controversies accompanying proposals to provide access to sexual and reproductive health education and services continue to delay government action and contribute to preventable morbidity and mortality for millions of young people, mainly in developing countries.

What can be done to rectify this situation? Most agree that multifaceted advocacy strategies coordinated among many actors from the community to global level are needed. Advocates for young people's sexual and reproductive health at all these levels can avail themselves of the same basic global policy instruments that are ratified or agreed to by governments. Using the examples of the advocacy goals of young people's access to sexual and reproductive health education and services and elimination of early marriage, the following sections will analyze these global policy tools: the political and legal instruments in UN consensus agreements and international human rights law.

The Right to Sexual and Reproductive Health Education and Services for Young People

Reading the international normative statements (consensus agreements, international human rights treaties, and General Comments to these treaties), an uninitiated reader might have the impression that there is widespread political agreement in the UN system on the needs and rights of young people with regard to accessing education and services for their sexual and reproductive health. This reader might also determine that the overwhelming majority of governments support actions that would fulfill these needs and rights. However, particularly in the consensus documents, a close look reveals the footprints of heated negotiations and concessions needed to reach agreement.

Consensus Agreements

At Cairo and then Beijing, the countries of the world committed themselves to provide sexual and reproductive health information, education, and services to adolescents. This commitment was renewed and strengthened in 1999 at the five-year review of ICPD (ICPD+5), when growing awareness of the HIV/AIDS epidemic lent greater urgency to the discussions. However, since 2000 Bush administration appointees to the U.S. delegations responsible for negotiating consensus agreement, along with a number of allied governments, applied intense pressure to reverse agreements reached in the 1990s (see Girard, this volume). The language of consensus agreements[5] has been weakened since 1999 by these concerted attacks in global policy venues. Because advocates at recent UN meetings have had to concentrate on blocking attempts to backtrack on earlier agreements, the pre-2000 ICPD and Beijing consensus agreements are more useful as advocacy tools to promote young people's reproductive rights.

However, disagreements on sexual and reproductive health issues show up consistently in the wording of the recommended actions, such that the Programme of Action seems to speak with two voices—one that respects adolescents' individual rights and freedoms, and another that allows for restrictions of these rights and freedoms, using words such as "appropriate" and "suitable" to provide the leeway demanded by conservative governments. This central passage on recommended actions illustrates the dual voices of the document—both enabling and potentially restricting fulfillment of young people's rights:

Recognizing the rights, duties and responsibilities of parents and other persons legally responsible for adolescents to provide, in a manner consistent with the evolving capacities of the adolescent, appropriate direction and guidance in sexual and reproductive matters, countries must ensure that the programmes and attitudes of health-care providers do not restrict the access of adolescents to appropriate services and the information they need, including on sexually transmitted diseases and sexual abuse. In doing so, and in order to, inter alia, address sexual abuse, these services must safeguard the rights of adolescents to privacy, confidentiality, respect and informed consent, respecting cultural values and religious beliefs. In this context, countries should, where appropriate, remove legal, regulatory and social barriers to reproductive health information and care for adolescents. (para. 7.45)

In the ICPD+5 review in 1999, political will to protect young people was stronger, mainly due to greater alarm about the expansion of the HIV/AIDS epidemic and growing recognition of young people's vulnerability to HIV. It is the only consensus agreement to establish specific benchmarks for coverage of sexual and reproductive health services for young people (15-24), including access to male and female condoms (UN 1999b).[6]

After the ICPD+5 review, opposition to the Cairo and Beijing agreements become more concerted, focusing on two hot-button issues— abortion and young people. Regarding young people's rights to sexual and reproductive health education and services, conservative forces use arguments that mistakenly equate protecting young people from morbidity and mortality with approval or even promotion of the behaviors that put them at risk. They assert parental "rights" to control what information adolescents receive and to which services they have access (UN 1999b).

As a result, negotiations in meetings since ICPD+5 have become extraordinarily intense. Post-ICPD+5 consensus agreements omit all mention of adolescents' access to condoms, and at best reaffirm the ICPD+5 benchmarks. The agreement from the 2002 UN General Assembly Special Session (UNGASS) on Children omits any mention of comprehensive sex education or reproductive health services for adolescents (UNICEF 2003).[7]

The outcome document from the 2001 UN General Assembly Special Session (UNGASS) on HIV/AIDS was more explicitly in the spirit of ICPD+5 but still speaks with two voices in many key passages. In response to pressure from some Muslim countries, the Vatican, and the United States, language was added to the document that opens the door for interpretations arguing that respect for "cultural values" could override the right to sexual and reproductive health information and services (see Girard 2001a). However, the language is balanced by a list of prevention interventions that includes "expanded access to essential commodities, including male and female condoms and sterile injecting equipment" (UN 2001b, para. 52). Likewise, the following target for near-universal access to sexual and reproductive health education and services is balanced by compromise language on a "full partnership" with parents and families.

By 2005, ensure that at least 90 per cent, and by 2010 at least 95 per cent of young men and women aged 15 to 24 have access to the information, education, including peer education and youth-specific HIV education, and services necessary to develop the life skills required to reduce their vulnerability to HIV infection, in full partnership with young persons, parents, families, educators and health-care providers. (UN 2001b, para. 53)

In summary, no agreements since 1999 unconditionally recognize governments' obligation to provide universal access to confidential sexual and reproductive health services, including condoms, to young people regardless of age, parental consent, or marital status. However, the ICPD and ICPD+5 agreements provide advocates with important advocacy tools. Using the ICPD+5 rights-protecting language and ignoring the ambiguities or absence of protection in later agreements have become a key strategy in global policy venues.[8]

Protections Under International Human Rights Law

While many advocates look to ICPD and other consensus documents, international and national advocates in general have not engaged intensively in country reporting to international human rights treaty monitoring bodies to pressure governments to provide sexual and reproductive health information, education, and services to young people. The one exception is where advocates have begun to engage in reporting to the Committee on the Rights of the Child (CRC). This notable gap is somewhat puzzling, since engagement with the international human rights system offers clear advantages over relying on the consensus agreements. The human rights system provides young people's sexual and reproductive health protections in its treaties and in their current interpretations, and in a key distinction, human rights treaties are binding on governments in ways that consensus agreements are not.

Much of the influence of the consensus agreements resides in the political process that led to their adoption, in which often intense negotiations among countries lead to commitments that everyone can agree on. While the language of treaties can also be fiercely negotiated, the language is crafted by lawyers rather than diplomats or technical experts. Once the country has ratified the treaty, the government is obliged to have national laws conform to the provisions of the treaty and to report periodically to the treaty monitoring body on progress toward national compliance with the terms of the treaty. Of course, there are loopholes in the system. Some countries do not ratify the treaties. Others ratify but express reservations to certain clauses in the treaty, and still others do not take the authority of the system seriously enough to make real progress toward compliance. However, the binding nature of international human rights law—and the process of reporting to the treaty monitoring bodies—provide a greater degree of legitimacy to stigmatized issues such as YPSRH by positing the policy goal as an international recognized human right. For this reason, the ICPD Programme of Action frequently cites international human rights conventions to back up assertions and recommendations.

Policy makers and advocates who support young people's rights to sexual and reproductive health information, education, and services are strengthened by ratification of the Convention on the Rights of the Child in all but two countries[9] and of the International Covenant on Economic, Social and Cultural Rights in all but six countries (UN 1966b, 1989). These treaties provide a solid basis for the ICPD and ICPD+5 commitments to promotion of adolescents' sexual and reproductive health.[10]

However, the subsequent interpretations of the treaties by their monitoring bodies provide much more explicit guidance on YPSRH issues than the treaties themselves. Although these interpretations, or "General Comments," are not binding, the authority of the committee members to interpret treaties in light of changing conditions and emerging issues is widely recognized. The contrast between the language of the consensus agreements and this General Comment from the CRC is striking:

the Committee is concerned that health services are generally still insufficiently responsive to the needs of human beings below 18 years old, in particular adolescents. . . . In the context of HIV/AIDS and taking into account the evolving capacities of the child, States parties are encouraged to ensure that health services employ trained personnel who fully respect the rights of children to privacy (article 16) and non-discrimination in offering them access to HIV related information, voluntary counseling and testing, knowledge of their HIV status, confidential sexual and reproductive health services, free or low cost contraception, condoms and services, as well as HIV-related care and treatment if and when needed. (UNCRC 2003a, para. 17)

In a subsequent General Comment, the CRC highlighted the obligation to ensure access to sexual and reproductive health information "regardless of marital status, and prior consent from parents or guardians" (UNCRC 2003b). The UN Committee on Economic, Social and Cultural Rights (CESCR), monitoring its associated International Covenant, has also emphasized state parties' obligations to guarantee confidentiality and privacy in adolescents' access to sexual and reproductive health services. The CESCR has also clarified that the right to health includes "the right to control one's health and body, including sexual and reproductive freedom" (UNCESCR 2000, para. I.8).[11]

In summary, the international human rights system offers stronger and more specific language for young people's rights to access sexual and reproductive health education and services. This advantage is also evident in the next example—early marriage. This issue excites less political controversy at the global level, but generates deep seated resistance at the community level.

Early/Child Marriage

Early marriage, also termed "child marriage," refers to any form of marriage that takes place before a child has reached 18 years.[12] Despite a worldwide shift toward later marriage and a minimum legal age of 18 in most countries in the world, more than 100 million girls under 18 are expected to marry in the next decade (UNFPA 2005e, 2004b).[13] According to UNFPA, the practice is still common among the poorest and in rural areas, and it is most prevalent in South Asia and Western and Middle Africa. In the less-developed world excluding China, 22 percent of women have given birth before age 18, with percentages ranging from 40 to 50 percent in the poorest countries of Africa and Asia.

The harm to girls caused by child marriage is well documented (see, e.g., UNICEF 2001; Bruce and Clark 2003). ICPD raised this concern as essential to achieving reproductive health in the context of the need for women's empowerment. Child marriage is prejudicial to girls due to their higher risks of maternal mortality and morbidity, the higher risk of mortality to their children, and because early marriage and early motherhood can "severely curtail educational and employment opportunities and are likely to have a long-term adverse impact on their and their children's lives" (para. 7.41). Later UN agreements and reports discuss the effects of child marriage with regard to social isolation, greater vulnerability to violence from husbands and extended family members, and higher risks of HIV infection, since the girls' husbands tend to be older and more sexually experienced. Recent studies in sub-Saharan Africa show that HIV incidence is growing fastest among young married women (Clark 2004; International Women's Health Coalition. 2005; UNFPA 2005e; Bruce and Clark 2004).

Consensus Documents

Most consensus agreements are equivocal on early marriage. For example, the consensus among ICPD signatories stated that countries should enforce laws against forced marriage, on minimum legal age of consent, and on minimum age at marriage, "and should raise the minimum age at marriage *where necessary*" (para. 4.21; emphasis added). Calling for enforcement of existing laws is inadequate, because it does not address the rights violations of girls in countries with insufficient or nonexistent laws. "Where necessary" is another phrase allowing for varying interpretations of the commitment. Many countries that specify 18 as the minimum age at marriage have lower ages with parental consent. Some countries do not have laws against forced marriage or a minimum legal age of consent, and in many cases, the minimum legal age is considerably below 18 (Shepard and DeJong 2005).[14]

In 1995, the Beijing Platform of Action noted the harmful consequences of early marriage and childbearing, and although it retained some of the ambiguity of the ICPD agreement, it added the crucial verb "enact": "enact and strictly enforce laws concerning the minimum legal age of consent and the minimum age for marriage and raise the minimum age for marriage where necessary" (UNDAW 1995, para. 274 (e)).

The Beijing+5 review (UN 2000b) and the preparatory document "World Fit for Children" (UNICEF 2003) for the UNGASS on Children have the strongest language of all the consensus agreements, explicitly calling on national governments to *eradicate* early and forced marriage. Both made an important policy advance by calling early marriage a "harmful traditional practice,"[15] thus including early marriage in the practices that are to be abolished under the Convention on the Rights of the Child (UN 1989).[16] However, both the Beijing+5 and UNGASS on Children agreements suffer from a lack of specificity and clarity. No consensus agreement explicitly recommends a minimum age of marriage of 18 for both sexes, with or without parental consent. By referring to "early marriage" and not "child marriage," these agreements leave room for varying interpretations regarding age and do not address the common practice of allowing earlier ages of marriage when there is parental consent.

The follow-up meetings to ICPD in effect ignored the issue of early marriage. The ICPD+5 resolution (UN 1999b), which contains important advances on the issues of access to sexual and reproductive health services, did not even mention early marriage, although it refers to "harmful traditional practices" prejudicial to the girl child, without naming them. Statements made at the time of the ICPD ten-year anniversary seemed even weaker on this issue than the original 1994 commitments, merely exhorting governments to address adverse consequences of early sexual activity, marriage, pregnancy, and childbearing.

At the time of the 2001 UNGASS on HIV/AIDS, the vulnerability of adolescent married girls to HIV infection was not as well publicized as it was five years later. However, in spite of numerous publications on the subject from the Population Council, the Innocenti Centre and others during the interval between the meetings, the five-year review outcome document UNGASS on HIV/AIDS does not mention marriage at all, much less child marriage, except for a brief reference to the vulnerability of married women when they cannot insist on condom use or faithfulness (Population Council 2004; UNICEF 2001).

Protections Under Human Rights Law

As with the case of young people's rights to sexual and reproductive health education and services, analysis of pertinent consensus agreements, human rights treaties, and their general comments on the issue of early marriage indicates that the international human rights system affords greater protection to girls than that afforded by consensus agreements. The Convention on the Elimination of All Forms of Discrimination against Women (UN 1979) states that any betrothal or marriage of a child should not have any legal effect.[17] The Committee on the Elimination of All Forms of Discrimination against Women in 1994 and the CRC in 2003 recommended that 18 be the legal minimum marriage age for both sexes, with the CRC stipulating that this minimum age should apply "with and without parental consent" (UNCRC 2003b, para. 20; UNCEDAW 1994).[18]

Why is the consensus language on HIV/AIDS and early marriage either weak or absent? First, socially conservative pressure groups at the UN and in many countries do not agree that child marriage is a harmful traditional practice. Rather, these groups see marriage as protective for young women. Underlying this view is a purely moral agenda, because the only protection afforded by early marriage is against pregnancy outside marriage. This protection relates to concepts of family and young women's "honor" rather than girls' health and well-being. The view of child marriage as protective rests on assumptions that have been shown to be false (UNFPA 2005e): that the husband will be free from STIs and HIV infection, that he will not force his young wife to have sex or bear a child against her will, that he will agree to use a condom, that he will not exercise violence against her, and that he and his family will encourage her to continue her education.

The references in UN documents regarding the rights and responsibilities of parents point to the other source of controversies. Resistance to official language calling for the elimination of child marriage is rooted in a reluctance to undermine parental authority. The family economics of poverty are linked to practices such as forced and arranged marriages and the dowry system. These practices are deep-rooted, as the term "traditional harmful practices" implies.

In summary, the most useful policy instruments for advocates seeking to end the practice of child marriage are the Convention on the Rights of the Child and Convention on the Elimination of All Forms of Discrimination Against Women, along with engagement in the country reporting processes. In countries where the law is in line with international human rights standards, the reporting process can highlight concerns and recommendations regarding inadequate enforcement of the law.

Looking to the Future

While reaffirming the importance of certain consensus agreements, particularly ICPD+5 and Beijing+5, this discussion clearly demonstrates that engagement with the international human rights system is an essential complement to advocacy strategies based on UN consensus agreements. The human rights treaties discussed here provide clearer and stronger language to use in YPSRH advocacy efforts. However, in spite of these protections, there is a notable gap between policy and reality. Many national governments ignore the injunctions of these treaties and of their monitoring bodies. At the national level, when governments have policies protecting young people, agencies on the ground often do not comply. How can advocates best use existing policies, agreements, and legal obligations to help remedy these inadequate responses to young people's sexual and reproductive health needs?

First, YPSRH advocates in many countries do not make full use of the reporting system to treaty bodies which provide regular institutionalized advocacy opportunities. In this system, a government's foreign ministry must organize the country's report to the treaty monitoring body. The ministry should ask for civil society participation or at least be willing to include advocates and young people's organizations, who can then work with the government to gather the relevant information on compliance with the treaty. When the government is hostile to such participation, advocates often organize "shadow reports" that are submitted directly to the Committee to ensure that the information will be taken into account in the final recommendations for the government (see CRLP 1999). Adding media coverage of the report and of the recommendations to this intervention can be effective in applying pressure on governments to fulfill their responsibilities to young people.

The efforts of YPSRH advocates would be greatly enhanced by increasing attention to the explicit obligations created by their governments' ratification of the Convention on the Rights of the Child and the International Covenant on Economic, Social and Cultural Rights in particular. When the Committee on the Rights of the Child is provided with adequate information on the subject, it has consistently enjoined governments to provide comprehensive sexual and reproductive health education[19] to adolescents, in defense of their right to scientifically accurate health information. The regular time intervals of reporting to the Committee allow advocates to use the recommendations in country-level advocacy after the meeting and to monitor the degree of compliance with the Committee's recommendations.

Consensus agreements while generally vaguer in language, have the advantage of stemming from a political process in which governments of the world reached consensus and agreed to invest in certain types of actions and programs. Many countries have created multisectoral committee to monitor progress on ICPD, as well as creating women's ministries that use Beijing as a basic reference document. For this reason, ICPD+5 and Beijing+5 are crucial complements to the more explicit obligations laid out in international human rights law.

Clearly, these official agreements and international legal instruments are crucial advocacy tools, but they are not sufficient to eliminate child marriage or provide rural adolescent girls with sexual and reproductive health education and services. There is no substitute for building allies; creating the political will and changing cultural attitudes within countries is the next step. At the national level, transforming the public discourse on YPSRH issues is needed, combined with increased citizen pressure to enact or enforce adequate laws and provide a sufficient budget for YPSRH program. In particular, advocacy to make governments accountable for protection of young people's health needs to focus not just on supply-side strategies, but also on advocating for investments in changing the demand side. The cultural barriers to young people's access to sexual and reproductive health education and services need to be faced head on. Government programs to eliminate child marriage, for example, need to invest in changing how these issues are framed in the public discourse, with social campaigns in the media, community-level social change initiatives, programs to remove the financial incentives to families leading to child marriage, and support to young people's organizations to enable them to mobilize on their own behalf. Global agreements and international treaties must be complemented by cultural change strategies, youth participation, and citizen oversight so that governments comply with their obligations to young people.

Chapter 9
Approaches to Sexual and Reproductive Health and HIV Policies and Programs: Synergies and Disconnects

Sofia Gruskin

The International Conference on Population and Development was a watershed for bringing human rights concepts and methods into sexual and reproductive health (SRH) and HIV work. Simultaneously, programs that want to be seen as having a strong technical justification with respect to sexual and reproductive health or HIV are distancing themselves from human rights both in their discourse and programming (Gruskin 2004). Given the increased discussion about integration and linkages between sexual and reproductive health and HIV, losing the common ground of human rights is worth examination. This chapter addresses these and other questions including: how did things get this way, and what are the implications for sexual and reproductive health and HIV going forward? Answers to these questions are particularly pressing given that the resources available for HIV-related programming have never been greater while those for sexual and reproductive health are shrinking. Although there have been periods of intersection and exchange between the worlds of HIV and sexual and reproductive health, the development of the two fields has often been on parallel tracks. This chapter traces the history and growth of efforts in both HIV and sexual and reproductive health and considers the extent to which several factors and events, from human rights to changes in donor priorities, have paved the way for joining efforts. The chapter ends by suggesting areas for future convergence.

Leading Up to ICPD: Lessons and Near Misses

The story of the relationship of those working on HIV on the one hand, and sexual and reproductive health on the other, is one of distance and proximity with change over time, although this change has not necessarily been in consistent or unidirectional ways. In part this story reflects its point of departure: the early focus of the response to HIV was predominantly on the care and prevention needs of men. These responses to HIV did not come from international or even national organizations but from men who were living with HIV and AIDS themselves, from their families and loved ones and soon afterward, from community-based HIV-oriented organizations. All recognized sexual and reproductive health concerns as closely tied to the ability of any HIV prevention effort to succeed (O'Malley 2004). While the very first organized activities focused on the immediate care needs of people with advanced illness, in promoting the concept of "safe sex" as the foundation of prevention, the HIV movement explicitly recognized the need to address issues directly linked to sexual and reproductive health. In the 1980s, the intersections between SRH and HIV were most visible in the way those working in HIV prevention adapted concepts and tools from the reproductive health and broader women's health movement. "Safe sex" as a cornerstone of HIV prevention was based on condom promotion and non-penetrative sex, both well-established efforts in contraception and prevention of sexually transmitted infections (STIs) (UNAIDS 2006b).

A well-known tenet of the HIV response continues to be the (greater) involvement of people living with HIV/AIDS in policy development and service delivery (the "GIPA" principle), a concept in many ways inspired by the women's health movement where the inclusion of women's voices in health care decision-making was understood to be central to effective health programming (Cornu 2002). So too was the recognition that a focus on the provision of services alone was insufficient. An effective response also required attention to the politics that influenced both the services offered and the ability of different populations to access them (O'Malley 2004). Thus, despite some concerns that working closely with those they perceived to be primarily engaged in sexual and reproductive health would reduce programmatic attention to sex and to sexuality simply to clinical functions, in general those working in HIV consciously learned from and engaged with the efforts of the sexual and reproductive health community.

The reproductive and sexual health needs of men are not high on the sexual and reproductive health agenda even today, but this history is relevant to any consideration of the conceptual, policy, or programmatic linkages between sexual and reproductive health on the one hand and

HIV prevention and care on the other. Despite the efforts of some forward looking activists, those involved in reproductive health policy and the delivery of services tended to shy away from HIV prevention or care. The reasons behind the lack of engagement of policy makers and program managers range from the technical to the political. For one thing, by the time HIV was understood to be an issue of global importance, those working on sexual and reproductive health were, quite understandably, not quick to jump on board an issue they thought could easily take attention and resources away from their hard-fought agenda. There were, however, other issues as well. HIV shed light on many thorny issues around sexual behavior and sexuality that the reproductive health community had been more than happy to keep off the table in order to engage more easily with governments and other conservative forces.

A practical example of this concerned the ways in which HIV prevention brought attention to condoms as both a preventive and a contraceptive strategy (WHO 1987). By the 1980s condoms were not a priority intervention within family planning circles, not only because new and more effective contraceptive technologies were available but because, even among some health professionals, discussion of their use raised issues still considered taboo, such as about how people have sex, not simply whether they have sex. At times it seemed as though services providers and programmers feared that attention to HIV would sully whatever sterility and cleanliness was coming to be associated with reproductive health; HIV immediately brought to the fore the need for frank talk about sex and about sexuality (ACPD 2006b). Reproductive health providers attended to reproductive behaviors but not to sexual behaviors or to sexuality (DeJong 2000). Unfortunately, the societal stigma around HIV infection, concerns about who was infected, and the behaviors that might have led them to become infected existed not only among government officials and conservative communities but among many of those involved in the delivery of family planning services (de Bruyn 2002). As a result, before the ICPD and for many years after, the individuals and organizations working in HIV and those working in sexual and reproductive health remained generally distinct.

As noted elsewhere in this volume, activism was crucial to the outcomes of the ICPD, and it is the one place where the sexual and reproductive health and HIV fields traditionally have comfortably come together. Activism in the area of HIV took place alongside activism that contributed to the shift from demographic population control models toward reproductive health. The relationships that existed between the activist communities in HIV and communities around women's rights allowed for some continuity of engagement between the fields, even when in the delivery of services and within institutional structures they functioned as distinct from each other. However, in the context of the ICPD negotiations themselves, the linkages between these activist communities were limited at best. At Cairo, despite the number of activists, nongovernmental organizations, service providers, program managers, government officials, and policy makers playing crucial roles in developing the final outcome document, few organizations and individuals engaged in HIV-related efforts were present or part of the negotiations. In fact, there were no organizations of people living with HIV present at the negotiations, and even organizations with a primary orientation to HIV were visibly absent (O'Malley 2004). It may well be that this lack of engagement from NGOs concerned with HIV is why, despite the generally progressive nature of Cairo's outcomes, the language and approach to HIV is distinct from that taken in the rest of the document.

Cairo is rightly recognized as a watershed in its recognition of the importance of human rights, health systems, laws, and policy, as well as underlying determinants, for the availability and use of sexual and reproductive health services as well as for moving beyond the confines of vertical family planning approaches. However, specific attention to HIV in the document is quite different from the tone and approach taken with respect to sexual and reproductive health issues more broadly. For example, the ICPD document generally affirms the rights of women and men to be informed of, and to have access to, safe, effective, and affordable family planning methods of their choice. The document goes further to state that the definition of reproductive rights "rests on the recognition of the basic rights of *all* couples and individuals to decide freely, and responsibly, the number, spacing and timing of their children and to have the information and means to do so, and the right to attain the highest standard of sexual and reproductive health" (para. 7.3, emphasis added). Paragraph 7.3 continues to "include the right to make decisions concerning reproduction *free of discrimination, coercion and violence*, as expressed in the human rights documents" (emphasis added). One can understand this language to imply that decisions concerning childbirth—whether or not one of the parents is HIV-infected—are to be made by couples and individuals, that population policies must allow individuals to decide whether they want children, and that the ability to do so should be free from government interference. When read against the sections of the ICPD document concerning HIV specifically, however, it is clear that when this section of the document was drafted, reproductive rights were not recognized to extend equally to everyone.

In contrast to the breadth of the language related to reproductive health, and even to reproductive rights, the HIV language focuses almost exclusively on prevention and control. Some explanatory language about vulnerability and the avoidance of discrimination in the context of HIV exists. However, the ICPD states as an objective that "sexual and reproductive health programs [must] address HIV infection and AIDS" (para. 8.29) but that this be limited to promoting "responsible sexual behavior, including voluntary [sexual] abstinence" for the prevention of HIV infection (para. 8.31). In addition to the obvious limitations of this approach, it is also worth noting that while attention is given to inclusion of prevention of HIV infection within the delivery of sexual and reproductive health services, attention to sexual and reproductive health within the delivery of HIV-related services is not even mentioned. Nevertheless, despite these obvious limitations, there is a great deal in the ICPD Programme of Action with respect to reproductive and sexual health and even with respect to reproductive rights more broadly that was able to be used effectively in the HIV context in the decade after Cairo (Gruskin, Roseman, and Ferguson 2007).

By linking governmental responsibility for sexual and reproductive health to a government's human rights obligations, Cairo's language and approach were directly applicable to many areas related to an effective HIV response. The broad concepts of reproductive and sexual health and rights could be understood to encompass HIV by virtue of how they were interpreted and applied, as well as to how HIV programming brought into play sexual and reproductive health concerns. This was true despite the fact that Cairo paid insufficient attention to HIV, and in particular ignored the rights and needs of people in relation both to the realities of preventing infection and to accessing needed services once infected. It nonetheless created a series of obligations for states, which in turn created obligations for the provision of health services, and those who provide them, with direct application to the context of HIV (Cook 1997). The international conferences that took place in the decade or so after Cairo all drew on this legacy and called attention to human rights in the international political commitments governments made in relation to health and development issues more broadly. Nowhere in these conference commitments is the obligation to promote and protect human rights in the context of HIV clearer than in the 2001 UN General Assembly Special Session (UNGASS) on AIDS. The 2001 UNGASS not only reaffirmed the links between human rights and HIV prevention and control, but signaled the increasing vulnerability of women to HIV infection as a major political and technical challenge for the years to come (UN 2001b).

The Legacy of ICPD for HIV: Legitimizing Use of Human Rights in Programming

Despite the limitations in its approach to HIV, Cairo was a landmark for people engaged in ensuring attention to human rights in both sexual and reproductive health and HIV programming. Not only a clarion cry for activists and academics, it signaled a time when governments and the United Nations system embraced (at least seemingly) the promotion and protection of human rights as crucial for effective action. As a result of the Cairo consensus, new resources were directed to previously existing "rights based" efforts, and projects sprang up in all corners of the globe that demonstrated the value of this wider conceptualization of health and development. Even as rhetorical attention to human rights had formed part of the global HIV strategy since its early days, ICPD was critical to HIV in that its general approach signaled the international political commitment of the governments of the world to actual incorporation of human rights norms in programming efforts. This in turn supported resources going to HIV-related programming that explicitly addressed human rights promotion and protection and supported organizations ranging from the International HIV/AIDS Alliance to the International Council of AIDS Service Organizations (ICASO) in their efforts related to human rights.

In the period after Cairo, the negative effects of violations of rights in relation to HIV prevention and care efforts (that is, ensuring the ability of People Living with HIV to live lives with dignity after diagnosis) was widely recognized and understood. Explicit recognition of these concepts found its way into the mission statements and strategies of organizations engaged in the HIV response, ranging from UNAIDS to bilateral donors including the UK Department for International Development (DFID) and Canadian International Development Agency (CIDA) and Swedish International Development Cooperation Agency (SIDA). Moreover, there were increasing examples of policy and programmatic efforts by NGOs, as well as by governments, where the use of key human rights principles, such as nondiscrimination and participation, seemed poised to help bring the epidemic under control (Hardee, Agarwal, Luke, et al. 1998). Discrimination based on HIV status, gender, sexual orientation, race, ethnicity, and other reasons (such as engaging in injection drug use or sex work) had been demonstrated to exacerbate vulnerability to HIV and thereby to hinder prevention efforts. People who engaged in sex work and those who injected drugs were understood to be particularly vulnerable both to infection and to inadequate access to needed services. Evidence was beginning to show that even when services were offered, if vulnerable groups were not part of the design of interventions they would not make use of the services, and it was therefore accepted that efforts were needed to ensure their active participation (UNAIDS 2000). Prevention strategies addressing not only risk of infection but the vulnerability of affected communities drew on the rights framework internationally endorsed at ICPD and became globally recognized as appropriate and useful to bring the impacts of the epidemic under control.

In the decade that followed Cairo, integration of human rights in HIV work necessarily brought attention to civil, political, economic, social, and cultural factors involved in the technical and operational aspects of HIV interventions—whether focused on prevention, care, and treatment or impact mitigation. The added legitimacy and visibility given to human rights through the international conference process also proved useful for HIV by highlighting the importance of the law, legal recourse, and the public accountability that governments and intergovernmental organizations have for their actions toward people in the context of HIV. Through this amalgam of factors, the place of human rights in the response became well established. Although the efforts needed to bring the epidemic under control globally were daunting, until recently some of the largest questions for the AIDS movement seemed to be about how to ensure the political will necessary to replicate successful interventions—despite their forcing attention to stigmatized and uncomfortable issues for politicians.

SRH and HIV Post-Cairo: Separate But Equal?

In the years following Cairo, the worlds of HIV and sexual and reproductive health can be seen to have developed along parallel lines, influencing each other in some ways but remaining distinct as well. There appeared to be little need and consequently, despite obvious points of contact, relatively little progress in linking HIV conceptually or operationally to sexual and reproductive health. A number of explanations for this slow progress, of different importance in different contexts, can be posited.

At the service delivery level, resistance from providers in both sexual and reproductive health and HIV to integration, or even to linkages, created formidable obstacles. In this debate, integration refers to settings where services are offered in the same location, and linkages occur when referral systems ensure that clients are directed to another location where the services they require are on offer. Even when there were good intentions, a number of problems presented themselves. SRH providers were already having difficulty delivering on the ambitious goals of the Cairo agenda, even when they fully believed in them. Many were reluctant to add yet another issue to their already burdened programs (Mayhew 1996; Lush 2002). In addition, some sexual and reproductive health providers, even if they did not personally resist integration, noted concern that their services would be stigmatized and therefore undermined through association with HIV-related services (Sai 2005). At the same time, those involved in the delivery of HIV services were concerned that sexual and reproductive health providers were inadequately skilled to deal with issues of sexuality, HIV care, and in particular marginalized populations. In addition, many HIV providers were concerned about the potential negative impacts of linkages for the well-being of their clients (O'Malley 2004).

One example to put these differences in perspective concerned the appropriate level of attention to give to married women of reproductive age, who formed the core clientele of many reproductive health programs. They seemed to those in the reproductive health community an easy group to target and prioritize for services, but many in the HIV field were concerned that an inordinate focus on this "safe" population would draw resources away from those vulnerable populations most in need of access to prevention and care. Academics and researchers also contributed to these divisions. A number of studies were published from the perspective of each field, pointing to a variety of operational risks of service integration. Despite a few good examples of how working together could be effective, studies drawing attention to the mixed results of attempts to integrate STI services effectively into family planning or maternal health settings were most widely cited (Askew and Berer 2003; Becker and Leitman nd). Furthermore, international conferences that convened actors from both fields were few.

The paradigms within which the fields operated also posed problems for building linkages, in particular in relation to the conceptual place they afforded each other in the hierarchy of issues and priorities. Observing how representatives of these two fields engaged with each other, it is probably a fair characterization to say that many of those whose work was primarily in sexual and reproductive health understood HIV to be a subset of reproductive health. In contrast, those working primarily in HIV tended to see reproductive health as only one small part of the many issues to be addressed with HIV. The implications of these conceptual differences should not be under-appreciated, as they may continue to impact how the fields understand each other and affect how they work together to this day.

Donor financing has also played a key role. In addition to the different levels of funding given to each area, the norm among many donors has been to finance separate, parallel programs and in so doing implicitly to discourage resources from being put toward integration

(Worthington and Kjaerby 2004). This parallel approach, in turn, was often mirrored in the programming structures of developing country governments and in front-line service provision. Thus, there were no obvious points of contact for institutions and people at policy or program levels in the two fields. Finally, the mainstream of international policy and technical guidance probably both influenced and reflected these trends, effectively keeping HIV and sexual and reproductive health separate in policies, programs, and practice. Taken as a whole, through the late 1990s, all these factors contributed to sharp divisions between reproductive health and HIV work at all levels of policy and program engagement.

Coming Together: Fortuitous and Not So Fortuitous Reasons

A variety of factors and events have significantly changed the landscape in the past few years, signaling interest from both the sexual and reproductive health and HIV fields coming together. The emphasis on vulnerability reduction in HIV prevention strategies, the use of syndromic diagnosis of STIs in men, the approaches to marginalized and underserved populations, and the innovations in social marketing in the HIV field have all played a role in attracting the attention of the sexual and reproductive health community. A few key developments are worth noting in detail and are briefly summarized below.

Politics and Access to Information

Beginning in the late 1990s, the sexual and reproductive health community has had to deal with numerous assaults on the Cairo consensus, ranging from the political to the financial. Those working in sexual and reproductive health have had to expend a great deal of effort not simply to improve their programs and services, but to react to political and ideological challenges threatening the core of their work (Center for Health and Gender Equity/Population Council 1998; Girard, this volume). Consequently, the sexual and reproductive health community has found itself needing to argue for the very existence of many of the components understood through the Cairo consensus to be key elements of reproductive health, many of which dovetail closely with concerns for the HIV community. As one particularly telling example, the Programme of Action recognized access to adequate health care information, counseling, and services as part of a government's responsibility for reproductive health. Yet in 2002 at the UNGASS on Children, the reproductive rights of adolescents to access scientifically accurate reproductive and sexual health information and services, as had been agreed to in Cairo, were seriously challenged by an improbable alliance of countries—including the United States, Sudan, and Iran, as well as the Holy See (UNICEF 2003). This was not an isolated incident at the global political level. Similar attacks on the reproductive rights of adolescents, and in particular on their access to appropriate information and services, have continued relentlessly since that time in relation to policy and program direction, as well as resource allocation. The sexual and reproductive health community has been forced to deal with the impacts of this in a variety of ways. At the same time, the HIV community has been struggling with how to deal with challenges to accurate information in its own sphere, in particular the inordinate emphasis and resources given to abstinence as a primary prevention strategy. The focus on abstinence, over information on condoms and safer sex, due in great part to the funding and other requirements imposed by the U.S. government, has the potential to undermine many of the gains in HIV prevention in countries throughout the world (Center for Reproductive Rights 2003; Bogecho and Upreti 2006). The need to ensure access to accurate and sound information and services goes to the heart of concern for both sexual and reproductive health and HIV. In many ways these attacks, whose results have been felt by those working in both areas, have resulted in a joining of concerns between activists, researchers, policy makers, programmers, and those involved in service delivery.

The Advent of AIDS Treatment

A number of changes in the response to HIV in recent years affect the linkages between the two communities, but none are as immediately important as the discovery and dramatic cost reduction of antiretrovirals (ARVs). With the advent of affordable therapy to tackle HIV, activist, government, and donor interest in HIV programming has shifted from an emphasis on prevention toward a strong focus on treatment and, over time, to care in a broader sense. Where previously it had been possible to consider governmental responsibility for HIV prevention and control as fairly distributed among all sectors, even if the health sector was in many ways front and center, this shift raised new issues. While the engagement of other sectors remains critical, services relating to treatment immediately draw attention to the need not only to deliver these services but for a functioning health system through which to deliver them, and therefore a need to strengthen the health sector more generally (Gruskin, Ferguson, and O'Malley 2007).

There has also been an unexpected shift in the use of human rights norms and standards in HIV programming efforts as a result of the increased focus on treatment. Even though attention to human rights has been a mainstay of treatment advocacy, the contribution of a human rights framework to delivery of services has been increasingly sidelined. Treatment programs have focused on ensuring the numbers of people in treatment, with insufficient attention to who those people are or what it will take to ensure that they can continue to access needed treatment and related services (Gruskin, Ferguson, and Bogecho 2007). Nowhere have the dilemmas raised by the limitations of this approach been clearer than in efforts focused on the prevention of HIV transmission from mother to child. There, the focus on providing drugs to pregnant women was initially only on preventing HIV transmission to infants. Little thought went into the woman's health needs: how she might live a quality life with access to the treatment she needed to stay alive over time. Over the past few years, based to a large degree on the success of a large-scale program that showed it was possible not only to reduce mother to child transmission but additionally to provide treatment to the mother over time, this has changed somewhat (Myer, Rabkin, and Abrams 2005). Globally, however, the emphasis unfortunately remains largely on preventing transmission, with insufficient focus on the health of the mother. As international guidance and increasingly the actions of national governments have spotlighted a range of issues in addressing mother to child transmission effectively, the need for increased engagement between the two communities has become clearer. These include the progress review of the Millennium Development Goals; the "Glion Call for Action" from WHO and other organizations; the "New York Commitment" from UNFPA and a group of high-level parliamentarians; the ICPD+10 declaration by a wide range of NGOs and civil society actors; and WHO guidelines for the "Integrated Management of Adult Illnesses."

The HIV community is beginning to take a hard look at antenatal services and the ways sexual and reproductive health services more generally are being delivered, while the sexual and reproductive health community is recognizing a need to more fully consider optimal approaches to working with HIV positive women, in the context of pregnancy and childbirth and beyond.

Women at the Center

Mother to child transmission is only one area that in recent years has brought attention to women in the context of HIV. Gradually recognizing women as a visible and affected population in all parts of the globe, HIV-related resources and programming are focusing on prevention activities that speak to the behavior and actions of women, especially on the ability, or lack thereof, to negotiate and enforce condom use. Nevertheless, the HIV community still by and large fails to address the complexities of what makes individual women vulnerable to infection and once infected to not receiving necessary care and support. Awareness of the gendered dimensions of the epidemic has grown. There has been increasing interest on the part of the HIV community to learn from the experience of family planning and those involved in the delivery of other sexual and reproductive health services, with respect to the effects on sexual behaviors and choices, as well as the ability to access and make use of services if they are offered.

To sum up, although sexual and reproductive health issues have not traditionally been a significant area of focus for the HIV community, the advent of treatment and recognition of the rights of positive people, both women and men, specifically in relation to bearing children, have made sexuality and reproduction significant areas of activism and concern (UNAIDS 2006). Recognition of women at the center of the HIV epidemic has resulted in a joining of interests between the HIV and reproductive health communities. This new dimension means a combined interest in focusing on sexuality, gender, and power differentials and all that is required to achieve gender equality, and for women and men to engage in healthy sexual relations, including as it relates to condom use.

Donor Funding and the MDGs

Development assistance for health remains inadequate overall, but dramatic shifts in donor priorities over the past few years have had enormous impacts on the interests of the two communities in working together, and consequently on the services delivered and approaches to their delivery. HIV work was severely underfunded through most of the 1990s. A shift in donor priorities has increased resources going in particular to antiretroviral treatment, and after 1999 has given the field of HIV unprecedented funding. This shift has also affected the relationship between sexual and reproductive health and HIV efforts in other ways, because as the funds available for HIV have increased the resources available for sexual and reproductive health have decreased (Druce, Dickinson, et al. 2006). The HIV world is flush with money and, as indicated earlier, a functioning health system, extending beyond simply the provision of treatment, is recognized as a top priority. The sexual and reproductive field, noticing attention and resources shifting to HIV, has recognized that joining with HIV efforts makes good sense not only in order to provide appropriate services as treatment becomes more available, but also pragmatically in order to access needed finan-

cial resources and harness political commitment to sexual and reproductive health concerns.

A related impetus for linking the efforts of the two communities has
come about as a result of the MDGs, arguably the development agenda
for this decade if not the millennium (UN 2001a). The MDGs contain
an explicit HIV goal and, due to political pressure, no explicit mention
of reproductive health. A target on Sexual and Reproductive Health was
recently incorporated into the outcomes of the 2005 World Summit, but
it is subordinate to the MDGs (Kaufman, this volume; IPPF 2006).
Nonetheless the goal on HIV/AIDS, with its specific focus on prevention, has been understood by all concerned to be directly linked to reproductive health concerns and is a major impetus for the development
of a common agenda (see Girard, this volume).

Many international donors have expanded their guidelines on HIV-
related funding to include investment in health systems development
with a view toward sustainable service delivery; sexual and reproductive
health concerns are increasingly seen to require attention to HIV in how
they are considered. Concurrently, international policy guidance is also
beginning to shift, which has helped the sexual and reproductive health
community, and over time both communities, to more carefully consider their intersections and commonalities (WHO 2004c).

The Current Landscape

The divide between sexual and reproductive health and HIV is decreasing in every way. The agendas of the sexual and reproductive health and
HIV communities are increasingly overlapping, with such shared concerns as gender dynamics, human rights, sexuality, pregnancy, childbirth, and breastfeeding. At a practical level, both communities are
beginning to give serious consideration to integration of services and
linkages between services. There is a recognized common need across
both communities for a functioning health system that can deliver both
HIV and sexual and reproductive health services. Larger questions are
now being raised related not only to how HIV and sexual and reproductive health are linked but to the ways in which sexual and reproductive
health services generally are being delivered and the extent to which
they engage with the specific sexual and reproductive health needs of
positive women and men, as well as whether they and other services are
cognizant of the HIV treatment needs of women outside the context of
pregnancy and childbirth. Convergence is increasingly recognized as an
imperative, and translation of this awareness into effective programming
with an appropriate balance of HIV and sexual and reproductive health
is therefore a top priority. Integration, or at least some degree of link-

age, therefore, is understood to be programmatically and potentially financially attractive, even as a number of issues remain to be resolved (Richey 2003).

Issues for the Future

Convergence of interest does not necessarily translate into a single obvious approach. Current debate is focused on whether integration of services or linkages between existing services is preferable and effective. Differentiation between physical integration and linkages between services raises critical differences. In some instances physical integration may seem to be preferable, but at other times it might seem best to keep services separate (Gruskin, Ferguson, and O'Malley 2007). More evidence is needed to assess which approaches are most effective in health and rights terms and therefore which will best serve the needs of their intended communities. Evaluation of these sorts of programs with attention to the core tenets of the Cairo agenda would seem to be a logical next step as the HIV and sexual and reproductive health worlds move closer to one another (Kitts and Lal 2006).

Physical integration, where services are offered in the same location, is often preferred by users, at least when the providers are trusted and the location is accessible and welcoming. These caveats are important, because providers that choose to physically integrate services must also decide whether to structure integrated services to cater to the population as a whole within a geographic area, or to provide a mix of general population "one-stop shops" alongside other services for specific population groups, such as youth-friendly clinics or specific services for sex workers.

The directionality of integration (whether HIV services are integrated into existing sexual and reproductive health services, or sexual and reproductive health services into existing HIV services, or both) also has important implications. Which populations will access services? What is the likelihood that health care workers will have the requisite training in all needed areas? How are the services perceived and used by the community? As large-scale roll-out of HIV treatment programs begins in resource-constrained settings, some countries are considering situating all HIV-related services and programs in existing reproductive health and maternal and neonatal health services (Lush 2002). While potentially laudable, this approach has important implications in terms of which populations will be able to access these services comfortably over time. Locating HIV services within these existing services would seem to facilitate the access of positive women interested in becoming pregnant to sexual and reproductive health services. However, recent studies indicate that positive women may prefer to access reproductive health services through HIV-related programs, to be sure that they do not face stigma or other problems connected to disclosure and to ensure that providers understand their health needs and concerns (O'Malley 2007). Furthermore, positive men may feel inhibited in this predominantly female environment, and positive women not interested in bearing children may also feel ill at ease using these services.

Despite much of this debate being focused on the appropriate way to offer services that engage with both HIV and sexual and reproductive health, health-related services are not delivered in a vacuum. Especially in the context of sexual and reproductive health and HIV, where taboos and stigma persist, the lessons from Cairo are particularly relevant. Cairo highlighted the ways the legal and policy environments shape the availability of services and programs and the degree to which they are responsive to the individual needs and aspirations of clients—in this case positive people. Cairo spoke to the need to address other cultural and social dynamics that affect demand, access, use, and quality of health and health services.

The sexual and reproductive health of HIV positive people is an area of activism and policy and programmatic change that was not imaginable even a few years ago. This is a welcome change requiring that more attention be paid to determine programmatically where efforts should be placed and how best to serve the reproductive needs of this growing population. In addition to its focus on the sexual and reproductive rights and needs of positive women, HIV is also bringing useful attention to the long ignored area of the sexual and reproductive health of men. All this is to say that it will be necessary to move beyond traditional conceptions of integration and linkages of sexual and reproductive health and HIV services to ensure that positive women and men have the requisite access to the services they require to go forward.

Unexplored areas of convergence in the interests of the HIV and sexual and reproductive health communities also exist in relation to people who are not infected or not aware of their status. Potential prevention technologies such as male circumcision are bringing new dimensions to consideration of the linkages between sexual and reproductive health and HIV, and the coming years will require attention as to how circumcision and other approaches will intersect with sexual and reproductive rights, needs, and choices (Sawires et al. 2007). As new technologies become more prevalent, policy and programmatic direction will be required. The basic principles of the Cairo agenda, in particular its general attention to reproductive rights noted earlier in this chapter, could usefully help guide programming approaches as well as the requisite monitoring and evaluation frameworks.

We have not done enough to provide the hard evidence of the difference the Cairo agenda can make to effectively address the reproductive and sexual health needs of all populations, particularly those living with HIV or AIDS. Improving the reproductive and sexual health needs of all people will require the sustained participation of affected communities, nondiscrimination in how policies and programs are carried out, and accountability with respect to the efforts of governments, intergovernmental and nongovernmental institutions, and the private sector. These are the basic human rights concepts understood in Cairo, which must not be forgotten. In the future, we cannot simply organize to keep the Cairo agenda alive because we believe in it. We must also do the additional work of gathering and publishing the evidence of rights-based approaches needed to inform beliefs, policies and practices.

The Cairo paradigm shift means the world will never again be as it was before 1994. Despite the challenges cited in this chapter and throughout the book, Cairo still has more weight for the conceptualization of issues than any international conference process before or since—even the MDGs. Cairo's basic messages are no less true now than they ever were, and its tenets can, in an evolving political climate, serve as the bedrock for all efforts going forward. It is no longer the specifics of Cairo so much as the basic messages it offers which are useful for efforts linking sexual and reproductive health and HIV as we move into the future.

Chapter 10
Technology, Reproductive Health, and the Cairo Consensus

Kelly Blanchard

The ICPD Programme of Action (UN 1995) includes both explicit and implicit references for investments in reproductive health technology development and increased attention to access to existing technologies. The Programme of Action provides a comprehensive vision connecting rights, technology, and the attainment of reproductive health. In Chapter 12, "Technology, Research and Development," the Programme of Action states the importance of research, in particular in giving more people access to safe and effective mean of regulating fertility. It recognizes that not all people find methods that suit them and that men in particular have limited methods of contraception. Specifically, paragraph 12.10 states in its call for improved collaboration and coordination that "Research needs to be guided at all stages by gender perspectives, particularly women's, by the needs of users, and to be carried out in strict conformity with internationally accepted legal, ethical, medical, and scientific standards for biomedical research" (para. 12.10).

To have meaningful choices, this formulation implies that men and women need the ability to access affordable, high quality technologies. The need for new family planning methods to meet a variety of user needs is clearly articulated, as is the need for research into new HIV/STI (sexually transmitted infections) prevention methods. This text highlights the need for affordable methods, and also the lack of family planning methods for men. Implicitly, development of new technologies and improved access to new and existing technologies are critical for women and men to be able to choose when they have children, reduce their risk of HIV/STIs, and reduce maternal mortality and morbidity. Asserting that women and couples have the right to control their fertility and childbearing is clearly an empty promise without the technologies and tools to implement their intentions.

This chapter addresses the question of whether these explicit and implicit references in the Programme of Action to reproductive health technology development did in fact lead to new technology development. Not all advances in reproductive health technologies are considered in this analysis, however. Clearly new contraceptives, new abortion technologies, and potential new HIV prevention methods, like microbicides and cervical barrier methods, are reproductive health technologies. For the purposes of this chapter we also include modifications of existing technologies—including simplified delivery systems or new evidence that supports improved access—to be part of reproductive health technology development. This chapter will not address assisted reproduction technology development, or other significant maternal health technologies due to space limitations.

This chapter primarily focuses on family planning, abortion, and HIV/STI prevention technologies. It argues that despite the focus on technology development in the Programme of Action, and the development of a number of new reproductive health technologies in the years since Cairo, ICPD arguably did not have a major impact. Rather, technology development has largely been driven by industry priorities, although HIV prevention technology development and research have received significant attention and funding and may well have incorporated some of ICPD's principles. The Programme of Action articulated the change in rationale for technology development. For contraceptive technologies, the driver had initially been population concerns, but with ICPD technological advances were increasingly seen as a way for women and couples to exercise their rights to achieve their desired family composition.

Negotiations at ICPD over the Programme of Action were significantly shaped by women's previous experiences of contraceptive technology, especially regarding abuses of women both in the name of developing new contraceptive technologies and in using contraceptive technologies to limit their ability to make choices about their reproductive health. This was critical to the overall paradigm shift in Cairo. Women's advocacy before and during Cairo also played a significant role in how the Programme of Action addressed technology and technology development. A full discussion of this history is beyond the scope of this chapter (see Hartmann 1995). However, the clear articulation of technologies as tools to exercise one's rights and the specific focus on ethical research and development for new technologies were a direct response to the abuse of women in unethical research and to programs that forced sterilization or contraceptive use for eugenic aims. The

Programme of Action and this paradigm shift provided new inspiration for technology development. ICPD highlighted the importance of contraceptives and HIV/STI prevention tools for individuals to actualize their reproductive and sexual health goals and provided a framework in which access to these tools became important health equity issues and a key component of being able to exercise one's reproductive rights.

Finally, this chapter concludes with a discussion about ICPD's continued relevance for the field. The Programme of Action's emphasis on the continued need for new technologies and the importance of acceptability and access remain critically important. However, reduced funding for contraceptive development in particular and waning attention to contraceptive access globally show that the international community's concern about access to and development of these technologies is lagging. The ICPD framework could be better leveraged to raise the issue of critical non-HIV/STI prevention technologies, and the general paradigm continues to be extremely useful for highlighting the need for public sector investment in technologies for women and men in low resource settings.

Reproductive Health Technology Development Since Cairo

In the time since Cairo there have been some significant reproductive health technology advances, including development and introduction of a number of new contraceptive methods, simplification of abortion technologies, and a significant increase in research on novel HIV/STI prevention methods.

Contraception

Several new hormonal contraceptive options have recently come on the market. Mirena, a progesterone-releasing intrauterine system (IUS), is an extremely effective contraceptive method (99 percent) (Trussell 2004). In addition, Mirena is a useful treatment for extremely heavy or painful menstrual bleeding and can provide an important alternative to hysterectomy in many cases (Pakarinen, Toivonen, and Luukkainen 2001; Fedele et al. 1997). The contraceptive patch, Ortho Evra, and the contraceptive vaginal ring, Nuvaring, are also now available (Ortho 2007; Organon 2007). Both methods effectiveness similar to that of the combined oral contraceptive pill (92 percent) (Trussell 2004) and are potentially easier to use and less prone to user-error since they do not require daily pill-taking. A new subcutaneous formulation (as opposed to the original intramuscular formulation) of Depo-Provera, the three-monthly contraceptive injection, has been approved (Pfizer 2005). The subcutaneous injection allows for a smaller dose, which may relieve some of the side effects associated with the injectable form, and also opens the door to further investigation of self-injection of injectable contraceptives, since subcutaneous injections are easier to administer. Self-injection or pharmacy injection could increase access to injectable methods and also improve user acceptability and continuation (Lakha, Henderson, and Glasier 2005). Finally, a single rod contraceptive implant is now on the market in a few countries (WHO 2003a), and was recently approved for use in the United States. Although no new male contraceptive method is yet available, research into male injectable methods continues, and recent increased industry interest in male methods will hopefully lead to a breakthrough in this area soon (Liu et al. 2006; Meriggiola et al. 2006).

Perhaps the most important advance in the delivery of an existing contraceptive method since Cairo is over-the-counter availability of emergency contraception (EC). EC is now available directly from a pharmacist or over the counter in 41 countries (OPR and ARHP 2007). In addition, recent research has shown that the progesterone only product has fewer side effects than the Yuzpe combined method and is at least as effective (WHO Task Force on Postovulatory Methods of Fertility Regulation 1998). EC has traditionally included two hormone doses twelve hours apart, but new evidence has shown that taking the two doses at the same time is equally effective, making the method much more user friendly (Ngai et al. 2005). Other significant contraceptive delivery advances include the increasing acceptance of quick-start method initiation, eliminating the need for the woman to wait for her next period and return to the clinic for her method (Westoff et al. 2002) and increased attention to pharmacy provision of contraceptive methods (Pharmacy Access Partnership 2007).

Abortion

Access to manual vacuum aspiration (MVA) for early abortion has increased dramatically since Cairo, and the MVA device itself has been updated to make it easier to use and reuse (Abernathy 2005). In addition, access to medication abortion technology has increased and mifepristone is now available in a significantly larger number of countries (Gynuity Health Projects 2005). Research on medication abortion has also led to simplified, less expensive, and easier to use regimens. Studies have shown that a reduced 200 mg dose of mifepristone is as effective as the original 600 mg dose (WHO Task Force 1993; Schaff et al. 1999), and home use of misoprostol, the second part of the most commonly used medication abortion regimen, has been shown to be safe and effective, eliminating the cost and inconvenience of a second clinic visit (Schaff et al. 1997). Continuing research on the use of medication abortion in rural areas and in facilities without access to ultrasound will hopefully further increase access to the method (Ellertson et al. 2000; Coyaji et al. 2001).

HIV/STI Prevention

Research on new HIV prevention technologies has greatly expanded since Cairo. Although already developed in 1994, the female condom has been introduced in a few countries and investigation of less expensive and new designs continues (Cervical Barrier Advancement Society 2007). Four microbicide candidates are now either in Phase III effectiveness testing, or scheduled for trials soon (Alliance for Microbicide Development 2007).[1] Nonoxynol 9 was tested as a potential microbicide and although results showed it was not effective (Roddy et al. 1998; Van Damme et al. 2002), results for second generation products will hopefully be available in the next few years. Third generation microbicide products, which include antiretroviral drugs, are now moving into human trials, although progress has moved in fits and starts. Preexposure prophylaxis with tenofovir or other antiretroviral drugs is also on the agenda, and despite the recently suspended tenofovir trials in Cambodia and Cameroon, new animal data indicate such approaches might be promising (Garcia-Lerma et al. 2006). Another microbicidal product, Ushercell, also moved into human trials recently, only to have the trials halted when women exposed to Ushercell faced an increased risk of HIV transmission compared to women receiving a placebo (Microbicide Trials Halted in Africa 2007). Cervical barriers including the currently available contraceptive diaphragm and new diaphragm-like devices are also being evaluated for HIV/STI prevention (Cervical Barrier Advancement Society 2007). Recent evidence indicates that a significant proportion of HIV infections likely take place at the cervix, and covering the cervix with a barrier may reduce HIV acquisition (Moench, Chipato, and Padian 2001). Most large microbicide and cervical barrier trials are also investigating prevention of other STIs including chlamydia, gonorrhea, trichomonas, herpes simplex 2, and the human papilloma virus. These STIs cause a significant burden of disease themselves, and also increase risk of HIV acquisition and transmission (Robinson et al. 1997). There is thus a great need for efficacious products, but trials of microbicides and other STI/HIV prevention technologies must as a necessity move cautiously in field-testing their products due to ethical considerations regarding informed consent and long-term access to care (Forbes 2006). Where research ethics for clinical trials in developing countries may have received somewhat short shrift in the past, the ICPD legacy has created an environment in which advocates and community groups can engage with researchers over the health needs and safety of trial populations.

Finally, we also now have access to a variety of antiretroviral technologies for prevention of mother to child transmission of HIV. Research has showed that a simplified nevirapine regimen could effectively reduce mother to child transmission by 50 percent, and this regimen is much less cumbersome and much more cost-effective than the more involved ones using AZT or multiple drugs currently in use in developed countries (Guay et al. 1999; Jackson et al. 2003). Nevirapine programs are now active in many developing countries, and access to these programs continues to increase (Kresge 2005).

Impact of the Cairo Programme of Action

How much of this increase in attention to reproductive health technologies is a result of the explicit and implicit call for increases in research in the Cairo Programme of Action? Arguably some. But global investment and attention to the need for the development of new reproductive health technologies falls short of the vision laid out in the Cairo consensus.

First, in terms of contraceptive developments, many of these advances are relatively minor improvements in the delivery of hormones and do not significantly address the need for a wider range of methods to meet the needs of men and women around the world. The technological improvements have been largely funded by the pharmaceutical industry and respond to developed world priorities and markets. The vast majority of these new methods are not available in developing countries. In most low-resource settings, family planning is targeted at women who still have access to only a few contraceptive options, usually an injectable and an oral contraceptive method, and perhaps an IUD.

Increased access to and improvements in EC have, however, largely been the result of international advocacy and were supported by public (government, multilateral, or foundation) funding. There has been relatively little industry interest in the method, although interest has grown significantly over the last decade. Part of the success of public funding for EC, though, is likely due to the fact that significant advances have been made with a relatively small investment. The changes in the EC regimen and delivery have been supported by a few significant studies, and the funding for these studies was significantly less than what is generally required for development of a completely new method. The lack of completely novel contraceptive methods, and the lack of progress in development of a male method, can be linked to the reduction in funding for family planning generally and the significant shortfall from the sums outlined at Cairo (Speidel 2005).

Similarly, the development of new abortion technologies has received relatively little public support. Only a few governments and foundations support work on abortion, and increased funding could significantly improve technologies and access to them around the world.

The HIV/STI prevention picture is different. Funding for new prevention technologies from both governments and private foundations has dramatically increased (AVAC 2005). But this increased funding and attention to the need for HIV/STI prevention technologies have not been argued from the Cairo framework, although significant gains have been made by interpreting the right to health as encompassing access to life-saving medication, such as antiretrovirals (Hogerzeil et al. 2006). Some aspects of the priorities outlined in the Programme of Action—including the need for attention to gender and user perspectives—are central to the rationale for increased attention to these technologies, especially to the development of new female-controlled HIV/STI prevention methods. However, as in the focus on HIV treatment and services, this effort has largely focused on HIV as separate from other reproductive health issues and has not embraced the Cairo definition of reproductive health (Kaufman and Messersmith 2006). Advocacy for increased investment in and attention to HIV/STI prevention technologies has largely not placed HIV/STIs within a reproductive health framework.

Although not the focus of this chapter, ICPD arguably has had a greater impact on access to existing technologies. Access to family planning globally has increased since Cairo (UN Department of Economic and Social Affairs 2003b), as has access to MVA, particularly for post-abortion care (Abernathy 2005). Integrated services in some countries may have unintentionally reduced access to family planning due to the loss of focus on the unique delivery of contraception in vertical family planning programs. But overall the Programme of Action greatly increased global attention to the need to provide family planning services and address other reproductive health service needs.

The Larger Context

The possible impact of the Programme of Action, though, is significantly limited by other forces and factors that affect the "if," "when," and "how" of technology development generally, and reproductive health technology particularly. Obviously, pharmaceutical companies are driven by profits. Profits in turn are determined by potential market and price. On a very basic level, market and price can be estimated by looking at consumer interest in and willingness to pay for a product. But other factors indirectly affect price. Potential legal liability and community attitudes toward a specific product can have a profound impact on the value of that product. The development of mifepristone (RU-486) for medication abortion illustrates the significant impact of attitudes toward the product, particularly in the U.S., which has a large effect on product development and international access—in large measure because of the size of the U.S. market and its influence in international family planning and other foreign assistance.

Mifepristone was developed in France by staff at Roussel-Uclaf in the early 1980s. Studies showed that mifepristone in combination with a prostaglandin was highly effective for termination of early pregnancy. Politics at Roussel-Uclaf, however, led the company to suspend promotion of the drug in France in the late 1980s. The French minister of health demanded that Roussel-Uclaf continue to make the drug available in France—declaring it the property of French women—and it was formally introduced in 1990. The company was increasingly the target of anti-abortion protesters and activists and refused, despite a letter from President Bill Clinton in 1993, to apply for approval for the drug in the U.S. The company decided instead to grant all rights to the drug to the non-profit Population Council, which had been extensively involved in mifepristone research. Continuing political interference in the U.S. and the lack of a corporate pharmaceutical sponsor dramatically slowed the approval process. The U.S. Food and Drug Administration (FDA) issued an approvable letter in 1996, but asked for additional information on labeling, manufacturing, and distribution. The original Hungarian manufacturer the Population Council had secured backed out in 1997. It took a number of years to identify another manufacturer and have it inspected and approved by the FDA. Continued pressure by U.S. antiabortion groups and the threat of boycotts and other activities like those directed at Roussel-Uclaf meant that no U.S. manufacturer was willing to produce mifepristone (and suffer boycotts of its other more lucrative products), and in fact the identity of the current manufacturer has not been disclosed. Finally, once the manufacturer was inspected and approved, mifepristone was approved for use by the FDA in September 2000. Since then, numerous bills have been introduced in Congress to try to remove mifepristone from the U.S. market or curtail its availability.

Other reproductive health products are subject to similar attacks in the U.S. efforts to make emergency contraception (Duramed's Plan B®) available over the counter have faced continued attack from conservative advocates and lawmakers. Despite overwhelming support from an FDA advisory panel for over-the-counter access, the FDA refused to approve Duramed's application for over-the-counter access, and a 2005 Government Accountability Office report found that the FDA did not follow its own procedures in the review of the application (Government Accountability Office 2005). Political interference in the decision clearly seems to have been a factor. Plan B® was finally approved for over-the-counter distribution in August 2006, when it became evident that the issue would hold up approval of President Bush's nominee to head the FDA. Conservative groups and lawmakers have repeatedly asserted that making emergency contraception available over the counter would encourage teenage sex, despite mounting rigorous evidence to the contrary. Conservatives have been successful at restricting access to abortion and contraception information and services and promoting abstinence-only sex education at both the federal and state level. In this climate, pharmaceutical companies weigh the costs not only of the research and development of the potential new drug, but also of a potential backlash related to the decision to develop controversial products.

Both mifepristone and emergency contraception have been made more widely available because of public sector funding and international advocacy on the part of women's health and rights advocates around the world. In both cases, foundation support of the commercialization of the product was critical, as was an active network of organizations willing to support the training, marketing, and legal functions normally carried out by an industry sponsor. Because major pharmaceutical companies were not willing to develop these products, the public sector needed to step in order to make them available.

Civil society advocates have played a similar role and have been much more successful in increasing access to HIV treatment in developing countries. Interestingly, many conservatives in the U.S. have been active supporters of these efforts. A number of factors probably account for the increased support for technology development for and access to HIV prevention and treatment compared to contraceptives and other reproductive health products. First, HIV threatens the health and has killed millions of people around the world. The HIV epidemic is a very visible problem in a way that poor reproductive health is not. Pitting children dying of AIDS against profits for big pharmaceutical companies is perhaps an easier sell than helping women and couples get access to contraceptives that work for them and help them plan their family size.

Second, the treatments that are now being made available through subsidized distribution and licenses to developing country companies are for the most part already available in developed country markets, and these regimens already bring large profits. Companies are increasingly donating their products for development and testing as potential microbicides or other prevention methods. However, they are not in general investing their own resources in product development, as they have determined that the profit-making possibilities are too small.

Third, access to treatment in particular has immediate and observable effects, with very visible short-term improvements that add to the good will generated for the company. In this manner pharmaceutical companies attempt to be seen as global good citizens. Increasingly, companies cannot afford to not participate in these programs because the treatment access movement has been so effective in working to shame those who will not help increase access to their products (e.g., Baker 2007).

Finally, public financing and support for these programs has grown immensely, and foundation and government support to increase access and help distribute these products has been critical to the success of the programs.

What might we learn from this that can be applied to other reproductive health products? Clearly, financial support is fundamental, and we will continue to depend on public financing for new technology development. We also would benefit from making a stronger case for the need for new contraceptives and other reproductive health technologies, highlighting the role contraception plays in development and poverty reduction, and telling the story of contraception more clearly and convincingly. Finally, HIV treatment activists globally have successfully used human rights claims and mechanisms to promote the agenda to increase access to health care. These tactics and achievements hopefully pave the way for similar arguments to be used to increase investment in other types of technologies. Politics in the U.S. and the lack of blockbuster profits from contraceptive and abortion technologies in the developed world will continue to hamper efforts to improve technology development and access, but other governments and advocates are increasingly stepping into the void. If motivated by a concern for developing country access, efforts must focus on critical actors in Europe as well as on encouraging international actors like the UN agencies and WHO to continue to advocate for reproductive health technology development.

Looking Forward

Many of the points raised in the ICPD Programme of Action are still vital today for the development of new reproductive health technologies. We still have too few contraceptive options, and many couples cannot find or access a method that meets their needs. A focus on understanding these needs and support for increased research on innovative ways to increase access to existing methods is critical to improve reproductive health around the globe. In addition, the need to consciously address gender and its impact on acceptability and the need for new technologies remains key to helping women in particular address their most pressing reproductive health needs and exercise their reproductive rights.

There is still clearly much work to be done to move forward the vision of reproductive health outlined at Cairo. In some ways we are coming full circle. The growing attention to the need to better integrate HIV and reproductive health activities and services seems to be bringing us back to the holistic vision of reproductive health that ICPD delineated. Increased attention to the reproductive health needs of women living with HIV, the need to integrate family planning into HIV services and vice versa, and the importance of family planning and safe abortion services for meeting the MDG on maternal health all point to the necessity of promoting the concept of reproductive health as it was outlined in the Programme of Action (Casterline and Sinding 2000; Myer et al. 2005; Miller, Shortridge, and Martin 2006; Center for Communication Programs 2007).

Finally, the fact that we have not met the technology goals laid out in the Programme of Action more than a decade later highlights the need for continued advocacy for public funding of reproductive health technologies. The ICPD document itself is a valuable tool as part of continued advocacy for increased investment in new and improved technologies. Questions remain, however, about how best to frame the points laid out in the Programme of Action and how to make the best case to funders and governments for increased investment in new reproductive health technologies. Advocates for new HIV prevention technologies have been very successful in documenting the potential impact of these advances while interest in access to contraceptive technologies has waned. The demographic target-driven population focus pre-Cairo provided a clear (though flawed) rationale for increasing access to contraceptives and it is not clear that the human rights approach has provided a compelling enough framework. ICPD focuses on rights and the need for equitable access to the tools to realize those rights. Increasingly a conceptual link between reproductive health, technology, and poverty alleviation and development is being made in an effort to bring focus back to the need for family planning. Innovative approaches for measuring the benefits of access to contraception, both individually and on the national and international levels, are needed to help document the successes of increased access and technology development and accurately describe the benefits that increased investment in new technologies and improved access will bring. It is also worth considering how to describe the variety of technologies—contraception, abortion, maternal and child health, HIV prevention, and others—which fall within the rubric of reproductive health technologies and whether a new frame is needed which looks beyond contraception and makes the case for development of and access to a larger range of technologies that can significantly improve reproductive health.

The Cairo Programme of Action both explicitly and implicitly called for the development of new and the improvement of existing reproductive health technologies. Significant advances have taken place since 1994, but ICPD was likely only a small factor, if any, in those advances. We need increased public funding for technologies to address the most pressing reproductive health needs of women and men in low-resource settings. The decade since Cairo has shown that without public commitment and support, technology development will be driven by industry, which will in turn be driven by developed country priorities and markets. Continued attention to the need for new technologies and improved access to existing technologies, and the potential for such technologies to improve reproductive health globally remain as important now as they were in Cairo.

Chapter 11
The Cairo "Compromise" on Abortion and Its Consequences for Making Abortion Safe and Legal

Marge Berer

The Programme of Action of the International Conference on Population and Development (UN 1995) is an extraordinary document. It is more than ten years since the conference, yet its comprehensive analysis of what constitutes sexual and reproductive health, reproductive rights, gender equality and equity, attention to the needs of adolescents and socioeconomic development as it relates to population health, and how these can and must be achieved, is unsurpassed. For those for whom the document itself is a distant memory, it is worth re-reading. There is one exception to its brilliance, however, which is the subject of this chapter, that is, how the document addresses induced abortion.

Induced abortion is referred to a number of times in the Programme of Action, either specifically (paras. 7.6, 7.24, 8.19, 8.25), by inference as a method of fertility regulation (paras. 7.2, 7.3, 7.5b), or in relation to unsafe abortion as one of the causes of maternal mortality and morbidity (para. 8.20).

The great contradiction contained in this document, and the reason why in the short run it was such a let-down on the subject of abortion, is that although it urged on page after page that reproductive health and fertility regulation were to be considered as reproductive rights, the safety and legalization of one of the most commonly used methods of fertility regulation—and a major cause of avoidable mortality and morbidity in women—was eschewed. All the negotiators managed to eke out in the effort to achieve a broad-based consensus was the proposition that "in circumstances where abortion is not against the law, such abortion should be safe" (para. 8.25).

What the Programme of Action Says About Abortion

The perception of abortion contained in the Programme of Action explains a great deal in relation to the continuing conflict that has taken place on the subject in the years since. In the paragraph defining what constitutes reproductive health, the Programme of Action calls for

the right of men and women to be informed and to have access to safe, effective, affordable and acceptable methods of family planning of their choice, and other methods of their choice for regulation of fertility which are not against the law. (para. 7.2)

From the perspective of what health services should be doing, it says that

Reproductive health care in the context of primary health care should, inter alia, include . . . abortion as specified in paragraph 8.25, including prevention of abortion and the management of the consequences of abortion . . . [and that] diagnosis and treatment for complications of pregnancy, delivery and abortion . . . should always be available, as required. (para. 7.6)

These first mentions in Chapter 7, having clearly been edited to reflect the more detailed text in Chapter 8, take an equivocal tone about abortion, not treating it as a means of fertility regulation or as a legitimate reproductive health service, but as something that must be prevented. In Chapter 8, the public health problem of unsafe abortion is stressed, but instead of recommending that all abortions should be made safe, which would resolve the public health problem fully, it recommends that all unwanted pregnancies should be prevented, as if this were feasible:

a significant proportion of the abortions carried out are self-induced or otherwise unsafe, leading to a large fraction of maternal deaths or to permanent injury to the women involved. . . . Greater attention to the reproductive health needs of female adolescents and young women could prevent the major share of maternal morbidity and mortality through prevention of unwanted pregnancies and any subsequent poorly managed abortion. (para. 8.19)

Thus, moral judgment on abortion constantly trumps the public health imperative to save women's health and lives. Safe abortion should be provided only if it is legal, on the one hand, and on the other hand, it should be prevented and recourse to it should be reduced, or better, eliminated. That women must be encouraged to use family planning is repeated time and again. Abortion is seen as a matter for governments only insofar as "Governments should take appropriate steps to help women avoid abortion" (para. 7.24), which is fine as far as it goes, but refuses to address what governments should do once a woman has an unwanted pregnancy and seeks an abortion. It is commonly known that contraceptive methods are not perfect and people are not perfect users of them, and that in some cases men stop women from using contraception, while in other cases rape, sexual abuse, and coercive sexual relations are the reason for unwanted pregnancy. Yet the document calls only for increased use of family planning (viz. contraception), as if contraception will eliminate "any subsequent poorly managed abortion" (para. 8.19).

Thus, women seeking abortion in countries where it is legally restricted and/or not provided safely are left with unsafe abortions. For them, the document recommends only "compassionate counselling" and "diagnosis and treatment of complications," in flagrant contravention of the duty on health professionals to "do no harm," one of the historical pillars of medical ethics.

Unlike the rest of the Programme of Action, the stance on abortion is not based on evidence of what is required to promote and protect reproductive health or to reduce maternal mortality, or on the right to decide the number and spacing of children. Instead, these paragraphs wash their hands of responsibility for the harm that results from unsafe and illegal abortion. Women living in countries where abortion is unsafe and illegal can only hope to be patched up after the fact.

The greatest impact, however, has been due to the following sentence, repeated in two different chapters:

In no case should abortion be promoted as a method of family planning. (paras. 7.24 and 8.25)

This statement, a masterpiece of equivocation, was originally imposed by the Reagan administration in the final recommendations of the 1984 Mexico City global population conference. It has proven to be a potent weapon in the hands of a right-wing U.S. government, which has used it to block work on making abortion safe and legal, in tandem with the threat of withholding funding. I well remember some of those who claimed to support abortion rights at the Cairo conference coming out of the negotiations saying that they "could live with" this phraseology. Many of them probably did not think abortion should be "promoted" either, as ambivalence about abortion among them was and perhaps still remains strong (Løkeland 2004). They were also willing to support the repeated references to preventing abortion, which they also agreed with, and they found it difficult to argue against respect for the law and the so-called "culture" in countries where abortion was illegal, even if the law and culture concerned were based on the oppression of women. This even though para. 7.3 says that the right to reproductive health also includes [women's] right to make decisions concerning reproduction free of discrimination, coercion and violence, as expressed in human rights documents. (para. 7.3)

The Programme of Action in fact never recognizes that for women living in poverty and young women, unsafe abortion is a form of economic discrimination, because women with money can pay for safe abortions; that abortion may be necessary as a consequence of sexual coercion;[1] and perhaps most important that because the means to provide safe abortions exist, making women have unsafe abortions is a form of violence against women (Amuchastegui Herrera and Rivas Zivy 2002). The anodyne term "unsafe abortion" makes it possible to forget the horrific morbidity and mortality that can result. Figure 1 is a reminder of what unsafe abortion actually means (Oye-Adeniran, Umoh, and Nnatu 2002).

This was the underbelly of the great compromise of Cairo, that with women's autonomy hanging in the balance, those who believe that motherhood should be forced on women had to be assuaged and were more important than women themselves. However, the longer-term out-

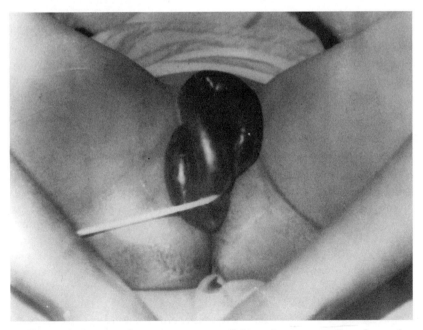

Figure 1. Loops of gangrenous small intestine protruding from the vagina, 20-year-old woman, Lagos University Teaching Hospital, Nigeria. (Oye-Adeniran, Umoh, and Nnatu 2002).

come of that fierce battle of wills and ideologies, which drew in people from all over the world, in spite of its equivocal outcome, put the public health problem of unsafe abortion on the global agenda in a way it had never been before. And on the agenda it has staunchly remained. The question of whether this has been a good thing or not, and whether what the document said would remain relevant, especially with the appearance of new politicians and governments with the passage of time, is the subject of the rest of this chapter.

The Compromise: Contradictory Stances

A compromise by definition ends up pleasing no one entirely. This compromise allowed the document to be passed by a large majority of countries, a major success for the thousands of people who worked hard for that goal. However, for a compromise to be workable, the terms cannot be so contradictory that implementing them is impossible. However, this is what has happened as regards abortion with the Programme of Action. Since 1994, both those who support safe, legal abortion and those who oppose it have focused only on the sentences and phrases in the Programme of Action that support their own position. Since ICPD, the Vatican has engaged in a proactive campaign against abortion that has been all the more effective in the context of the rise of religious and political fundamentalism in all world regions and religions. From the day George W. Bush took office in 2001, he added fuel to that campaign. On the other hand, for those who support women's right to safe abortion, outrage and dismay at the terms of the compromise in many cases motivated a renewed effort to campaign for safe, legal abortion.

Both sides remain uncompromising, though there have been recent efforts on the part of some pro-choice activists in the U.S. to seek another sort of compromise position, based on so-called "fetal value" and "prevention of abortion." Unfortunately, this did not arise in response to a comparable willingness to compromise by anti-abortionists, and I believe it is doomed to failure (Kissling 2005). Yet all anti-abortionists have not supported the same goals either, and the various anti-abortion partners during the Cairo negotiations did not all have the same ends in mind, nor the same ends as the Bush administration. The Vatican was and remains opposed to the whole concept and practice of fertility regulation, not just abortion, while the then largely pronatalist Latin American governments that had weak family planning programs or sided with the Vatican in 1994 today mostly have far more substantial family planning programs and many are actively debating abortion law reform. The countries where a conservative interpretation of Islamic law is dominant were opposed to the legalization of abortion on the grounds of "culture" and support for "the rights of the family" over the rights of the individual (woman). This was both a pronatalist and anti-women's rights position rather than a strictly religious one. Indeed, a number of theological interpretations of Islam and a number of Islamic countries permit abortion in the first months of pregnancy (Serour, Ragab, and Hassanein 1996).

The Bush administration has had to take a complex stance, because it has had to engage internally with almost 40 years of U.S. government support for family planning programs at the global level and a long-standing commitment to reducing maternal deaths, which has included support for post-abortion care programs. The upheaval caused by the changes in leadership, senior staffing and policy in key U.S. government offices, such as the United States Agency for International Development (USAID) and the United States Food and Drug Administration (FDA), that have emerged under Bush will, I believe, prove disastrous for the United States in the long run. Most countries have made efforts, both large and small, to incorporate the ICPD Programme of Action into their national policies, programs, and services (Haslegrave 2004), while the biggest donor in the field before 1994 has rapidly been backpedaling. This has caused havoc in countries where long-standing U.S. funding was withdrawn or threatened with being withdrawn (Crane and Dusenberry 2004).

The bullying that has accompanied U.S. efforts to derail the implementation of the Programme of Action is thought to be unprecedented. At first, it was only whispered about in the corridors but then it was confronted openly, and anti-ICPD resolutions put forward by the U.S. were roundly defeated in every post-ICPD-related international meeting (UNFPA 2005). While the Bush administration has certainly succeeded in stopping work being done in the short term, it is also causing great resentment.

However, USAID under Bush has a right to claim that it too is implementing the ICPD Programme of Action, as regards the stricture that "In no case should abortion be promoted as a method of family planning" (paras. 7.24 and 8.25). This is the basis for the memorandum containing the Bush version of the Global Gag Rule. In it, neither financial support nor technical assistance for activities related to abortion is permitted.[2] In this memorandum, abortion was considered a method of family planning when it was for the purpose of spacing births. This includes, but is not limited to, abortions performed to protect the physical or mental health of the pregnant woman. It does not include abortions if the life of the woman would be endangered if the fetus were carried to term or abortions following rape or incest (since abortion under these circumstances is not considered a family planning act). Also excluded from this definition is the treatment of injuries caused by an abortion; thus, post-abortion care is explicitly permissible, and again is a Programme of Action goal (Global Gag Rule Impact Project 2003).

In addition to refusing to fund abortions as a method of family planning, the Gag Rule's definition of promotion of abortion includes, but is not limited to, operating a family planning counseling service that includes advice and information regarding the benefits and availability of abortion as a method of family planning; providing advice that abortion is an available option in the event other methods of family planning are not used or are not successful, or encouraging women to consider abortion; lobbying a foreign government to legalize or make available abortion as a method of family planning or lobbying such a government to continue the legality of abortion as a method of family planning; and conducting a public information campaign regarding the benefits and/or availability of abortion as a method of family planning (Global Gag Rule Impact Project 2003). All NGOs in countries who are recipients of USAID funds have been required to sign the Global Gag Rule before their grants are approved or continued. Not having an alternative source of funding, most of these NGOs are believed to have signed (Crane and Dusenberry 2004; Global Gag Rule Impact Project 2003). There are also notable exceptions, such as that of the International Planned Parenthood Federation (IPPF 2007).

The problem with all this is not what "promotion" of abortion means, since abortions will be needed regardless f whether anyone promotes it, but also what "family planning" means. The fact of the matter is that the practice of family planning and abortion can never be separated. In this, the Vatican at least has a consistent world view, while the Gag Rule is contradictory. But the Bush government is not interested in philosophical or linguistic debates. It is the very ambiguity inherent in its policy that gives the Gag Rule power, because if USAID even thinks an NGO has transgressed (and it has people tasked with watching for this at country level), it can cut their funding off. The threat alone has worked very well in stopping NGOs that are dependent on USAID from doing anything related to abortion, for fear that they will be defunded (Crane and Dusenberry 2004).

Whither the Right to Safe, Legal Abortion

As powerful as the alliance against abortion was in 1994, the momentum generated by ICPD and the overwhelming acceptance at country level of the need to protect and promote sexual and reproductive health and rights has been far stronger. In the Soviet Union and Eastern Europe, abortion had been legalized in the 1950s and in some cases even earlier. In the U.S. and Canada, most of Europe, New Zealand, and Australia, the main battles for legalization of abortion had taken place and been won by the end of the 1970s. However, in 1984 at the Fourth International Women and Health Meeting in Amsterdam, many of the women from developing countries said they could not participate in a network if the word "abortion" was in the name and could hardly raise the issue aloud in their own countries. In the more than twenty years since then, a sea change has taken place; unsafe abortion is a public health problem being raised in country after country in the developing world.

The language of ICPD+5 on abortion in 1999 was the basis for the WHO Safe Abortion guidance document (WHO 2003b) and the lever for more work on abortion on the part of governments. It also spurred an increase in funding for making abortion safe on the part of several European donors, especially Sweden, the Netherlands, and the UK.

All over Latin America and the Caribbean, abortion is the subject of public debate, in which the supporters of safe abortion are becoming far more numerous. The Mexico City legislature has made abortion legal during the first trimester, although it is being appealed to the Supreme Court (Billings et al. 2002; *The Guardian* 2007). In Cuba and Guyana, the laws are liberal. In St. Lucia and Trinidad, the law has been changed, and Jamaica is considering legal reform as well (Center for Reproductive Rights 2007). A parliamentary bill to make abortion legal up to 12 weeks of pregnancy in Uruguay in 2004 was lost by only four votes, although some 63 percent of the population support law reform (Hierro López 2004), and in Brazil a bill has also been tabled though the outcome is currently uncertain (Adesse and Campello Ribeira de Almeida 2005). Campaigns for health services to provide legal abortion under existing laws, such as those allowing abortion on grounds of rape, are ongoing in Mexico and Brazil ("Brazil to Ease Abortions for Pregnant Rape Victims" 2005). Clarifying the legal situation to allow abortion when the fetus is unviable is being supported by obstetrician-gynecologists in Peru and Brazil (Catholic World News 2004; Ferreira da Costa et al. 2005). In Colombia, a human rights lawyer successfully challenged the law on abortion in the Constitutional Court as a violation of several of the human rights instruments signed by the country. The court situated its decision in the tradition of ICPD and Beijing, and subsequent interpretations of human rights by international human rights bodies. Abortion is now legal to save the life and health of the woman, in cases of rape, and when the fetus is not viable (Women's Link Worldwide 2005, 2006).

In Africa, abortion has been legal in Tunisia, Zambia, and South Africa for some time. Ethiopia recently liberalized its law as well. Campaigns are taking place for liberalization in Kenya, Nigeria, and Ghana. Mozambique is also planning legal reform. In Asia, Nepal's Family Planning Association defied the Global Gag Rule and worked for legalization of abortion, with law reform succeeding in 2004. Abortion services are being made available through the health system (Shakya et al. 2004; Thapa 2004) and through several nongovernmental clinics (Barbara Crane, Ipas, pers. communication 2006). Cambodia has also liberalized its law. India, in spite of a long-standing liberal law, is often held up along with Zambia as the exception to the rule that where it is legal, abortion will be safe, but efforts to tackle morbidity and mortality from unsafe abortions are growing (Hirve 2004).

Safer surgical methods of abortion, particularly manual and electric vacuum aspiration, are more widely available and training in using them has been carried out in a growing number of countries thanks to NGOs like Ipas (Hessini 2005), Marie Stopes International, and a growing number of private providers. At the same time, women's access to medical abortion in legally restricted settings, using at least one of the two types of abortion pill that have been included on the WHO List of Essential Medicines since mid-2005, is reducing many first trimester abortion deaths, according to providers of post-abortion care.[3]

At the ICPD, it was agreed that where abortion was illegal, post-abortion care services ("management of the consequences of abortion," para. 7.6) should always be provided. Many hospitals are more willing and better equipped to treat women with incomplete abortions than in the past, when the morbidity from dangerous invasive methods was far worse than it is today. Progress has been made in Mexico, Brazil, Bolivia, Peru, Nicaragua, El Salvador, and Guatemala, among others, in increasing the availability of post-abortion care, but a recent review of post-abortion care initiatives in public hospitals in seven Latin American countries shows that much work remains to be done (Billings and Benson 2005). In Guatemala, for example, post-abortion care has recently been scaled up and is available in the majority of district hospitals. Unfortunately, at least in the first two years of this program, mortality from unsafe abortion had not been reduced (Kestler et al. 2006).

In Africa, "a recently developed model of costs for abortion care shows that treating incomplete abortions in tertiary facilities costs ten times more than providing elective abortion in a primary health centre" (Johnson 2004). Moreover, in 2006, a paper examining the extent of hospitalization for abortion in 13 developing countries where abortion is still illegal reported that hundreds of thousands of women are being treated each year, taking up hospital beds and resources that could be used to improve women's health as well as make abortion safe (Singh 2006).

Thus, there is a long way to go, and all is not rosy. Fundamentalism grows apace and the gulf between fundamentalist and secular world views is widening, with women's rights hanging in the balance. The situation for women needing an abortion in Poland is dire (Polish Federation for Women and Family Planning 2005), and the battle to legalize abortion at a woman's request will be uphill for decades to come in many countries. The problem of morbidity and deaths from unsafe second trimester abortions is often hidden, as has been shown in Mexico (Walker et al. 2004), and even in the developed world second trimester abortions are less accepted than those in the first trimester. As one Norwegian author has argued, even in Europe "the legal right has been won, but not the moral right" (Løkeland 2004).

On the other hand, in the now ratified 2003 African Charter on Human Rights and Peoples' Rights on the Rights of Women in Africa, states are called on to protect women's reproductive rights by authorizing abortion in cases of sexual assault, rape, incest, fetal impairment, and where continuing the pregnancy would endanger the life or mental or physical health of the woman (African Union 2003). Rulings on the part of several UN treaty bodies have also supported abortion rights. For example in November 2005, the United Nations Human Rights Committee, which monitors countries' compliance with the International Covenant on Civil and Political Rights, decided its first abortion case, brought by a woman who had been refused a legal abortion and forced to carry a nonviable fetus to term. The Committee established that denying a woman access to legal abortion violates her most basic human rights. This was the first time an international human rights body has held a government accountable for failing to ensure access to legal abortion services (Center for Reproductive Rights 2005).

In 1994, the same year as the ICPD, Jain and Bruce proposed some sensible indicators to measure whether women were achieving their reproductive intentions in a healthy manner. These included the extent to which women are able to have a desired pregnancy that results in a positive outcome, prevent an unplanned pregnancy, terminate an unwanted pregnancy safely, achieve the desired interval between two consecutive births, and prevent any associated reproductive morbidity (Jain and Bruce 1994). These acknowledge, simply and without compromise that safe, legal abortion is a central aspect of fertility control.

It is time for unsafe abortion, and the ICPD compromise on abortion with it, to become an anachronism. In a few short years, the 20-year period originally set to achieve the goals of ICPD 1994 will be upon us. It would be too optimistic to say that the trend toward greater access to safe, legal abortion is inexorable. History is cluttered with political backsliding and stalled initiatives, especially when it comes to implementing verbal support for women's rights. However, the Vatican and the current, and not necessarily enduring, fundamentalist stranglehold on U.S. politics notwithstanding, the trend is that unsafe, illegal abortion is on its way out, not least because low fertility is here to stay for the foreseeable future—with a two-child norm for the majority of the globe, many one-child families, and a growing number of people who have no children. More and more women are being educated and are in paid employment. Although access to contraception is still limited for many and unsafe abortions still take place, more women and men are practicing fertility regulation. With fewer children to raise, they have time for doing other things with their lives as well. The right to family planning has been accepted by most women and men—and almost all governments—and has been accepted as a socially acceptable, legitimate practice, even in some conservative societies. Efforts on the part of those who would turn the clocks back are unlikely to succeed in the long run, whether those who, as anti-abortionists, would rescind all access to contraception and safe abortion or those who are proposing to push the fertility rate back up where it has fallen below replacement level, e.g., in Europe, while claiming to be pro-choice.[4]

Would women be worse off insofar as abortion is concerned if the Cairo compromise had not taken place? Yes, without a doubt, which is why the pro-choice government delegates and NGO representatives at the conference spent so many grueling hours hammering it out. However, the terms of the compromise do not support making all abortions safe and legal.

As is common with extremists, the Bush government has gone overboard in its efforts to limit sexual and reproductive rights. Like all donors, however, the U.S. needs to give financial support to other countries both in order to assert its leadership in the world and to have influence over the policies and programs of those countries. Recipients of funding need to recognize their collective power and refuse, individually and collectively, to accept the Gag Rule, just as governments overwhelmingly voted no when Bush administration representatives at the UN Special Session on Children in May 2002 (Girard 2002) and regional ICPD+10 meetings in 2003 and 2004 tried to introduce clauses to undermine the 1994 Programme of Action (Haslegrave 2004).

A women-centered perspective considers abortion legitimate not only if it is to save the life and health of a woman, or as a consequence of rape or incest, or because of fetal impairment, but also on social and economic grounds, to protect a woman's existing children, and as a method of birth spacing or limiting births. A woman's reasons for abortion always come back to the fact that she does not wish to carry a particular pregnancy to term. A women-centered perspective considers the need for abortion to be a necessary part of sexual and reproductive life. The legalization of abortion is fundamental to the long-term safety of abortion and the ability of health services to provide it as a legitimate procedure.

Making abortion legal is the only way that morbidity and mortality from unsafe abortions have been reduced historically, as evidenced in an analysis of national data from more than 160 countries (Berer 2004). If women are to have not only the inalienable right to life, but also the right to life on their own terms, the argument for making abortion safe, legal and accessible is unassailable.

Part III
Challenges to Institutionalizing Reproductive Health and Rights

Chapter 12
Advocacy for Sexuality and Women's Rights: Continuities, Discontinuities, and Strategies Since ICPD

Françoise Girard

On 13 December 2002, day three of the Fifth Asia-Pacific Population Conference at the UN Economic and Social Commission for Asia and the Pacific (ESCAP) in Bangkok, more than 30 governments from Asia and the Pacific, along with a number of former colonial powers that retain membership in ESCAP, assembled in a large conference room to review regional progress on the implementation of the Programme of Action of the 1994 International Conference on Population and Development (ICPD) (UN 1995).

The atmosphere was extremely tense. The U.S. plans for war in Iraq were already palpable, and some countries of the region were being courted heavily by the U.S. for their support. Even before delegates began discussions, Bush administration officials announced that the U.S. could no longer fully support the ICPD Programme of Action, and needed "clarifications" about whether reproductive health included abortion. The Cairo consensus was in danger of being rolled back.

In Bangkok, the U.S. delegation was composed of well-known right-wing negotiators, such as John Klink, a former member of the delegation of the Holy See at the ICPD and Beijing Conferences. Under his guidance, the U.S. delegation objected to previously agreed upon terms such as "reproductive rights" and "sexual health," obstructed the desire of all other governments present to reaffirm the ICPD consensus, made threats to withhold U.S. Agency for International Development (USAID) funding to recipient countries of the region, issued ultimatums, and threw procedural wrenches in the works at every turn. Yet the effect was not to divide and cow Asia-Pacific governments, on the contrary, they were uniting to stand by the goal of reproductive health for all as laid out in 1994.

On that day, Elaine Jones of the U.S. State Department took the floor to make a statement about the Billings ovulation method, a "natural" method of family planning. Stating that she was married and had been using the Billings method successfully for ten years, she described how to use it to determine the consistency of vaginal mucus. She then indicated that the U.S. would insist on inclusion of the term "natural family planning" in a paragraph of the draft Plan of Action on research priorities.

A moment of silence ensued. Asia-Pacific delegations were astonished. Did the U.S. mean that one American women's experience should guide Asian priorities in contraceptive development? The Thai delegate politely responded that the Billings method would not be very useful for women who have reproductive tract infections. But one of the delegates from Iran, a fully veiled obstetrician, could not contain herself. Turning around to address the U.S. delegation, she vehemently questioned the rationality of the U.S. insistence on "natural" family planning, "Mr. Chair, natural methods have a high failure rate! If you are so concerned about abortions, why do you insist to include natural family planning methods in the same document? It does not make sense to my delegation!" (see Block 2003)

When the Chair adjourned the session, as he would many times over the next few days, all delegations but the U.S. left the hall to meet in a small side room, where they strategized to preserve ICPD. India, China, the Philippines, Indonesia, Iran, Pakistan, Turkey, and others were determined that ICPD must stand. The U.S. delegation was becoming isolated, and its lack of interest in good-faith negotiations was apparent to all. Its extreme positions served as a uniting factor for other countries, even for governments that held conservative views on some aspects of sexual and reproductive health.

In the end, the Plan of Action adopted by the Fifth Asia-Pacific Population Conference reaffirmed the ICPD Programme of Action. Delegates also defeated every U.S. amendment that sought to weaken its content (UN Economic and Social Commission for Asia and the Pacific 2003). They handed the U.S. resounding defeats (31-1 and 32-1) when forced by the U.S. to vote on the sections on Reproductive Rights and Reproductive Health and Adolescent Reproductive Health. But the Bangkok Plan of Action did not advance the overall Cairo agenda. Nor were any of the seven days of the negotiation devoted to reviewing progress and discussing challenges in implementation. It had taken concerted effort by the delegates merely to save the concept of "reproductive health."

That scene, or ones similar to it, would play out repeatedly over the next years, as the ICPD+10 and Beijing+10 reviews unfolded at the regional and international levels between December 2002 and April 2005. In only a few years, the context for international negotiations on women's health had shifted from the mood of optimism in the post-Cold War era that gave rise to the cycle of international conferences of the 1990s to a feeling of embattlement generated by the Bush administration's hostility to sexual and reproductive rights. Women's health activists had grappled for years with the Vatican's opposition to sexual and reproductive rights in the context of international diplomatic negotiations, but U.S. opposition was a new development. The leadership role of the U.S. in Cairo to advance reproductive rights, and to support international consensus-building generally, was a thing of the past. The activism on combined fronts—gender justice and economic justice—that lay at the heart of the ICPD Programme of Action and the Beijing Platform for Action seemed something of a distant memory. While structural adjustment programs, unsustainable consumption, and neoliberal policies had been important subjects of debate in Cairo and Beijing, negotiations had now narrowed to the ever challenging questions of sexuality and reproduction.

Meanwhile, on the development front, the Millennium Development Goals adopted by the General Assembly in September 2000 (UN 2000a), and their indicators adopted a year later (UN 2001), had left out the ICPD Programme of Action goal of reproductive health for all by 2015 (para. 7.3).

Yet while progress on the ICPD agenda could not be achieved in intergovernmental negotiations, neither could the right-wing elements that now dominated U.S. foreign policy on reproductive health and women overturn the Cairo Programme or the Beijing Platform. In many ways, the ICPD+10 negotiations in Bangkok were a harbinger for events to come at the UN and elsewhere.

The "Paradigm Shift" Confirmed—ICPD and Beijing

As noted elsewhere in this volume, the ICPD Conference, held in Cairo in 1994, was a watershed in the field then called "population." The international women's health movement organized as never before and forged a pragmatic if uneasy alliance with family planning and environmental groups interested in maintaining strong support for contraception in the final agreement. Thus equipped, women's health advocates prevailed on governments from the North and South to adopt a human rights-based approach to women's health and reproduction (Programme of Action 1994).

This "paradigm shift" was accomplished by means of a solid critique of two essential elements of international development policy at that time, population control and structural adjustments. Population control programs, which were then heavily promoted by donors such as USAID, were shown to condone human rights violations. Activists also pointed out the great and growing impact on the environment of Western and Northern patterns of production and consumption. Structural adjustment programs and neoliberal policies, which were supported by the United States and put forward by international financial institutions such as the World Bank, were denounced by Southern governments and the global women's movement; they highlighted the devastating impact these policies had had on health and education systems throughout the developing world.[1]

Many of the government delegations in Cairo were headed or staffed by population and health specialists, who proceeded from knowledge of conditions in their country rather than a purely ideological mindset. Many of them had been approached at home by women's health activists and had become concerned that "population policy" was characterized by practices that were coercive and negated women's ability to decide on family planning methods for themselves. This insight provided considerable opening for activists to maximize gains for women's rights and fairer economic policies, in a context where those governments then most supportive of sexual and reproductive rights (Europe, U.S.) were also the most opposed to reviewing neoliberal economic dogma.

For similar reasons, women's health activists would also prevail over organized religious opposition, embodied in the Holy See's refusal to join the political consensus on reproductive rights.[2] Gita Sen observed as much, adding that "considerable advances were possible on reproductive and sexual health and rights during the 1990s because of the limited control over state power by religious fundamentalists" (Sen 2005a: 2).

However, religious fundamentalisms as political forces in international negotiations were on the rise after ICPD as was the development of new alliances at the international level to fight the very notion of gender equality. The "unholy alliance" of the Holy See, conservative Catholic countries, and Islamists did not ultimately hold in Cairo, since Muslim leaders held more moderate views than the Catholic Church hierarchy on contraception and abortion. But avenues of collaboration were laid out, which would be used again at Beijing and thereafter.

Cairo was also characterized by the fact that no attempt was made to forge a unified developing country position on social issues. The "G-77" group of developing countries at the UN negotiated traditionally as a bloc on economic issues only. In Cairo, therefore, it did not seek to reach an internal consensus on issues such as abortion or adolescents' access to reproductive health services, leaving each country free to express its views on these matters. Rather than racing to the lowest common denominator on topics such as the definition of "family" or whether the word "sexuality" should be included in the Programme of Action, health specialists expressed diverse points of view based on their national realities.

The same dynamic prevailed at the Fourth World Conference on Women in Beijing in 1995. The final Platform for Action reaffirmed the ICPD Programme of Action in spite of opposition by religious conservatives. It also significantly pushed the agenda forward on women's right to control their sexuality, unsafe abortion, and violence against women. The continued strength and presence of the women's movement, from the South and the North, played a crucial role in Beijing, in spite of attempts by the Chinese hosts to isolate women's groups in Huairo, more than an hour away from the Conference site.

The Beijing Conference also benefited from the visible leadership of delegates from sub-Saharan Africa and the Caribbean, including a large numbers of women members of government delegations. While the U.S. played a more discreet role in Beijing due to the domestic electoral considerations of the Clinton administration, the EU jumped in and was very active in negotiations to reaffirm ICPD and to secure the right of women to control their sexuality.

The Plus 5s, Economic Justice, and Women's Rights in the Balance

The ICPD+5 (1999) and Beijing+5 (2000) reviews took place in a different and already changing environment. Preparatory negotiations took place at UN headquarters in New York, a venue ill-suited for a review of implementation at the national level. Professional diplomats, rather than health experts, handled matters they knew little about.

North American right-wing groups attended in large numbers to oppose the ICPD Programme of Action and seek to weaken its provisions. Whereas the ICPD Programme of Action dealt with a range of interrelated issues, such as migration, consumption patterns, and sustainable economic development, the ICPD+5 negotiations focused very quickly on the "controversial" topics of reproductive and sexual rights, notably abortion.

Given this and the New York UN headquarters context—where developing countries had been feeling increasingly disempowered on economic issues—G-77 developing countries chose to speak with one voice as a way of obtaining further concessions on economic justice issues, such as structural adjustments and debt relief. Developing countries' growing frustrations regarding trade, debt, and development assistance, while genuine, provided convenient support to conservative forces seeking to beat back sexual and reproductive rights. This meant that Southern governments that held progressive views on issues such as adolescent health were effectively silenced, since they were part of the G-77 bloc, for much of the negotiation.

As a result, the ICPD+5 negotiations proved extremely difficult and were marked by renewed debates on previously agreed concepts such as "reproductive rights." But, after weeks of negotiations in New York in March and June 1999, Latin American leadership set a path forward. To begin with, the group of conservative Latin American Catholic countries was already smaller than in Beijing (it now basically consisted of Argentina, Nicaragua, and Guatemala). The eventual willingness of key Latin American countries, notably Peru and Brazil, to speak separately from the G-77 on abortion and adolescent health and take the lead on this issue led to important advances on unsafe abortion and to a renewed consensus on all other matters (UN 1999a).

A year later, a similar scenario unfolded at Beijing+5 in New York. While many issues were on the table as had been the case in Beijing, sexual and reproductive health and rights quickly became the dominant topic. The alliance of right-wing groups and conservative governments seized on abortion, "the family," sexual orientation, and adolescent sexuality as subjects on which they hoped to make gains. Once again, large numbers of North American right-wing activists were in attendance, particularly at the March 2000 Preparatory Committee meetings.

This time, Latin American and Caribbean countries worked as a progressive bloc from an earlier point in the negotiations. They showed that it was possible to support women's health and at the same time to take a firm stand on issues of economic justice (Sen and Correa 1999). ICPD and ICPD+5 were reaffirmed in the final document, and advances were made on violence against women and adolescent health programs (UN 2000b). But the strong North American right-wing presence and a reinvigorated unholy alliance of the Holy See and Islamists prevented further gains on sexual rights and sexual orientation. And the continued opposition of the Clinton administration to language critiquing neoliberalism and unfettered globalization also prevented agreement on those fronts.

The Plus 10s—Resisting the Bush Administration

Ten years after Cairo and Beijing, the UN would normally have been expected to call a major global conference on each agenda. While Cairo set a twenty-year program, and therefore did not technically require a new conference at the ten-year mark, there had been a major intergovernmental gathering on "population" every ten years since 1974. A major ICPD+10 conference in 2004 could, in theory at least, have been used to assess progress at the national and international level. Beijing's agenda was not time-bound, so there was arguably even more need for a large global meeting in 2005, both to review progress and to reach additional agreements. Some in the family planning and feminist communities argued that large intergovernmental conferences were essential to renew momentum and recommit resources, and bring in new actors and activists.

Instead, regional reviews were used, and the relevant functional commissions of the UN—the Commission on Population and Development (CPD) and the Commission on the Status of Women (CSW)—were tasked with adopting resolutions on the ten-year anniversaries. Why was this course chosen?

The Bush administration's extreme hostility to sexual and reproductive rights was a crucial factor in the decision by governments not to hold major conferences in 2004 and 2005. In this changed context, those women's health and rights advocates[3] who had been most closely associated with the negotiations in Cairo, Beijing, and at ICPD and Beijing+5 strongly opposed holding a global conference on reproductive health or women. Many progressive governments in the EU (notably the Netherlands and UK), as well as Canada and others, shared that view, as did the leadership of UNFPA. All had had a chance to evaluate the extreme tactics of the U.S. at the UN Special Session on Children in 2002, where an extremely arduous negotiation had ultimately yielded only a barebones reference to ICPD and Beijing (UNICEF 2003, para. 37.3). They had thus become persuaded that the risk of "reopening" ICPD and Beijing in large intergovernmental conferences was greater than the potential benefits.

At the same time, decisions to hold regional meetings to review implementation had already been made in some regional Economic and Social Commissions of the UN, notably the Economic and Social Commission for Asia and the Pacific. The choice having already been made in some respects, activists and progressive governments mobilized around the regional events, in the hope that these events could be more substantive than a global political meeting.

As planning progressed, not much coordination or overall strategy was in evidence. Different meeting formats were adopted by each Commission, with ICPD+10 and Beijing+10 effectively overlapping in some regions. ICPD+10 and Beijing+10 negotiations were held in Asia-Pacific, Latin America, and Africa, while Europe/North America and Middle East/West Asia preferred to hold expert meetings.

At the global level, the CPD held two sessions to reaffirm the ICPD and ICPD+5 agreements, in March 2004 and March 2005, while the CSW 2005 held its own in March 2005. For its part, the International Planned Parenthood Federation organized a Global NGO Round Table in London in August 2004, with a view to reenergizing action on ICPD implementation (Countdown 2015 2007).

As in Bangkok for ICPD+10, the Bush administration took an aggressive stance at all the meetings where they were present (the U.S. is not a member of the Economic Commission for Africa). Throughout the negotiations, U.S. positions mirrored those taken by the Holy See since Cairo on abortion and reproductive health. In particular, the U.S. repeatedly objected to the expression "reproductive health services" by claiming that this would force countries to offer abortion services. At times, the U.S. even adopted the Holy See's views on contraception, for example when it promoted natural family planning methods at the Bangkok ICPD+10 meeting, or stated—also in Bangkok—that the U.S. "supports innocent life from conception."[4]

But the regional meetings proved a different environment from that in New York. Progressive forces were able to defend all the key concepts in the ICPD Programme of Action, including reproductive health, sexual health, reproductive rights, and reproductive health services. Each ICPD+10 regional agreement reaffirmed the reproductive rights of adolescents, and the need to ensure adolescents' access to reproductive health information and services that are youth-friendly, age-appropriate, evidence-based, and respect adolescent confidentiality. For example, the Asia-Pacific Plan of Action calls for HIV prevention programs that include provision of male and female condoms and promotion of consistent condom use (UN Economic and Social Commission for Asia and the Pacific 2003, paras. H3 and H4).

In Bangkok, concepts the U.S. had insisted on were struck out or not included in the final text, including "abstinence as the healthiest choice" for adolescents; "minimizing the incidence of abortion"; "abortion-related mortality and morbidity" (as opposed to mortality resulting from unsafe abortion); "untimely" pregnancies (as opposed to unwanted); and "adoption" as an alternative to reliance on abortion. Mention of "cultural values and religious beliefs" without the corresponding reference to human rights in a paragraph on family planning was also removed—with the agreement of governments such as Iran and Malaysia, who usually insist on affirmation of "cultural values."

All three negotiated ICPD+10 documents (Asia-Pacific, Latin America and the Caribbean, and Africa) reaffirmed the ICPD Programme of Action and the ICPD+5 agreements.[5] In Asia and Latin America, the final documents even called on governments to address unsafe abortion as a major public health concern through appropriate strategies, explicitly referring to paragraphs of the ICPD Programme of Action (paras. 7.24 and 8.25) and ICPD+5 (para. 63) on unsafe abortion (UN Economic and Social Commission for Asia and the Pacific 2003, para. F6; UN Economic Commission for Latin America and the Caribbean 2004a, para. 4xi).

Similar patterns were in evidence at the Beijing+10 reviews. In Latin America and the Caribbean, the U.S. delegation, led by Ellen Sauerbrey, U.S. ambassador to the Commission on the Status of Women, mounted a sustained attack on sexual and reproductive rights at the June 2004 progress review in Mexico. Many Mexican right-wing groups never seen before at a UN meeting were in attendance. While the U.S. positions on reproductive health did not find much favor with the Latin American and Caribbean government delegates, the virulent and unexpected U.S. attack on Cuba's alleged promotion of sex tourism further united opposition to the U.S. The final result was not only reaffirmation of the Beijing Platform for Action, the Beijing+5 agreements, the ICPD Programme of Action, and the ICPD+5 agreements (UN Economic Commission for Latin America and the Caribbean 2004b),[6] but an explicit mention of "sexual rights," in spite of vehement objections by the U.S. and Holy See delegations.

6 xi) Review and implement legislation guaranteeing the responsible exercise of sexual and reproductive rights and non-discriminatory access to health services, including sexual and reproductive health, in accordance with the Lima Consensus.

The Asia-Pacific Beijing+10 meeting in September 2004 issued a report and brief communiqué that reaffirmed the Beijing Platform for Action and called for reproductive health services (UN Economic and Social Commission for Asia and the Pacific 2004), while the African meeting in October 2004 adopted a series of measures to accelerate implementation of Beijing and issued a renewed call for access to sexual and reproductive health care services and education as a condition of achieving the Millennium Development Goal (MDG) on HIV/AIDS and ICPD target on maternal mortality (UN Economic Commission for Africa 2004, para. 28).

As the regional reviews progressed, women's health activists increasingly focused their attention on the need to improve the MDG framework, in order to remedy the Millennium Summit omission of the ICPD goal of reproductive health for all by 2015. Key work was done through the UN Millennium Project—which had been tasked by UN secretary general Kofi Annan to develop strategies for implementing the MDGs—

to ensure that its Task Forces recognized the contribution of sexual and reproductive health services to the eradication of poverty.

The report of the UN Millennium Development Project issued on 17 January 2005, which reflected the excellent research and policy work done by the Project's Task Forces, did indeed include prominent recommendations on sexual and reproductive health and rights as essential elements of planning for development and poverty reduction (UN Millennium Project 2005a). The hope was that this technical work, coupled with negotiated language affirming the importance of ICPD to achieving the MDGs, would eventually lead to a revision of the MDG Road Map to include targets that measured sexual and reproductive health services. This seemed a tall order, not least of which because the climate for agreements of this kind had become even worse in New York. At the April 2003 session of the Commission on Population and Development, reaffirmation of ICPD and ICPD+5 had been achieved with some effort (and thanks to the remarkable negotiating skills of the representatives of Peru, Brazil, and the Netherlands) (UN Commission on Population and Development 2003).

A year later, at the March 2004 CPD session, the negotiation initially failed to reach a consensus on that basic subject. The U.S. and its allies made renewed use of issues such as homophobia, fear of family breakdown, and panic about pre- and extramarital sexual activity. U.S. strategists were particularly active in stoking these fears with conservative Islamists. Suddenly the reaffirmation of the ICPD Programme of Action was described as tantamount to support for same-sex marriage. Not coincidentally, the March 2004 CPD session took place at the same time as (and in an adjoining conference room to) a meeting of the UN Fifth Committee, where UN internal policy on granting benefits to same-sex partners of UN employees was being discussed. Meanwhile, at the UN Commission for Human Rights in Geneva, Brazil had presented a resolution against discrimination on the basis of sexual orientation. Sensing the impending damage and with hysteria mounting in the room, the chair of the CPD decided to adjourn the meeting without an agreement. It was only after a resumed CPD session in May 2004 that reaffirmation of ICPD and ICPD+5 was agreed upon. The U.S., Egypt, and Nicaragua reserved (UN Commission on Population and Development 2004).

Importantly, the 2004 CPD Resolution also insisted that the implementation of ICPD and ICPD+5 make an essential contribution to the development goals included in the Millennium Declaration. The CPD went further in 2005, to "*Emphasize* the importance of integrating the goal of universal access to reproductive health by 2015 set at the International Conference on Population and Development into strategies to attain the internationally agreed development goals, including those contained in the Millennium Declaration, in particular those related to improving maternal health, reducing infant and child mortality, promoting gender equality, combating HIV/AIDS, eradicating poverty, and achieving universal access to primary education" (UN Commission on Population and Development 2005). British and Dutch leadership were essential to this particular agreement.

Yet more hurdles were to be overcome. At its March 2005 session, the CSW sought to simply reaffirm the Beijing Platform for Action and Beijing+5 agreements. The chair of the CSW had prepared a one-page Political Declaration to that effect, in the hope of avoiding negotiations and the predictable debates on abortion and sexuality matters. This tactic was foiled by the U.S., which on the first day insisted on a negotiation and presented an amendment to the paragraph that would reaffirm Beijing and Beijing+5, "while reaffirming that they do not create any new international human rights, and that they do not include the right to abortion." The U.S. amendment caused much consternation and blocked discussions for a week. It was only after the U.S. was denounced by women's groups in the international press for seeking to overturn Beijing that the U.S. withdrew the first part of its amendment (on "no new rights"), and eventually the entire amendment. Regrettably, the chair of the CSW and some progressive government delegations felt compelled to state the obvious and reassure the U.S. that the Beijing Platform for Action was not a binding document and could not create new rights—thereby allowing the U.S. to claim to have obtained statements "clarifying the intent and purpose of Beijing" (UN Commission on the Status of Women 2005). Fortunately, the final resolution stated that implementation of the Beijing Platform for Action is essential to achieving the international development goals (2005).

This painstaking preparation work, and intense lobbying of UN diplomats over the summer of 2005 by women's groups, bore fruit at the UN World Summit in September 2005. There, heads of state committed themselves to

57 (*g*) Achieving universal access to reproductive health by 2015, as set out at the International Conference on Population and Development, integrating this goal in strategies to attain the internationally agreed development goals, including those contained in the Millennium Declaration, aimed at reducing maternal mortality, improving maternal health, reducing child mortality, promoting gender equality, combating HIV/AIDS and eradicating poverty. (UN 2005a)

Interestingly, the U.S. delegation, led by newly appointed U.S. ambassador John Bolton, did not take aim at this language, even as it sought to overturn and amend many of the other provisions of the draft outcome document. In preparation for the World Summit, women's rights advocates had sought to reinvigorate the links between economic and gender justice and established a broad coalition on all issues of interest to women. This coalition then supported other constituencies pushing for advances on the environment, overseas development assistance and debt relief, trade, disarmament, peace building, humanitarian assistance, and human rights. It was no comfort to women's rights groups that, while good new language on gender and reproductive health remained in the final text, no progress was possible on debt relief and fair trade, the environment, or disarmament.

In August 2006, Kofi Annan, in his progress report on the work of the UN, recommended the incorporation of the new commitments made at the 2005 World Summit into the existing MDG framework, including the establishment of a new target for universal access to reproductive health (UN 2006, para. 24). This recommendation was approved by the General Assembly in October 2006. The technical work to select the appropriate indicators for this new target has been undertaken by the Inter-Agency and Expert Group on Millennium Development Goal Indicators.

Reflections

Nearing the end of the Bush administration, activists can take pride in the fact that the ICPD and Beijing agreements have been preserved. Women's health advocates and progressive governments weathered the storm, and successfully pushed back attacks on sexual and reproductive health. Moreover, they were able to reinstate the ICPD goal of universal access to reproductive health by 2015 within the MDG framework, as a target, if not as a full-fledged goal.

Against the Bush administration's determined attempts to roll back the ICPD Programme of Action and the Beijing Platform for Action, resistance strategies proved most effective at the regional level. Committed implementers and technical experts demonstrated that they actually cared about the content of the agreements and understood the implications of words such as "services." This kind of experience was in short supply in New York, where negotiations remained difficult and acrimonious.

Resistance to the U.S. and its allies was achieved by significant mobilization of experienced feminist activists, and the initiation of new activists into negotiations as well as intensive work with progressive governments. In Asia-Pacific, India, China, Indonesia, Thailand, Turkey, and the Philippines played important roles in supporting Cairo and

Beijing. In Latin America, Brazil leading Mercosur (Argentina, Uruguay), Peru, and Bolivia were instrumental in preserving the agreements. Threats by the U.S. to withhold foreign or military assistance to try to force developing countries to acquiesce to its views were ultimately unsuccessful, but they caused much consternation and anxiety. Gita Sen aptly stated, "It cannot be forgotten that, for a small country, contradicting the Vatican is one thing and standing against the United States is entirely another thing" (Sen 2005a: 14).

It is also important to note that the UNFPA capacity to brief governments in-country, while slow to activate itself before the ICPD+10 Bangkok negotiations, proved extremely useful once in action. UNFPA was also able to produce good first drafts of negotiation documents and to advise governments on procedural matters during negotiations.

Notwithstanding the considerable energy expended to defend the conceptual and material gains heralded by the decade of ICPD and Beijing, little or no advances on sexual and reproductive rights were possible even at the regional level. Certainly there were no gains on the rest of the ICPD agenda (migration, consumption, trade, and macroeconomic policy). The regional meetings were nevertheless beneficial in other ways, as they saw the active participation of youth in negotiations and the inclusion of new activists. The U.S. positions proved so extreme that they served as a uniting factor at the regional level, even for conservative countries such as Iran.

For the activists and governments involved, there was no choice but to stand up and defend ICPD and Beijing. But devoting resources to these processes took away from national efforts that might have been more productive. The same "sexual and reproductive rights troops" have been called upon to advocate and lobby at the UN since the early 1990s, and some, if not all, are clearly exhausted and weary.

To conclude by way of prognostication, looking forward to a period of relative calm on the UN negotiation front, and in light of the Democratic-controlled U.S. Congress and Democratic presidency, where should reproductive health and rights advocates now focus?

First, we may well have to conclude that new, bolder agreements are not likely in the near future. There is little or no appetite for them at the intergovernment level. This much was clear at the 2005 UN World Summit. Not surprisingly, the UN High-Level Meeting on HIV in May 2006 did not generate significant new commitments. As the UN considers other reforms, including that of its gender architecture, more institutional energy appears to be directed toward structure and form, rather than advancing content (see Larson and Reich, this volume).

Activists may therefore consider returning to implementation matters.

The reproductive health community continues to be in disarray over the large sums of money going into HIV programming, to the detriment of integrated sexual and reproductive health services (see Gruskin, this volume). In many cases such as India, Ministries of Health are separating or consolidating HIV services from the rest of sexual and reproductive health, "National AIDS Councils" are flourishing, and health professionals are moving over.

Yet the continuing increase in HIV incidence among women and youth (girls particularly) in some areas of the world underlines the need for the reproductive health community to reach out to the HIV community to find a path to cooperation. Sexual and reproductive health services and maternal care remain an important point of access to health services for women and girls. More will need to be done to foster dialogue with health authorities, to secure investment for HIV prevention and care in sexual and reproduction health facilities. In that respect, it is surprising to realize that few reproductive health organizations have paid any attention to the Global Fund to Fight AIDS, TB, and Malaria—an organization that has disbursed over $3 billion for evidence-based health programs since its creation in 2002. Proposals for integrated services could be included into the overall national proposals put together by the Country Coordinating Mechanisms.

Moreover, rather than accede to its tendency to retrench into its specialized work and narrow its field of action, the reproductive health community needs to get reinvested in broader debates over macroeconomic policy and poverty eradication, as it was in Cairo. The MDG framework, for all the travails it put reproductive health activists through, made it clear that the connections between poverty, income inequality, and sexual and reproductive health need to be continually underscored. As noted by the Millennium Project Report on Sexual and Reproductive Health, "The record of incorporation of population dynamics and reproductive health into poverty reduction strategies to date is disappointing" (Bernstein and Juul Hansen 2006: 105). Much work has to be done to ensure that developing countries include a sexual and reproductive cost and benefit analysis in the course of their national development strategy exercises, and to persuade "poverty NGOs" to take sexual and reproductive health on board.

Finally, macroeconomic policies that stop greater investments by poor countries in health and other social sectors, thereby threatening already weak health systems, need to be challenged by the reproductive health community. In this respect, the Report of the UN Millennium Task Force on Maternal Mortality made clear that, without functioning health systems and a "health system response," maternal mortality and morbidity will not be eliminated (Freedman et al. 2005a). Sexual and reproductive health requires, by its very definition, a complex set of multisectoral interventions. The advocacy communities for reproductive health and for poverty reduction would achieve much more through joint and systematic effort. Without a systemic approach, the ambitious goals set in Cairo and Beijing will remain elusive.

Chapter 13
Situating Reproductive Health Within the Academy

Alaka Basu

If reproductive health is an academic field, what does its core curriculum, or even its core course look like? This chapter examines the potential for and the problems with designing an academic course on reproductive health. Such an examination is important because, while reproductive health may be a legitimate concern of academia in principle (and even that is debatable), it has not received serious attention as a field of study in practice, although ad hoc courses on reproductive health have become common in many institutions. In addition, quite apart from the substantive content of a course (or series of courses) on reproductive health, one needs to think about the potential audience for such courses—who are the students of reproductive health? Indeed, the content of pedagogy on reproductive health will crucially depend on the backgrounds and professional interests of the students to whom it is addressed.

As a point of departure, it is worth considering whether reproductive health is a legitimate field of pedagogical activity at all. Should attention be paid to the *teaching* (as opposed to the *training*) of the subject. Teaching here refers to imparting critical methods of analysis and research, while training refers primarily to imparting the technical ability to deal with the medical recognition and treatment of reproductive health problems. Especially given that the larger framework of the reproductive health paradigm is political rather than intellectual, are the immediate interests of reproductive health best served by biomedical training and the longer term interests best served by social activism rather than abstract research in the academy? These are not questions that were asked by the fledgling Cairo Programme of Action at the International Conference on Population and Development (ICPD) (UN

1995). But answers to these questions are necessary now that the reproductive health paradigm has become mainstreamed in our language, even if it still has a long way toward achievement.

Indeed, there is some concern that the abstract research of the academy and the institutionalization of reproductive health as one more field of study will add very little to the political agenda that originally energized the subject and may actually detract from this larger agenda for social change. This kind of criticism has been voiced more than once in recent times against the parallel field of women's studies. For example, in a scathing critique of the preoccupations of contemporary U.S. academic feminism developed in the course of a sharper critique of the iconic status of Judith Butler's work, Nussbaum (1999) lamented the retreat from effective political action and indeed the cynicism about the *possibilities* for effective political action that modern pedagogy in the subject transmits. That is, in Nussbaum's framework, not only are the theorizing and elaborating and nitpicking of contemporary theoretical women's studies divorced from the realities of poor women's lives, the field's self absorption leads it to promote an unwarranted pessimism about the original feminist project of social transformation itself. Add to this the demands of professional ladder-climbing through teaching and research lines in universities, and women's studies in the U.S. may as well be little more than yet another somewhat marginal academic discipline.

Yet one can think of the tension between political activism and academic theorizing cutting both ways. It is not surprising that Brown (1997) frames her critique of women's studies in reverse terms—her complaint is that women's studies in the academy is informed so exclusively by political considerations that it is bound to fail the academic tests of scientific and intellectual rigor that are supposed to define research and pedagogy. Brown therefore questions the value of institutionalizing feminism as a separate academic field built around a singular identity (gender). Instead, women's studies should incorporate gender and its complexities into academic disciplines that are distinguished by their modes of analysis (that is, by genre) rather than by the identity of the objects of their enquiry.

Carrying this analogy to the field of reproductive health pedagogy, one might ask, in the spirit of Nussbaum's critique, if the reproductive health paradigm is best suited to pragmatic action on the ground, rather than to abstract theorizing in the academy. This question is important both when directly addressed to dealing with the literal problems of reproductive health or more broadly addressed to the problems of discrimination and marginalization. In the spirit of Brown's critique, one may also reflect on whether reproductive health studies need to be housed in and across more than one kind of academic discipline, such as medicine, anthropology, demography, or political science.

Experience suggests that teaching and research in reproductive health, even though abstract and theoretical at times, is a legitimate activity because reproductive health is not simply a matter of treating infections and disabilities of the reproductive health system, however important these are. More often than not, such illnesses are outcomes of much larger socioeconomic and political arrangements that differentially influence the exposure to as well as the outcome of reproductive health problems. Even more pertinently, reproductive ill health, as we understand it today, is much more than infection. Good reproductive health implies both the absence of illness as well as the presence of a satisfactory and autonomously determined sexuality. By extension, as defined in the Programme of Action, the right to reproductive health implies the right to reproductive health services certainly, but it also implies the right to autonomy and choice in the matter of preventing poor reproductive health and ensuring good reproductive health. The issue becomes even more complicated when reproductive health is defined in its fullest sense to refer to matters of healthy sexuality and to control over the timing and numbers of births. All these are outside the purview of a generally trained medical or paramedical practitioner. They require an understanding of and commitment to issues of ethics and equality that are not taught in a standard medical program, and therefore they require continuous reflection on and research on these larger questions in ways that go well beyond the powerful but introductory discourse on the subject in the Programme of Action.

As for Brown's question to women's studies programs, Weigman (2005) responds with a question of her own. She asks why privileging academic disciplines like anthropology or sociology (into which Brown would like to introduce a strain of gender studies) is any more legitimate than privileging women's studies (or some form of identity studies in general), in which the methods of sociology and anthropology are then incorporated. Brown's criticism is less relevant to reproductive health because it has not (or at least not as yet) sought independent disciplinary status for itself. Indeed, the very nature of reproductive health pedagogy will be heavily influenced by its parent department or institution.

Who then will we be teaching when we design our courses on reproductive health? And equally important, to whom *should* we be teaching reproductive health? And *where* will these courses be taught, both in terms of institutions as well as geographical location? Given that reproductive health is not a formal discipline of study and that, more often than not, it is a subject in which any teaching will have to be tightly connected to policy, field action, and field activism, the *who, where,* and *why* questions will have important bearings on the *what* and *how* of reproductive health pedagogy.

The possibilities are daunting. Students taking a course in reproductive health may be undergraduates or master's or doctoral candidates, may be based in schools of public health or in social science departments of universities, may be located in the Western world or in a variety of Third World settings. Indeed, they may not be students in the formal sense at all—they might well be policy makers, health workers, or administrators of nongovernmental health organizations, who need to be introduced, or reintroduced, to the possibilities for improvements in reproductive health or the possibilities for activism around reproductive health matters.

Depending on the nature of the above scenarios, a basic course in reproductive health could take one of three dominant forms. Dominant in the sense that while the primary focus in each case will be on one of the forms discussed below, each kind of course will also draw more or less heavily on the methods and materials of the other two. Before examining these three potential perspectives in the teaching of reproductive health, it is useful to reflect on some important topics that *any* perspective on reproductive health pedagogy should include.

The first perspective has to do with semantics. Given the highly politicized nature of the field and given the disrespect shown for language in most political discourses, a careful student of the central questions in reproductive health needs a sharp ear. There is a gulf of difference that separates the term reproductive health as used by a health activist compared to the same word bandied by a population scientist (whose allegiance to population control has not been fully shaken off), or its use by a religious conservative who coopts the language of reproductive health to stress the *health* (breast cancer, for example) consequences for women of abortions (see, e.g., Coalition on Abortion/Breast Cancer 2006).

The student of reproductive health also needs a sharp eye. Definitions and meanings of popular terms are fluid and political and a reading of the literature on matters related to reproductive health requires an ability to seek exact definitions, to search out footnotes, and to examine author credentials. Not because these credentials will expose dishonesty or plagiarism. Rather prior beliefs and agendas greatly influence the meaning imputed to words and phrases even when the language of discourse is ostensibly a common one. This careful attention to language (and to something as crucial but routinely ignored as footnotes) is analogous to efforts to teach students in sociology to "read" statistical tables; less important are the techniques of analysis used. There must be, however, critical attention to definitions and in particular what the units of measurement refer to, what the denominators are, and what has been excluded.

A good course in reproductive health, in whatever home department and addressed to whatever constituency, should pay much attention to the meanings of ostensibly simple words. This exercise is particularly fraught as more comprehensive definitions of reproductive health now include things like sexuality and sexual rights, as distinct from reproduction and reproductive rights. Moreover, the master-narrative of sexuality (heterosexual marital sex), for example, is so entrenched that the political consequences of support for sexual rights tends to be conservative rather than liberational. In other words, when sexual rights are appropriated by authority (or even by an unthinking public), most of the radical language of the reproductive health discourse is muted and adumbrated.

Second, reproductive health pedagogy, like pedagogy in women's studies, cannot escape at least a partial .empirical and experiential framework. That is, abstract theory cannot be the beginning and end of the subject. The topics included in reproductive health are too close to home for teachers and students. Using this closeness to reflect on real life experiences in the classroom can only enrich the subject. Much of the pedagogical material will strike a chord in many minds, especially in multicultural classrooms. Students should be encouraged to include in dialogue the knowledge gained from personal experience or from the experience of others—the latter either directly or more tangentially, including through literature and travel.

Finally, any teaching on reproductive health must recognize the importance of diversity of the reproductive health experience. Just as biology is not destiny for women as a whole, *within* women too, the commonality of biology must not be allowed to hide the wide variations. There is diversity among women with regard to the problems of reproductive health and access to good reproductive health that exist across world regions (Olatunbosun and Edouard 1997), as well as between different groups of women within individual regions. This theme of the differences in the female experience in general (that is, not in the context of reproductive health per se) has already occupied large amounts of space in women's studies. Not only are there a First World and a Third World that differ in radical ways as far as women are concerned (see among the numerous studies, Mohanty 1988), but even within the developed world, the middle-class white female experience is not at all representative of either the reality or the normative standards of women's lives (once again, in the large literature, see Mohanty 2002; hooks 1981). Moreover, it is not enough to acknowledge differences in experience. It is also important to acknowledge and sometimes (but not always, one cannot carry cultural relativism too far, especially on questions of something as basic as the right to good health in general and good reproductive health in particular) accommodate differences in desired outcomes in reproductive health, even on matters as apparently universal as the need for sexual relations.

There are many other less central commonalities in the three kinds of perspectives in reproductive health pedagogy. These perspectives expand in scope to move from reproductive health as largely a problem of public health to look at reproductive health as a more comprehensive aspect of population issues, and finally to reproductive health as a symbol of even larger matters of equity and discrimination and justice.

Reproductive Health as "Reproductive Health"

A course designed from this perspective would focus on the clinical components of reproductive health and the medical solutions (both clinical and public health related) to these problems. Such an approach is not something to be dismissed lightly. As we know from several studies, there is a real and large reproductive health problem in women in all parts of the world. Whatever its deeper sociocultural and political origins, there is no doubt that this problem causes much physical and emotional distress at the individual level and has important implications for productivity and welfare at the societal level. Therefore, even simply identifying, diagnosing, and treating common reproductive health problems is something that a good course on public health must give priority to teaching.

More than a decade after ICPD, it is disappointing that reproductive health pedagogy is not commonplace in this basic form even in schools of medicine and public health. Indeed, given that many reproductive health issues are indeed *health* issues, it is surprising that except for the Commonwealth Medical Association, no representatives of associations of medical educators or medical practitioners attended either ICPD in 1994 or ICPD+5 (Haslegrave and Olatunbosun 2003). The recognition that reproductive health is something separate from and in addition to obstetrics and gynecology does not seem to have translated into much curriculum design for the teaching of reproductive health to medical or paramedical practitioners. The training of paramedical personnel in reproductive health is even more crucial in this because they are often the first and often the only contact that women in poor countries have with the medical system.

A good basic text that one might use for designing such a course on reproductive health as a medical and management subject might be the report prepared by the National Research Council (NRC) (1997). It would need much supplementation, of course, with later research on more precise measurements and definitions of the components of reproductive health that allow comparisons across regions, as well as provide tools to monitor and evaluate interventions (see Fortney 1995). More conceptual frameworks that place reproductive health in its larger socioeconomic context, along the lines of Mosley and Chen's 1984 framework for understanding the determinants of child mortality, would also need to be developed and taught. A background text like the NRC report would also allow the instructor to develop ideas on larger operational matters as well, to include questions about the relationship between services for reproductive health and those for health in general, the role of clinical versus community based services, the most cost-effective ways to provide services for reproductive health, and so on.

And here it should be mentioned that an important source of information on all these matters is the large and often meticulous family planning literature of the pre-Cairo period. There is no need to throw the baby out with the bathwater. Many of these very questions have already been debated (sometimes ad nauseum) in the context of providing family planning services to otherwise underserved populations; many of the lessons from this research and analysis are relatively easily extrapolated to apply to the post-Cairo paradigm. A good course in reproductive health would be conscious of the potential contributions of this older literature even while it searches for new ways of addressing the reproductive health problem.

At the same time, reproductive health problems and solutions are not merely matters of medical or even traditional public health concern. A minimum amount of supplementation of the basic material in the NRC volume is essential. Important sociocultural questions to do with norms and beliefs about and constraints on the acknowledgment of reproductive health, the ability to seek treatment, and the knowledge and space to follow treatment procedures need to be covered in a course that is serious about reducing the physical burden of reproductive disease. Obviously, this would by no means be solely a course in biomedicine.

Two examples are illustrative of how a good public health course on reproductive health would take sociocultural and larger political factors into account. The first concerns domestic and sexual violence as a part of reproductive health. If violence is a problem of reproductive health (and most would agree that it is), a good reproductive health course, even one that is aimed primarily at health workers, must transmit not merely the treatment of the physical outcomes of such violence, but the methods of preventing it in the first place. These methods are hardly in the same class as the immunizations that protect child health. At the very least, they require debriefing health professionals so that they can step back from their own cultural assumptions about and tendency to implicitly condone such violence (and even experience it themselves, as did the nurses in rural South Africa described in Kim and Motsei 2002).

A second example relates to what reproductive health policy must do about the vexing question of female genital circumcision (FGC); calling it female genital *mutilation* is already taking an aggressive political stand on the matter that may well be ineffective given that the subject matter has more nuances than the international movement against FGC is sometimes willing to concede. In particular, students would need to reflect on the relative virtues of zero-tolerance versus harm-reduction strategies in this case (see, e.g., Shell-Duncan 2001). The answers are far from clear in either direction. Local circumstances must certainly be invoked in deciding if national policy must be pressured to clamp down completely on all forms of FGC (and thereby very likely drive them underground) or create an alternative ritual (a light nick with a sterile needle to draw a drop of blood, for example).

Even if the safety and relative superficiality of the procedure are ensured, one may of course nevertheless object to the very idea of FGC as a patriarchal imposition and as an invasion of bodily integrity. Alternatively, one may now work toward gradually reducing its significance to a cultural symbol with no real larger subtext. In any case, invoking a rights approach to eliminating FGC may be more useful than focusing on health consequences, given the limited data we have (see Snow 2001) on short or long term reproductive morbidity of the different degrees of FGC. But there are no easy answers to these questions and a good course would not seek them. Instead students would be encouraged to debate the possibilities and to enlighten themselves with the universal as well as local ethics of these practices: how can or cannot they be reconciled with larger questions of autonomy and bodily integrity; what about girls and women who *choose* to undergo a circumcision; what does choice mean in their circumstances; how may one influence this so-called choice?

Reproductive Health as a Paradigm

Reproductive health pedagogy centered on the reproductive health paradigm that came out of ICPD is what is best suited to teaching in the traditional departments of demography. Here the focus on reproductive health would go beyond the physical parameters of reproductive and reproductive tract problems. It would deliberate about an alternative way to describe the "population problem" that has formed the basis of most studies of population in the developing world historically and is today also (albeit in different form, the population problem here being low fertility) a central question in population studies of the developed world. The focus here would be on an approach that looks at the problem of population as an issue of reproductive health, with the client audiences consisting of individuals with reproductive health related needs rather than nations with too many or too few people. However, underlying this approach are politically correct, but far from proven, assumptions that taking care of reproductive health will also take care of the larger macro-population questions of fertility (high or low) and mortality. An honest reproductive health course would critically examine some of these assumptions, with a stated goal of promoting good reproductive health in its own right rather than for instrumental reasons to do with national needs (see Basu 1997).

Given that we are talking here of teaching and not the political advocacy that was necessary to get reproductive health on the agenda in 1994, a good course on reproductive health for students of demography and population studies (as well as for those in gender studies and public health) would in fact go beyond the old reproductive health versus population antagonism to make peace with the international population movement. While the population paradigm may have become disreputable (at least in some quarters) after ICPD, so too the reproductive health paradigm is contentious in some circles. Interestingly, it is not the old population control lobbies that present the greatest challenge to the reproductive health paradigm; instead both the reproductive health paradigm and the population paradigms are jointly under assault by powerful conservative, right wing forces, especially those with a religious agenda, in many parts of the world. This is primarily because, even if for different reasons, both the reproductive health and the population perspectives depend on easy access to contraception as well as access to abortion when such contraception fails.

Indeed, it is not necessary for the population and reproductive health movements to stand in opposition to one another, even if the original relations between them were set up as adversarial.[1] There is enough common ground once both sides acknowledge that reproductive control is a matter of women's rights and that the timing and number of births is something that women not only need to be able to decide for themselves, they also have the right to claim the services to operationalize these decisions. This is not as strange a conjoining of agendas as it might sound at first blush. The population control lobby is not, in principle, only about numbers even if its arguments did often deteriorate into a focus on numbers of births, births averted, and the larger national economic and social consequences of these matters. An important section of the international and local population movement was deeply concerned with the individual benefits of access to information about and

services for birth control as well. The old maternal and child health programs for example were predicated on the belief that fewer and well-
spaced births were good for the health of women and children and that
withholding these rights from women was in fact a way of entrenching
existing patriarchies even more solidly (Basu 1996).

It is these commonalities that will have to be stressed as the pre- and
post-Cairo population and reproductive health lobbies jointly take on
the might of the anti-women and anti-reproductive health movement
that is gathering force in public life, especially in the United States, the
country with the single largest influence on population and reproductive health policies worldwide. This common platform would stress also
that the losers are once again going to be the most marginalized
women—whether regionally or within individual regions and countries.
The better off will always find the contraception and abortion services
they need, at least for the moment. "For the moment" because eventually "all" women will pay for this steady erosion of reproductive health
rights by the power and money of the neoconservative movement.

Reproductive health pedagogy with this kind of focus on both the differences and the commonalities between the old population and the
new reproductive health paradigms would also pay serious attention to
the role of the state. While population control policies were certainly
state sponsored and state controlled in most parts of the world, now that
the language of individual rights and individual choice has entered the
subject, governments have become far too willing to leave the actual access of services for contraception and reproductive health in general to
individual initiative. The timing of the reproductive health paradigm
has made this abdication of responsibility easier. All over the developing
world, neoliberal economic policies and the pressures exerted by international institutions have made health (and education) services one of
the first casualties; and in fact a supposed concurrence with the reproductive health paradigm has facilitated state withdrawal from family
planning and reproductive health activities in the name of respecting
women's choices. In India, for example, the giving up of the infamous
target approach to population policy now often means the absence of information on or services for birth control by government health agencies even when women seek such services. So it is the private sector or
else the nongovernmental sector that steps in to fill this gap—both
these sectors have immense difficulties with outreach, motive, and resources. No pragmatic pedagogy on reproductive health can leave out a
critical reexamination of the role of the state.

The study of the state as actor assumes particular importance in the
framework of reproductive health and reproductive *rights*. Hoarsely asserting rights is little more than a parlor game if there is no entity

responsible for ensuring these rights and no mechanism for holding such an entity accountable. In most cases, this entity will have to be the state, whether through its executive, legislative, or public services function. A good course on reproductive health would cover some of the debates on the state and civil society in the context of human rights in general and reproductive health rights in particular.

Any course on reproductive health rights would not be complete without a consideration of the responsibilities that must accompany the entitlement of rights. That is, in what ways are individuals who claim rights also to accept responsibility in the exercise of these rights? What kinds of questions of individual and collective rights and responsibility are implied in the reproductive health rights paradigm? Even when there is no physical coercion by an outside agency, how do education and information on the meaning of responsible rights tread the fine line between genuine education and psychological manipulation? What is the meaning of informed choice? These are all philosophical issues at one level, but their understanding and interpretation have important real world consequences. They cannot be left out of the academic discourse on grounds of unnecessary abstractness.

Reproductive Health as Metaphor

This is the most ambitious (and perhaps most contentious) approach to reproductive health pedagogy. The central premise of this approach is that reproductive health is best conceived as a metaphor for the problems of marginalization and exclusion that exist for all kinds of subgroups in a population, not just for women. Thus gender and reproductive health issues would serve as an entry point to develop theoretical and empirical methodologies to examine socioeconomic and political inequalities in general. Academic methods and arguments from feminist and gender studies would be stretched to apply to studies of other kinds of marginalization instead of focusing exclusively on women.

In particular, a course like this would pay much more attention to the reproductive health concerns of poor men (see, for instance, Basu 1996). The language of the reproductive health discourse is still too fixated on the notion of either men's *responsibilities* for or, more generously, men's *involvement* in women's reproductive health improvements. What is lacking is an interest in men's reproductive health as an end in itself, for men's own welfare. Referred to here are not only the physical problems of male reproductive health—the infertility or the enlarged prostates or the erectile dysfunction, but also the larger questions of male sexual identity and male sexuality. The cultural as well as political frameworks for understanding these subjects and the expectations they generate are as limiting and strangulating for men as they are for women. They are particularly strangulating for poor men in all parts of the world, where the emasculation caused by poor physical reproductive health is strengthened by extra-domestic economic and political structures over which they have little control. That is, reproductive and sexual rights and choices need to be stressed for men as much as they are for women, even if the current domestic imbalance gives men an edge.

In addition to serving as an entry point to study marginalization in general, the field of reproductive health research, as it has currently developed, also has much to offer to surrounding disciplines. While the methods and theories of, say, women's studies or anthropology or general public health can inform research and teaching on reproductive health, reproductive health studies also has an independent stream of research techniques that can strengthen these other fields. For example, feminist research and action related to side effects and abuses of contraceptive methods can be very usefully extended to developing commercial research protocols and marketing by the pharmaceutical industry in general (Correa 1997). This is especially true with countries like India now making it much easier for multinational pharmaceutical companies to conduct clinical trials (see Nundy, Chir, and Gulhati 2005). This strand of research in reproductive health can be introduced into pedagogy in a variety of social and economic development fields.

Similarly, studies on differentials in reproductive health and especially on the medical "ills of marginality" (to borrow from Ecks and Sax 2005, a special issue of *Anthropology and Medicine*), provide interesting hints to probe the nonmedical ills of marginalized groups as well. Indeed, in many ways, it appears that analytical research on something as real-life and policy sensitive as reproductive health can feed into new paradigms of theoretical and abstract research in a variety of disciplines. It would be doing a great disservice to the field to position the study of reproductive health as merely something to do with schools of public health and largely concerned with design of effective health policy, however important this singular motivation is.

The ICPD Programme of Action has virtually nothing to say explicitly on pedagogy as an integral part of furthering the reproductive health paradigm. But there are implicit references to it in at least two contexts: in the emphasis on training staff to address the problems of reproductive health, and in the demand for more data collection and research on the biomedical as well as the social and political underpinnings of reproductive health. The question of training immediately implies some form of education, even if the language in Chapter 13 of the ICPD Report seems to stress more the need for technocratic training to provide and manage reproductive health services. In fact, this chapter does use the word education, not in the context of education on reproductive health but rather as a call for education and productive advancement of women to overcome general gender biases in education.

The need for trained personnel is also implied in ICPD's call for better reproductive health information for vulnerable groups, especially adolescents. Presumably the disseminators of such information will first need to be educated on reproductive health matters themselves.

Chapter 12, on data collection, analysis, and research, certainly implies research *capacity*, something that cannot be conjured up without at least some prior education (as opposed to medical training) in both empirical techniques and more substantive interpretative analytical methods. In this sense, it is not surprising that the report in paragraph 12.6 calls for "training programs in statistics, demography, and population and development studies" to be "designed and implemented at the national and regional levels." The word "training" here is certainly misused—it is pedagogy rather than training that is required for the research expertise that the report seeks. But what is more surprising is that this paragraph does not mention reproductive health at all; it must be that at the time of the drafting of this report, it was still too early to reflect on the intellectual project of producing a body of specialists educated in reproductive health in the broadest sense.

What is also surprising is the finding that this lack of emphasis on pedagogy in ICPD has not led to more widespread post-ICPD reflections on and suggestions for developing reproductive health as an academic field. As discussed in an earlier section, the little there is on this subject refers to reproductive health education in the medical school curriculum. One is therefore forced to wonder whether the neglect of reproductive health as an explicit goal in the Millennium Development Goals is only consistent with this lack of attention *within* the field of reproductive health to creating a systematic body of evidence-based knowledge on the subject. The best form such a systematic body of knowledge would take would arguably be a pedagogical endeavor that describes, analyzes, and criticizes the field in the best traditions of academic scholarship. Really to take the subject of reproductive health seriously, one needs a professionalization of the field in terms of both trained practitioners on the ground and educated researchers who carry the intellectual understanding of the field forward.

This chapter has expressed some preliminary thoughts. It has focused on some philosophical and conceptual possibilities; it has not gone into the nitty-gritties of course *content* and teaching *methodology*. Because this is such a new field, for the moment, it would be expected that such content and methodology issues in reproductive health pedagogy would be as variable as the individuals teaching such courses and the students taking them. But these initial attempts to develop a larger framework for such pedagogy can be seen as a plea for greater collaboration and consultation among the teachers, funders, academic departments, and university administrators who all have a stake in developing programs of teaching in an area that is immediately consequential for all people's lives.

Chapter 14
The Political Limits of the United Nations in Advancing Reproductive Health and Rights

Heidi Larson and Michael R. Reich

The United Nations has played a critical role in both advancing and con-
straining reproductive health and rights around the world in the late
twentieth and early twenty-first centuries. These dual effects are a result
of the nature of the United Nations—the politics of its member states,
on the one hand, and the politics of its many institutions, on the other—
as the UN has sought to address substantive issues related to reproductive health and rights. This chapter considers the limitations of the UN
system for promoting reproductive health and rights in light of the
UN reform agenda and suggests future avenues of engagement with the
UN for advocates and practitioners.

The UN engagement with reproductive health and rights reflects the
broader debate over the effectiveness of the United Nations. This debate
has a long history, going back to the founding of the UN, and indeed
back to the earlier efforts at creating the League of Nations. But the debate became particularly heated in the late twentieth century, following
the UN fiftieth anniversary in 1995. Even enthusiastic supporters of the
UN agreed that the organization needed a period of reflection, reform,
and reinvigoration. For example, Bruce Russett, a Yale political scientist
who has written extensively on this issue, identified ten "balances" for assessing different UN reform proposals (Russett 1996). Meanwhile, critics of the UN have attacked the legacy of former secretary general Kofi
Annan as one of "monumental failure" and called the UN an institution
filled with "mismanagement, corruption, and anti-Americanism" and
dominated by "scandal, division, and failure" (Gardiner 2006).

In March 2005, the secretary general issued his own report that re-
stated the core mission of the United Nations as freedom from want,

freedom from fear, and freedom to live in dignity. The report also proposed a series of strategies for strengthening the institution, seeking to identify "reforms that are within reach—reforms that are actionable if we can garner the necessary political will" (UN 2005b: 3).

In an effort to catalyze these reforms, Kofi Annan appointed a High Level Panel on UN System-Wide Coherence in early 2006 to look at coordination across UN agencies in areas of development, humanitarian assistance, and the environment. The final report of the Panel, titled *Delivering as One*, proposes a number of bold recommendations which, among the various reform initiatives, probably have the most relevance to how the UN will continue to address reproductive health. Among the various recommendations, the report calls for the establishment of "a dynamic UN entity focused on gender equality and women's empowerment." It notes, "While the UN remains a key actor in supporting countries to achieve gender equality and women's empowerment, there is a strong sense that the UN system's contribution has been incoherent, under-resourced and fragmented" (UN 2006b: 34-35).

Although the High Level Panel Report was prepared under former secretary general Kofi Annan just before the end of his term, the demand for UN reform became compelling enough to remain high on the agenda of incoming secretary general Ban Ki-moon. Soon after his appointment in early 2007, the new secretary general endorsed the principles of the High Level Panel report, including acknowledging the need to "strengthen the Organization's gender architecture":

I am in full agreement with the Panel's assessment of the need to consolidate and strengthen several current structures in a dynamic United Nations entity focused on gender equality and women's empowerment. (UN 2007, para. 17)

Current UN reform trends are aiming to move toward comprehensive development frameworks at the country level, with country "ownership" and "One UN" (program) with "One Leader" overseeing and representing the various UN agencies such as UNFPA, UNICEF, UNDP, and UN-AIDS. Other reform proposals at the global level include one central fund and one Sustainable Development Board that would oversee the combined work of the agencies and move them toward a common development agenda.

What, though, are the implications of these reforms for politically sensitive issues such as reproductive and sexual health and rights? Without a separate, distinct advocate and fund for reproductive health, will the critical issues raised in the ICPD agenda be in jeopardy? Will donors who do not want to invest in reproductive health concerns cut their overall contribution to the proposed development fund? Most importantly, who will decide, in an overall development budget, the proportion of funds allocated to reproductive and sexual health concerns? Will some of the UN policy advocacy for reproductive health be lost?

This chapter examines key expectations of the UN following the ICPD, critical constraints to the UN's capacity to address reproductive health and rights, and finally implications of the current UN reform efforts for reproductive health and rights. Three key expectations of the UN following ICPD, as outlined in the Programme of Action, were: first, to advocate widely for the ICPD program; second, to improve action on reproductive health across the UN agencies and improve the coherence of these actions; and finally, to review and monitor progress against the ICPD agenda.

At the same time, three particular constraints limited the capacity of the UN to make real advances toward these expectations. First is that international agreements, goals, and conventions developed under the auspices of the United Nations are largely driven by the geopolitical context outside the UN, reflected in evolving trends in development and population debates. In other words, the UN does not have a separate voice. Rather, its voice is defined by the views and actions of its member states and increasingly by non-state actors. The second key constraint is that, while the UN fosters the development of new international commitments and conventions, those who sign on to the key principles of these international agreements also have an option—through "reservations"—to opt out of specific commitments that conflict with their cultural, ethical, or religious mores or political concerns. Consensus is achieved by allowing assenters to avoid specific words, concepts, even chapters. The consensus around international agreements, then, is more around principles and aspirations, with the implementation being highly dependent on the specific national setting. Finally, a third constraint is the influence of the national policies and politics of some individual member states, especially the United States, who seek to shape UN actions and policies through the use of economic and political pressure.

Expectations of the UN After ICPD

In order to take a critical look at what the UN has delivered against the ICPD goals, it is important to look back at what was expected of the UN. While there have been a range of expectations expressed by countries as well as by activists and other non-state players, the ICPD Programme of Action (UN 1995) outlines explicit roles for the UN in the follow-up to ICPD. It calls for a proactive role for the UN in three key areas: advocacy (para. 16.8); implementation of the Programme of Action (paras. 16.16,

16.29); and monitoring of the implementation (para. 16.23). Across these three areas, the Programme of Action also expects the UN to look inward at its own effectiveness and coherence, echoing other calls for a reformed UN, this time through the lens of reproductive health.

In the area of advocacy, the Programme of Action looks to the UN along with governments and NGOs to promote the ICPD Agenda and engage widespread public support:

Governments, organizations of the United Nations system and major groups, in particular non-governmental organizations, should give the widest possible dissemination to the Programme of Action and should seek public support for the goals, objectives and actions of the Programme of Action. (para. 16.8)

The Programme of Action also expects the UN to support implementation of the Programme by providing support to countries, through national and regional mechanisms, but also by looking internally at strengthening the capacities of various UN agencies to provide appropriate follow-up to the Conference:

All specialized agencies and related organizations of the United Nations system are invited to strengthen and adjust their activities, programmes and medium-term strategies, as appropriate, to take into account the follow-up to the Conference. Relevant governing bodies should review their policies, programmes, budgets and activities in this regard. (para. 16.29)

The language of the Programme of Action reads very much like the language used in the UN reform process. The calls for "a more coherent reporting system" (para. 16.24), for "improving efficiency and effectiveness of the current United Nations structures and machinery" (para. 16.25b), and for a clear recognition of "the division of labor between the [UN] bodies concerned" (para. 16.25c) resonate strongly as objectives of the UN reform process.

Last, in sections on follow-up to the Conference, the Programme of Action looks to the UN Economic and Social Council and the General Assembly to provide "system-wide coordination" of monitoring implementation of the Programme of Action. In other words, across the various UN bodies and the wide range of actions called for in the Programme of Action, the UN should ensure that there is a coordinated monitoring effort:

The Economic and Social Council . . . should assist the General Assembly in promoting an integrated approach and in providing system-wide coordination and guidance in the monitoring of the implementation of the present Programme of Action and in making recommendations in this regard. Appropriate steps should be taken to request regular reports from the specialized agencies. (para 16.23.)

A number of UN entities are involved in addressing the expectations in the follow-up to the ICPD. While the UN Commission on Population and Development[1] is officially responsible for conducting annual reviews on the progress on the ICPD Programme of Action, UNFPA is the lead advocate across the UN system and also plays a role in reporting progress against ICPD goals through its State of World Population Report[2] as well as through other ICPD-specific documents (UN 1999b; UNFPA 2005c,d).

At the country level, UNFPA is the independent voice to speak out and influence policy on sensitive issues around reproductive and sexual health. Internationally, it is one of the few UN bodies—along with UNAIDS and WHO—still willing to talk about condoms and sexual health despite increasing conservatism among some member states.

Other UN bodies, such as WHO, UNAIDS, UNICEF, and the World Bank, contribute in different ways toward the ICPD agenda, some more explicitly than others. UNAIDS, for example, is a unique UN entity called the Joint United Nations Programme on HIV/AIDS, established one year after ICPD, which works with ten UN bodies to ensure coherence in the global AIDS response. In the area of sexual and reproductive health, UNAIDS produces technical guidelines and policy guidance as sexual and reproductive health issues pertain to HIV/AIDS. UNICEF, on the other hand, has focused its programmatic response to ICPD more explicitly on the promotion of women's health and safe motherhood (UNICEF 1998). Overall, the different UN bodies provide technical and training support, policy advocacy, monitoring and evaluation and to a certain extent, funding, with the World Bank carrying the most weight in the area of funding.

The World Health Organization (WHO) has been a key partner with UNFPA in addressing the ICPD Programme of Action. As the UN specialized agency on health, WHO is the lead agency in setting international standards and norms, establishing global indicators against which to measure progress, and providing technical advice and training guidelines to countries. In 2001, WHO published a set of reproductive health indicators to monitor global progress:

During the international conferences of the early and mid-90s, such as ICPD, countries endorsed a number of global goals and targets in the broad areas of sexual and reproductive health. A proliferation of indicators to monitor these goals ensued, proposed by a range of agencies. In 1996, WHO took the lead in organizing an interagency technical process that led to the selection of 15 global indicators for monitoring reproductive health targets. (WHO 2001: 1)

And, in 2004, ten years after the Cairo Conference, WHO launched its first reproductive health strategy, which was adopted at the 57th World Health Assembly (WHO 2004b). Although the UN and its various agencies have delivered concrete advances on some key ICPD expectations, particularly in providing technical and policy guidance and monitoring support (as discussed above), the extent to which it has been able to advance implementation of the ICPD agenda has been limited by a number of constraints, many of which are political.

The UN as Geopolitical Mirror

The history of how reproductive health and rights have been addressed by and through the UN reflects broader trends in the external, geopolitical environment. As one commentator stated in a panel reflecting on ICPD+10 in 2004, "The Programme of Action reflects what the political conditions allowed us [the reproductive health community] to achieve at that point. . . . The documents went as far as they could at the time they were created, and they are better than the political reality today" (Correa et al. 2005: 110). But who creates the "political reality"? It is in part created by many of the same member states that sign onto these international development goals and commitments.

In 1993, Lynn Freedman and Stephen Isaacs published an article that captured the historic shifts in the development and population debate in the decades before ICPD. The article also reveals the role of UN agencies as conveners of conferences that reflect political trends at particular historical moments:

The first comprehensive statement of human rights, the Universal Declaration of Human Rights, adopted by the UN General Assembly in 1948, failed to mention reproductive rights at all. . . . In 1974 . . . at the World Population Conference in Bucharest, Romania . . . the western-oriented population movement was confronted by a third world challenge. . . . [T]he priority given by western governments controlling population growth appeared more like a plot to ensure their own primacy in the international order. . . .

When the next international population conference was held a decade later in Mexico City, the world had changed dramatically yet again. . . . Rather than urging developing countries to take strong measures to curb population growth, as the U.S. had regularly done in the past, their representatives of the Reagan administration now declared that "population growth is, of itself, a neutral phenomenon." . . . Something else was operating in Mexico City. That "something else" had ominous implications for reproductive autonomy. The "right-to-life" movement had expanded internationally. (Freedman and Isaacs 1993: 20–22)

One of the biggest challenges to the ICPD agenda today has its roots a decade before ICPD existed. The "Mexico City Policy," or the "Global Gag Rule," was announced by President Reagan in 1984 and stated that

U.S. foreign assistance would not be given to any organizations that provided any information about abortions or made abortion services available. In 1993, one year before the Cairo Conference, the political environment had changed, and President Bill Clinton rescinded the Mexico City Policy. The International Conference on Population and Development in 1994 thus reflected a time of change and opportunity. But that window of opportunity was not long open. In January 2001, President George W. Bush fully reinstated the Mexico City Policy immediately after his inauguration.

Today, over 10 years after the Cairo conference was held, the "right-to-life" movement, growing neo-conservatism, and Islamic fundamentalism have come together to challenge the reproductive health and rights agenda in even bigger ways. Just over five years after ICPD, at the 2000 Millennium Summit, the decision to exclude a reproductive health goal in the Millennium Development Goals signaled a retreat from key parts of the ICPD agenda and reflected the limits of the UN consensus approach. A few scholars have noted that

The exclusion of the reproductive health goal from the MDGs was a matter of political expediency. . . . Opponents of the goal had characterized it as promoting abortion and undermining family values by calling for sex education for adolescents. They threatened to block agreement on all the MDGs unless the reproductive health goal was eliminated. United Nations officials were under enormous pressure to have the Millennium Summit participants reach a consensus on the goals and relented to the demand of the few countries involved in the threat. (Campbell et al. 2006: 5)

In many ways the ICPD agenda was a precursor to the MDGs (UNFPA 2004b). The Programme of Action situated reproductive health and rights squarely in broader development concerns, such as sustained economic growth, gender equality, health, and education. The MDGs, though, focused on broader development concerns, dropped reproductive health due to its political sensitivity. Five years later at the 2005 World Summit, which was organized to review progress toward the MDGs, a new turn occurred. "Achieving universal access to reproductive health by 2015, as set out at the International Conference on Population and Development" was added as a commitment to the World Summit Outcome document (UN 2005a). A new MDG on reproductive health was not added, but this commitment to universal access represented a new win in the tug of war over international development goals, as an important ICPD goal was reaffirmed on the global agenda.

The Limits of a Global Consensus Process

One of the core tensions for the UN is between the preservation and the erosion of state sovereignty (Russett 1996). Especially in the social sectors, the UN can convene international conferences that generate global agreements and goals and establish standards and global policy, and its specialized agencies can provide technical guidelines and advice on meeting these objectives. But the UN has no legal authority over member states for enforcing those goals, standards, and policies. This tension appears in the UN's engagement on reproductive health and rights, with implementation clearly assigned to individual states. In 1999, the General Assembly reiterated this protection of state sovereignty for reproductive health and rights in its report on key actions for implementation of the ICPD:

The implementation of the recommendations contained in the Programme of Action and those contained in the present document is the sovereign right of each country, consistent with national laws and development priorities, with full respect for the various religious and ethical values and cultural backgrounds of its people, and in conformity with universally recognized international human rights. (UN 1999b, para. 5)

When global goals and conventions are agreed to through the United Nations, member states have the option to endorse but not fully agree with the document under consideration. This process allows global agreements to be officially agreed upon and consensus produced on the overall principles, while allowing member states to opt out of agreeing to specific clauses, articles, or even words that, for religious, cultural, or state sovereignty reasons, they are not able or willing to endorse.

In some cases, delegations can express reservations about entire chapters of an internationally agreed upon goal or program, as the Holy See did in expressing a general reservation on the chapter on International Cooperation in the ICPD Programme of Action. Other examples of reservations of the ICPD Programme of Action illustrate how a UN consensus process works in practice:

The delegation of Afghanistan wishes to express its reservation about the word "individual" in chapter VII [the chapter on reproductive rights and reproductive health] and also about those parts that are not in conformity with Islamic Sharia. (Delegation of Afghanistan, UN 1995: 149)

The terms, "family composition and structure," "types of families," "different types of families," "other unions" and similar terms can only be accepted on the understanding that in Honduras these terms will never be able to mean unions of persons of the same sex. (Delegation of Honduras, UN 1995: 150)

The delegation of Jordan understands that the final document, particularly chapters IV, V, VI and VII, will be applied within the framework of the Islamic Sharia and our ethical values, as well as the laws that shape our behaviour. We will deal with paragraphs of this document accordingly. Therefore, we interpret the word "individuals" to mean couples, a married couple. (Delegation of Jordan, UN 1995: 152)

Especially broad-sweeping reservations came from the delegation of Yemen, which, in addition to joining other Islamic nations in their reservations "on every term and all terminology that is in contradiction with Islamic Sharia," expressed concerns relating to para. 8.24 of the Programme of Action. They were particularly concerned about the last sentence of the paragraph, which reads, "Adolescent females and males should be provided with information, education and counseling to help them delay early family formation, premature sexual activity and first pregnancy." In short, they noted, "Actually we wanted to delete the words, 'sexual activity'" (UN 1995: 155).

The practice of allowing reservations reveals the limits of the UN consensus process. Global agreements are constructed around broader principles, not specific actions, so that implementation, in the end, is limited by "the sovereign right of each country" and "with full respect for the various religious and ethical values and cultural backgrounds of its people" (UN 1995: 7).

In addition to the reservations expressed by individual countries, groups of purportedly likeminded countries often align together to block or limit the scope of international agreements that are not in accord with their beliefs. Similar to the group of countries that agreed to the Programme of Action only to the extent that it fit within "the framework of the Islamic Sharia," the Holy See played a proactive role in liaising with conservative countries that think similarly about what is acceptable—or not—around reproductive health and rights. As described by Gita Sen,

the Holy See, though only an observer state at the UN, has played a key role in developing both strategy and tactics for the opposition to gender equality and women's human rights. By creating alliances with conservative governments across traditional religious divides, and by bringing its skills to bear on coalescing a non-governmental opposition as well, the Holy See played a critical role throughout the first decade after the ICPD. Part of this role has recently been taken over by the neoconservative U.S. administration. (Sen 2005b: 49)

Restricting the language in international agreements and lobbying to limit the extent of freedoms are common tactics of UN member states (and even observers). Another tactic is to restrict the resources for the implementation of commitments made. In the discussion below, we examine how UNFPA's experience with the loss of financial support from the United States is a poignant example of an attempt to use financial weight to limit the ability of the UN to support realization of ICPD goals.

The Opposition of the U.S. Government

While a number of UN entities have worked on aspects of the ICPD Programme of Action, UNFPA has the most explicit mandate to support the ICPD agenda and particularly its reproductive health and rights goals. And, of all the UN agencies, UNFPA has most directly embraced the ICPD agenda as its guiding mandate. The positions of UNFPA, therefore, aroused the direct and public opposition of the U.S. government under President Bush.

Speaking out on increasingly "sensitive" issues around reproductive health has cost UNFPA financial support from the United States. In a speech at the founding conference of the United Nations Organization, President Harry Truman stated, "We all have to recognize—no matter how great our strength—that we must deny ourselves the license to do always as we please" (Annan 2006: 3 online version). Yet, years later, the United States has refused to allocate its agreed upon commitments— reaching over 150 million dollars in the course of five years—for UNFPA. The United States is trying to change UN policy and program choices by making financial commitments conditional on its own value-based political agenda. As reported by Americans for UNFPA:

For the fifth year in a row, the Bush Administration announced September 13th its decision to withhold the $34 million appropriated by Congress to UNFPA, the United Nations Population Fund. This makes $161 million denied to proven programs that reduce maternal mortality, provide millions of women with contraception and prevent the spread of HIV. (Americans for UNFPA 2006, para. 1)

The U.S. rationale for refusing to provide committed funds to the UNFPA was the U.S. government's claim that UNFPA was endorsing a "coercive" one-child policy in China by supporting reproductive health activities in that country. This claim persisted even after an independent assessment team of three UK parliamentarians (from the Labour, Conservative, and Liberal Democrat parties) found no evidence to support it. According to the McCafferty report,

The UK MP delegation concluded that the work UNFPA does in China, is playing a positive and important catalytic role in the reform of RP/RH services in China . . . .The UK MP delegation was convinced that the UNFPA programme is a force for good, in moving China away from abuses such as forced-family planning, sterilization and abortions. (McCafferty et al. 2002: 10, online version)

Furthermore, the report recommended that "It is vitally important that the UNFPA remains actively involved in China, with continued financial support from the UK and other Western Governments" (McCafferty et al. 2002: 11, online version). In the end, although the U.S. withdrawal of funding took a toll on UNFPA, in many ways the U.S. administration's efforts also partly backfired. Not only did UNFPA continue its program in China, but the number of new national donors to UNFPA increased dramatically. The U.S. government refusal to provide financial resources to UNFPA provoked an outpouring of support from other countries as well as private U.S. citizens who formed an NGO to raise funds for UNFPA from the American public. This led UNFPA executive director Thoraya Ahmed Obaid to comment to reporters that in response to these actions UNFPA had received more donations from more countries in 2005 than since its founding in 1969 and that its regular resources increased to almost $350 million, from around $322 million (Deen 2006).

Although the funding cut by the U.S. curtailed some programming, UNFPA today has more donors than any other UN agency, even though many of them have smaller resources to give compared to the U.S. The outpouring of support by other countries in response to the U.S. pullout reflects the tension between the U.S. and its opponents over reproductive health policies.

In a somewhat ironic way, the UN mechanism has worked. Although the U.S. withdrawal of funding affected UNFPA's capacity to deliver its programs, other UN member states weighed in to publicly support UNFPA and its mission. Despite the U.S. position, the China program was not stopped.

Another instance of U.S. funding flows reflecting changing political trends is outlined in the UN Population Fund 2004 *State of the World Population* report (UNFPA 2004b), where the financial and political trends around contraceptives are discussed. The Report points out that the U.S. Agency for International Development (USAID) had "dominated public sector contraceptive supply since the 1960s, [and] was the largest, accounting for almost three fourths of the $79 million in reported donor support for 1990." Furthermore. by 2000, "the number of active donors had grown to 12 or more, but total donor support remained relatively flat during the decade. The USAID share fell to 30 percent, while that provided by UNFPA grew by 40 percent. These agencies and four others (PSI, World Bank, German Federal Ministry for Economic Development and Cooperation, and DFID) accounted for 95 percent of contraceptive commodities provided to developing countries" (UNFPA 2004b: 47).

U.S. political and financial bullying around reproductive rights is not limited to the UN stage. The Mexico City Policy has led to significant financial cuts for a number of important NGOs, taking a serious toll on reproductive health services in many developing countries. Furthermore, the impact has grown beyond the specific restrictions initially stated in Reagan's Mexico City Policy. An article on the Global Gag Rule notes, "It is pertinent to note that even though the provision of certain abortion services is allowed on paper, in practice the policy has had a tremendous chilling effect on providers who choose not to discuss abortion at all rather than risk losing their funding" (Bogecho and Upreti 2006: 18). The "chilling effect" of U.S. policies did not stop the efforts of the UN and its member states from achieving the ICPD goals, but it did produce political and financial limits that are still being felt today in the implementation of reproductive health and rights programs around the world. A change in administration may help turn the tide.

Looking across the activities of the United Nations in response to the ICPD reproductive health and rights agenda, we have examined three key expectations and three key limitations. The three key expectations were to advocate widely for the ICPD Programme of Action; to improve action and coherence on reproductive health across UN agencies; and to review and monitor progress against the ICPD agenda. The three limitations are the geopolitical context that restrains the voice of the UN; the reservations that allow member states to agree without fully agreeing; and the financial pressures some countries use to push their political agendas. Despite these significant constraints (and indeed sometimes because of them), various UN agencies have promoted the ICPD agenda and helped catalyze changes in discourse and action around reproductive health internationally.

In reviewing ten years of implementation since the 1994 ICPD, the 2004 *State of the World Population* report acknowledges a number of positive achievements. "Reproductive health has been advanced in policies and institutions," the report notes. "Topics that were previously ignored in policy discussions—like harmful traditional practices, gender-based violence, adolescent reproductive health, post-abortion care, the health needs of refugees and people living in emergency situations, the security of supplies of reproductive health and family planning commodities, and the role of culture as a vehicle for advancing basic human rights-are now routinely addressed and acted on" (UNFPA 2004b: 92).

But the report also underlines that action by the UN (as well as others) has been far too limited. The report identifies a number of areas with a "long way to go" (7), including addressing pregnancy-related deaths. Over 529,000 women die of pregnancy-related causes each year, with 99 percent of the deaths in the developing world. According to estimates by WHO, UNICEF, and UNFPA, this estimate has not changed significantly since ICPD (UNFPA 2004b: 51.) In the developing world more than one-third of all pregnant women receive no health care during pregnancy. Another area of need that remains is serving the more than 350 million couples that still lack access to the full range of family planning services. The report also notes that nearly one-fifth of the global burden of illness and premature death—and one-third of illness and death among women of reproductive age—are due to gaps in reproductive and sexual health care.

Persistently high maternal mortality rates speak to the limits of real progress. As the World Bank publication *Reproductive Health: The Missing Millennium Development Goal* concludes, "Absolute failure may be a fair way of describing how badly public health care systems have performed in the area of reproductive health, especially for poor and vulnerable people" (Campbell et al. 2006: 8). WHO expresses a similar theme of limited progress in a blunt question raised at the start of the 2005 *World Health Report* in a section called, "Patchy Progress and Widening Gaps— What Went Wrong?":

Why is it still necessary for this report to emphasize the importance of focusing on the health of mothers, newborns and children, after decades of priority status, and more than 10 years after the UN ICPD laid out access to reproductive health care for all firmly on the agenda? (WHO 2005: xiv)

Such questions, posed by UN entities themselves, speak to the limits of what the UN can achieve on the ground. Although these reports repeatedly state that the needed knowledge and tools are available, and conclude that they "just" need to be scaled up, the official reports rarely talk explicitly about the political constraints to action. Yet these constraints often create real barriers to tangible achievement. The UN system is highly political, affected by both external and internal politics in its language, allocation of resources, and scope of work. It can play a critical role as a convener, advocate, and independent monitor, but expectations of what it can actually deliver need to be seen through a political lens that is focused on practical reality.

Among a number of recommendations made in the Report of the Secretary General's High Level Panel on UN System-Wide Coherence was a proposal that the UN establish a new entity for gender equality (UN 2006b). There is no question that the world needs a higher level of attention to one of the biggest drivers of poor reproductive health— gender inequality—given the limits of UN mechanisms. But is a new UN entity on gender equality the answer? Probably not; what is needed is significantly more than a new UN entity. Aside from the risks of marginalizing a critical issue that needs attention by *all* UN bodies, there are a number of other ways in which the UN can better leverage its existing mechanisms and resources.

Consider, for example, UNAIDS. No other UN entity serves such a cross-cutting function, rallying disparate UN bodies, including the World Bank, around a common cause and exemplifying the potential for a reformed UN system. According to the UN organizational chart, UNAIDS is listed under "Other UN Entities" along with the UN University, UN Office of Project Services, UN System Staff College, and Office of the UN High Commissioner for Human Rights. As noted above, UNAIDS is defined as the "Joint UN Programme on HIV/AIDS," "co-sponsored" by ten different UN bodies and is unlike any other UN entity. Ironically, although it is "co-sponsored," one of its key functions is to raise funds for its ten co-sponsors to strengthen the global response to AIDS.

Although UNAIDS is burdened with layers of internal transaction costs, it has had a significant role in rallying UN agencies around a common UN response to AIDS and has had a particular impact in looking beyond the UN system and opening its doors to civil society, brokering relationships across governments, businesses, researchers, and community-based groups. It is the only UN entity that has invited NGO members to its Board. While UNAIDS is not perfect, and would not work as a model for every new significant issue that emerges, a number of its mechanisms and tactics push the limits of the UN system in areas where the ICPD agenda could learn and benefit.

The current trend in the latest wave of UN reform, at least in the area of development, is toward "Delivering as One" through one common program, one common leader, and one common fund. While there are potential strengths in bringing together the collective work of different UN agencies into a cohesive whole, there are also risks. Some of the more politically sensitive issues—such as reproductive and sexual health and rights—could be submerged or subverted by the search for commonality. Without a separate, distinct advocate and fund for reproductive health, some of the critical issues of the ICPD agenda could be pushed off the policy agenda at country level. Perhaps effective UN reform will need both "One-ness"—reflected in the pursuit of coherence in data, policies, and programs—and room for distinct advocacy efforts around critical issues such as reproductive health and rights.

Ten years after the Cairo Conference, achievement of the ICPD agenda is facing a number of persistent as well as new challenges, including growing conservatism around the world. The principles around which international consensus is gained will not, by themselves, make a positive difference, especially when the most powerful countries in the world try to use financial bullying to impose their policies. International agreements such as ICPD can be powerful levers for change, if they are owned and championed by a multitude of players including, but well beyond, the UN system.

As imperfect as the UN system and its wider response to ICPD have been, consider for a moment what the current and future state of reproductive health might have been, had there been no International Conference on Population and Development or UN mechanisms to support it. While the impact of the current UN reforms on reproductive health and rights remains to be seen, the UN must continue to be supported in its advocacy, implementation, and monitoring role for achieving the important goals borne at ICPD.

Chapter 15
Examining Religion and Reproductive Health: Constructive Engagement for the Future

Frances Kissling

The oppositional role to the International Conference on Population and Development (ICPD) played by conservative religious groups, especially the Vatican, has been well chronicled (see Girard, this volume; Kissling 1999), although not always well understood. That opposition has not diminished since the conference took place in 1994. Rather, it has awakened an international consciousness among conservative religionists, especially fundamentalist Christians in the United States, and subjected developing country reproductive health programs to ongoing criticism. It has also frightened UN officials and other multinational agencies, encouraging them to mute their voices in support of the goals of the ICPD Programme of Action (UN 1995).

The vehemence and sometimes viciousness with which conservative religious groups still struggle against public policies that support the rather modest reproductive health objectives developed at the ICPD is a primary obstacle to improving services and creating political will in favor of sexual and reproductive health and rights worldwide. At the same time, it has also awakened an interest among some reproductive health advocates in better understanding religious beliefs about reproduction and facilitating the participation of religious leaders in promoting reproductive health services and rights. This chapter examines both religiously based opposition as an obstacle to achieving the ICPD goals and analyzes the potential that religious values might have in developing ethically based reproductive health policies that favor a woman-centered approach to reproduction.

Determining the meaning and purpose of sexuality and reproduction has been a central preoccupation of many of the world's religions, particularly those in the Abrahamic traditions (Judaism, Christianity, and Islam). All these religions have highly developed codes of behavior related to sexuality and reproduction that are proscriptive in regulating marriage, sexuality, gender relations and roles, and procreation within the faith group. At times, these religions have sought to influence public policy related to these issues, seeking legal conformity with their own moral codes and believing that their positions derive from a common moral sensibility that transcends sectarian beliefs and expresses a universal and timeless understanding of the purpose of sexuality and procreation. This view has especially dominated Roman Catholicism, which is the most centralized of the Abrahamic faiths. It has also engendered hostility from more secularized forces in international politics such as the European Union, and from feminist groups who have experienced the negative effects of discrimination against women in the world's religions and want nothing to do with religious groups, however benign.

No official religious institution is more identified as hostile to sexuality and reproductive rights than the Roman Catholic church. Through its UN status as a non-member state permanent observer, it has been active on questions of population policy and reproductive health since the 1974 Bucharest World Conference on Population. At that conference, which focused predominantly on population policy, its delegation's views were largely ignored. The dominant view that population size and growth needed to be controlled if poverty was to be alleviated created almost no dissent at that time. The church's opposition to family planning was of course well known, but not shared by most of the world's faiths and certainly not by governments. Religion had not yet emerged as a dimension of statecraft. Pope John Paul II, who played a major political role in the downfall of communism and thus gained a respected position as a world leader, had not yet been elected pope. Within the UN itself, religious organizations had historically opted for low key supportive roles focusing on peace and poverty alleviation and avoiding controversy. In the global North, religious practice was on the decline, and rumors that God was dead were on the rise.

Ten years later, the 1984 UN Conference on Population in Mexico City fell hostage to American fundamentalist Christian thought, especially about women, sexuality, and reproduction, issues that had provided the margin of victory for Ronald Reagan. Fundamentalist Christians had historically avoided entanglement with politics, preferring to establish insular communities where they avoided social and cultural trends that deviated from their beliefs. The liberal movements of the 1970s, which led to women gaining many rights in the workplace, sexuality education in the schools, and legal family planning and abortion, changed that. It was no longer possible to send one's children to school or listen to television and not be assaulted with ideas that contradicted one's world view. These Christians "struck back" and organized for conservative Republican candidates in unprecedented numbers. The easiest way for the administration to reward them for their support was by enacting restrictions on reproductive health in international policy. While these groups viewed the UN with suspicion and were not involved as NGOs, the Reagan administration, in an alliance with the Vatican, pushed for a strong antiabortion plank in the Mexico City conference document. The statement was ambiguously worded, asserting, "In no case should abortion be promoted as a method of family planning" (UN 1984). This phrase served as the cornerstone of U.S. international family planning policy and became known as the Global Gag Rule or Mexico City policy.

Throughout the 1980s the influence of conservative religion in politics grew. Roman Catholicism under the Polish pope, John Paul II, flourished due to his role in the downfall of communism in eastern and central Europe. American fundamentalist Christians continued to dominate Republican Party politics and the U.S. airwaves with televangelists. Muslim conservatives at both the governmental and nongovernmental level from the Taliban to the Muslim Brotherhood overshadowed moderate voices in the Muslim world. While these groups had strong differences on many political and theological issues, including deep seated hostilities toward each other, they were united in their view of men's role as head of both family and society and in upholding prohibitive views on a woman's right to reproductive freedom. The articulation of a conservative vision of sexual, reproductive, and family life united them.

At the same time as these conservative religious groups were gaining ground at the national level, a new consensus on human rights and freedoms related to women and reproduction was developing, and new approaches to population policy were emerging. Many of these trends are described in other chapters in this book. Here it is sufficient to say that we were brought to the verge of a new way of conceptualizing "the population problem" and designing solutions by two trends: the realism of the population establishment that further reductions in population growth were unlikely to result from the singleminded approach to supplying family planning methods and the idealism of the women's health movement's focus on comprehensive quality of care and respect for the right of each woman and couple to freely decide on methods of fertility control.

The 1990 election in the United States of Bill Clinton, a pro-choice president, led to an immediate change in U.S. international family planning policy. Simultaneously, the UN was planning an unprecedented round of international policy meetings aimed at thorough reviews of key concepts and human needs. The issues in the round of five conferences to be held between 1992 and 1997 were the environment (the Earth Summit, in Rio in 1992) human rights (World Conference on Human Rights, Vienna, 1993), population (International Conference on Population and Development, Cairo, 1994), women (Fourth World Conference on Women, Beijing, 1995), and social development (the Copenhagen Social Development Summit, 1995). Each of these conferences would subtly influence the others. For population and development, this would mean a diminution of emphasis on demographics and a greater emphasis on human rights, a holistic model of health care, and attention to women's empowerment.

One would think that religious institutions would be ecstatically supportive of such a value oriented approach. One might even hope the Vatican—which had consistently criticized population programs for ignoring economic development as a solution to the problem associated with population growth and for coercion in government population programs—would find something to support.

The first hint that this would not be the case surfaced during the 1992 Rio Earth Summit. Vatican officials vigorously opposed any effort to include population growth as a factor contributing to environmental degradation. The arguments were well known and long standing. Church officials claimed that linking these two issues had led to an excessive focus in the environmental movement on population control as the solution to environmental problems rather than efforts to control corporate misuse of environmental resources and overconsumption in the North. With feminists making similar arguments, some leading environmentalists and members of the population establishment became alarmed at what they feared would be an alliance between feminists and the Vatican at the 1994 ICPD. In fact, Jessica Matthews, then vice president of the World Resources Institute, wrote a scathing op-ed in the *Washington Post*, blasting a "small but noisy" group of women's advocates for lining up with the Vatican. Matthews claimed that feminist opposition to linking environmental problems with population was "playing into the hands of people who really are the enemies . . . like the U.S. government, Jesse Helms and the Vatican" (Matthews 1992: C7).

Far more important than the unwarranted fears that feminists and the Vatican were in bed together was the simple fact that the Vatican presence in Rio and the extent to which they lobbied to keep population concerns out of the Earth Summit document put the ICPD community on notice that serious Vatican opposition to ICPD would emerge.

And it did. In the process, any idea that feminist perspectives on population and reproductive health and those of the Vatican were similar was disproved. In fact the Vatican and other conservative religious groups seemed more opposed to a human rights, woman-centered, re-productive health perspective on population growth than they were to the older demographically driven approach.

Vatican opposition to ICPD has been well covered in both scholarly articles and the popular press (see Religion Counts 2002). The Vatican and its allies opposed in Cairo and in follow-up meetings proposals that would recognize the right of individuals as well as couples to decide on family size, the right of adolescents to confidential information as well as family planning services, efforts to prevent unsafe abortions or ad-dress the public health problems associated with unsafe abortions, ac-cess to condoms as a way to prevent the transmission of HIV and AIDS, and sexuality education that was not exclusively focused on abstinence. At the 1995 Fourth World Conference on Women, they opposed even the concept of women's rights preferring instead to speak of women's dignity and questioning whether women's rights constituted the cre-ation of a new right. Similar opposition was raised at the 1993 Vienna Human Rights Conference. No opportunity over the last 21 years has been missed to attempt to undo the progress made at Cairo. In deliber-ations over the establishment of an International Criminal Court Vatican, officials opposed efforts to declare enforced pregnancy an in-ternational crime. As an indication of its vehemence, UNICEF has been consistently attacked by Vatican officials who in 1996 withdrew their an-nual contribution of $2,000 and threatened to boycott school-based fundraising initiated by UNICEF, claiming the agency is pro-abortion.

Numerous conservative NGOs, particularly those from the U.S., seemed to "discover" the UN during these meetings and actively lobbied during ICPD and other conferences against the Programme of Action and reproductive health and rights, creating a highly contentious atmo-sphere, intimidating other NGOs and even delegates. Two factors killed the possibility of a formal 10-year follow up to evaluate the Programme of Action: fear of the positions that would be taken by the U.S. under the George W. Bush administration and fear that conservative religious NGOs would dominate the meetings in an alliance with the Vatican and the U.S.

Perhaps most disturbing is the fact that no official religious denomi-nations associated with the UN were actively and openly supportive of the Programme of Action, even when the denomination had a positive position on various reproductive health issues. This is in sharp contrast to the participation of many denominations at the Fourth World Conference on Women and the other major conferences mentioned above.

Religious institutions worldwide are rife with internal debate about women, sexuality, and reproduction and are reluctant to speak out on these issues. One need only look at the way the ordination of women bishops and gay clergy has led to massive defections in the Episcopal Church to see the problem (Markham 2007). Every pro-choice on abortion denomination in the U.S. has a pro-life pressure group that regularly seeks to overturn the position. And no denomination wants to be in open disagreement with the Vatican.

Recognizing the enormous negative influence the Vatican and some U.S. fundamentalist Christian groups have had on stifling support for ICPD within the UN and a number of developing country missions, UNFPA and some major international NGOs have attempted to reach out to the religious community (UNFPA 2007). This is motivated not only by a desire to respond to conservative religious critics at the policy level but by a recognition that religious organizations are major providers of health care, educators of women, and a major factor in the way many—but not all—believers make decisions about reproduction. It is assumed that the world's religions could be one of the most significant forces for the implementation of ICPD rather than the most significant obstacle.

Is this assumption reasonable? Yes and no, as those who fully support the concept of women-centered sexual and reproductive health policies will readily grasp.

First, to the extent that mainstream Northern religious denominations have supported international family planning, they have often done so out of a commitment to the old paradigm of benign population control. Denominational publications and statements are filled with concern for the environment and with a belief that there are just too many people for there to be enough food, jobs, health care, and shelter. These concerns are not malevolent; they are rooted in a commitment to social justice, but simply not well developed in relation to gender and certainly subject to traditional religious beliefs that link sexuality and procreation to marriage.

In almost all the world's religions, current official teachings hold that the only legitimate expression of sexuality is within heterosexual marriage. Any aspect of ICPD that stretches that notion is hard to address and almost impossible for an official religious body to support in a public statement. A few individual religious leaders have developed arguments in favor of condoms to prevent the spread of HIV and AIDS (see the example of the Reverend Gideon Byamugisha, Anglican Church of Canada 2002), access to contraceptives and even abortion in some circumstances, for adolescents who might have sex anyway, and even abortion in some circumstances, but official groups are silent. For example, the World Council of Churches has no position on most sexual and reproductive health issues and dropped its support for family planning two decades ago in deference to a minority of members who were opposed to it.

Many religious denominations also lag behind the UN consensus and positions on women's rights. While most denominations claim that men and women are equal before God, they view equality in limited ways on a day to day basis. Most still hold patriarchal views of men's role within the family and give preference to men in many areas of life. Girls' education still lags behind that of boys in countries where religion is a dominant provider of education or influences public education policy. Religions worry that recognition of the equality of men and women in society will lead to demands that women be treated as equals within the religion itself. Sharia law also affects the status of women and girls relative to the power of husbands and fathers. This is not to suggest that advances have not been made on these issues by many religious leaders, but to note that in the mainstream of practice and religious education serious differences exist between the values laid out in UN documents and official teachings.

The ability to establish partnerships with religious groups on the full Cairo agenda is clearly limited, as the experience of the last 15 years demonstrates. The number of religious groups in opposition to sexual and reproductive health has grown since Cairo, although modestly. The election of George Bush, the reinstatement of the Global Gag Rule which prohibits U.S. funding of overseas groups working on abortion, and newly relaxed U.S. rules on funding religious agencies in the U.S. and abroad have provided substantial funding for conservative religious groups who provide substandard reproductive health care in the developing world. These include programs focused on abstinence-only sexuality education and programs that do not provide condoms to prevent the transmission of HIV (Global Gag Rule Impact Project 2003; PEPFAR Watch 2007). Even within the European Union, religious groups are actively lobbying against reproductive health funding.

Efforts to work with mainstream religious denominations are limited and sporadic. There is still ambivalence in secular circles regarding religion, which is treated with either suspicion or disdain. The attitude of the UN toward religion is complex and changing. Over the last decade, religious NGOs have sought a greater role in support of the UN. Several large major religious meetings have been held within the UN. There have been magnificent displays dominated by male clerical leaders, resplendent in flowing robes and focused on matters where there is little dispute among the world's religions. It does not take much courage for a religious leader to speak out in favor of the alleviation of poverty, protection of mother earth (the only strong female presence in many religious gatherings), and peace. Divisions emerge over questions of the balance of power among participants, but issues such as women's rights, sexuality, and reproduction are taboo, controversial, and unimportant. UN religious meetings are usually addressed by the secretary general and other high ranking officials, but an arm's length approach is maintained. A case in point is the Millennium World Peace Summit of Religious and Spiritual Leaders, which although it was held in August 2000 at the UN in New York, was never an official UN event. In addition, when its organizers asked for official status as an advisory group to the UN Secretariat, their request fell on deaf ears.

A counter-effort to convene women in religion at the UN was undertaken and funded by the UN Development Fund for Women (UNIFEM). Criteria for participation in this meeting politely excluded women whose focus of work was change within their denominations. A review of the profiles of religious groups that belong to the UN Committee on Religions and lists the issues and conferences member organizations are involved in showed not a single member involved in ICPD or the five-year review process.

Within UNFPA, a serious effort to address culture and religion has been undertaken, but it is still woefully inadequate and in some aspects poorly constructed. UNFPA has sponsored a number of meetings at the regional and local level with religious leaders and a few have resulted in positive statements on less controversial aspects of the ICPD Programme of Action. Thoraya Obaid, the head of UNFPA, has gone out of her way to address religious groups and meet with religious leaders. However, there has been very little effort to bring religious leaders into the mainstream of UNFPA's work and into constructive engagement with family planners, women's groups, or government officials. A review of invited experts to UNFPA technical and expert meetings since Cairo shows almost no representation from the religious community. It is as if religion is viewed in a vacuum. There is a fear that if religious leaders engage directly with family planners or feminists or demographers on a regular basis, something bad will happen.

Finally, one can evaluate the importance of an effort by the resources allocated to it. The amount of staff time and resources allocated to religion and culture in UNFPA is minuscule. Modest efforts like this will not serve to counter the massive efforts of those religious groups who have made opposition to the Cairo paradigm central to their agenda.

There is also an understandable desire for the UN and governments to use religion as a credentialing factor rather than in genuine engagement regarding both agreement and conflict. Instead, one simply seeks "respectable" religious figures—almost always male and relatively conservative theologically—the very figures that want to avoid speaking out on sex and reproduction. Little effort has been made to reach out to and promote more likely allies—women working within denominations and in interfaith settings who are sympathetic and knowledgeable. Groups like Sisters in Islam, Women Living Under Muslim Laws, the International Association of Buddhist Women, the Circle of Concerned African Women Theologians, and the Ecumenical Association of Third World Theologians are almost invisible. Religious sisters in Catholic orders have extensive experience working with poor women and are often meeting their reproductive health care needs, yet little outreach to them occurs. A woman-centered reproductive health care paradigm must include the strong involvement of women religious leaders in interpreting religious teachings and moving them forward. One should no more see a panel composed of all male clerics than one should see a panel comprised of all male parliamentarians or all male doctors.

The largely negative and oppositional role played by conservative religionists combined with the reluctance of those in favor of reproductive choice to speak out makes it difficult for supporters of the Cairo consensus to craft a positive strategy of engagement. Yet such a strategy is critical to working with many women. Muslim feminist scholar Riffat Hassan has noted that it is far easier to go into a Muslim village and assure women that the Qur'an supports their right to reproductive health than it is to tell them a UN document will make them free (see Hassan 2007). Advocates of choice need to balance a constructive critique of inappropriate attempts by religions to limit reproductive choice with support for the renewable moral energy liberating religious thought can bring to the development of reproductive health policy that furthers human dignity.

In looking forward in reflection on ICPD, four simple rules should govern the involvement of religious groups and beliefs in the work toward achieving the Cairo consensus.

First, government officials and those in multilateral agencies need to overcome their fear of criticizing religious practices and positions that are dangerous to women's health. Religious groups have every right to express their views, even to seek to see them enacted in civil law. It is the obligation of government and public health officials to evaluate these positions by standards of care and principles of human rights rather than as sacrosanct religious teachings. A perfect example of courage by government has been the reaction of UNFPA, WHO, and UNAIDS to claims by Vatican officials that condoms have small holes through which the HIV virus can pass. These three agencies promptly and publicly refuted these claims and called them irresponsible and dangerous (WHO, UNAIDS, UNFPA 2004).

Second, legislators in Catholic countries need to educate themselves about their rights as Catholics and make a distinction between what their religion might demand and what their oath of office demands. The refusal of Colombian parliamentarians to acquiesce to the church's demand that they overturn the Colombian Supreme Court's ruling that abortion should be decriminalized in a number of circumstances or face excommunication is exemplary.

Third, providers of reproductive health services need to build bonds with sympathetic religious leaders. These leaders can help providers respond to women's moral concerns about family planning and abortion. In turn, the religious leaders will learn more about women's actual experience as mothers and as women. Over the years, I have been impressed by the strong advocacy of Catholic religious leaders who work directly with the poor make for family planning. There is no substitute for direct experience of people's needs.

Fourth, the articulation of a woman-centered approach to reproductive health is fragile. Religious leaders have something to offer in terms of an understanding of ethics and respect for persons, and their views should not be automatically dismissed.

Collaboration between religious groups and advocates of full sexual and reproductive choice will always include an element of tension. The sexual teachings of most of the world's religions lag behind the moral insights of their own members and current ethical theories that evaluate the goodness of sexuality and reproduction by standards of justice rather than by marriage. The challenge for all is to find ways to talk to each other that assume good will, focus on the desire to understand and respect the other, and where all parties are willing to be changed by contact with each other. Our common commitments to human dignity and poverty alleviation can forge some of these bonds.

Chapter 16
Conclusion: Conceptual Successes and Operational Challenges to ICPD: Global Reproductive Health and Rights Moving Forward

Rebecca Firestone, Laura Reichenbach, and Mindy Jane Roseman

Despite the diverse disciplinary perspectives and experiential backgrounds of the contributors to this volume, when read as a whole this set of essays suggests important mutual understandings and areas of convergence around ICPD. This concluding chapter summarizes these points of consensus regarding the conceptual underpinnings of ICPD as well as its operational challenges based on the organizing premise of this volume—that conceptually, ICPD still has great resonance, even in the face of the obstacles related to institutionalizing the Programme of Action and the complexities of realizing the human rights principles of the ICPD. We then use these common reflections as a springboard to propose areas where proponents of the reproductive health and rights agenda of ICPD can take action to overcome the obstacles in the years to come.

Conceptual Foundations of ICPD

There are a number of points upon which nearly all the contributors agree. First, Cairo represented a reorientation in population and development policy—the "Cairo paradigm." While some contributors believe the extent to which governments and other actors have adopted this paradigm varies, most agree that conceptually ICPD brought an important and enduring shift in policy and programming. This concept still has resonance across the disciplines represented here, and countervailing international trends notwithstanding, ICPD remains foundational to the achievement of global health and development goals.

However, when looked at descriptively the ICPD Programme of Action overwhelmingly reflects the political process out of which it was born and which resulted in the compromises required to achieve the Cairo consensus. As Marge Berer notes in her chapter, a compromise, by definition, pleases no one. This displeasure is most evident in attempts at operationalizing ICPD. Conceptually, diverse actors and governments could buy into ICPD's broad agenda; operationally, this same compromise has created problems as it purposefully left significant room for interpretation on particular issues, such as abortion or young people's sexual and reproductive health.

The chapters in this book illustrate that ICPD holds different meanings based on an individual's disciplinary and experiential location. The conceptual underpinnings of ICPD can be successfully incorporated into public health, human rights, demographic, development, and empowerment arguments—all of which are propounded in this book. This diversity of meaning is a reflection of the strength and wide-reaching impact of ICPD. It also calls attention to the fact that ICPD was not minted overnight but rather reflects a long and rich conceptual history fostered by a range of movements—human rights, population, development, and social justice, to name a few. The analyses in this book remind us that while ICPD remains foundational, it does not operate in isolation from other policy paradigms. More than ten years on, ICPD may be seen as a necessary but not sufficient condition for achieving particular health and development goals, whether it is support for young people's sexual and reproductive health or more fruitful interaction between the HIV/AIDS and sexual and reproductive health communities.

The contributing authors are in agreement that despite formidable challenges, the ideas bound up in the words "reproductive health and rights" have made, and will continue to make, important improvements in the way development and health research, policy, and programs are designed and implemented. What Cairo got right was not unsubstantial: that economic and technological development requires governments and other appropriate parties to ensure that individuals can make meaningful and informed choices. Furthermore, because women bear the physical burdens of reproductive choices differently from men, it is their individual and informed decision making capacities which were and remain Cairo's priority. Empowerment through education and legal and policy reforms, as well as the provision of a range of health services and information related to reproduction and sexuality, comprise many of the action points in the Programme of

Action. If we are to move the reproductive health and rights agenda forward, we must be up front about the enduring value of ICPD's legacy.

Realizing Human Rights and ICPD

While ICPD's core principles remain intact, the chapters on human rights in this volume suggest that human rights alone are neither a quick fix nor a silver bullet, but a long-term project. While embedding the analysis of reproductive health in the language of human rights has given powerful impetus to the field, it has not been sufficient. Human rights claims do not magically stop harmful practices, overcome discrimination, build services, or allocate adequate resources. The invocation of human rights principles and mechanisms is not a trump card and will not lessen the hard work needed to put rights-based approaches into action. As a discourse and a claim, human rights have moral and legal force, but human rights operate in an environment of competing claims that must be taken into consideration even as rights are progressively realized over time. To that end, knowledgeable advocates and scholars, committed activists, and an organized social movement are necessary to sustain the reproductive health and rights nexus of ICPD.

Political Challenges Since ICPD

As many of the contributors describe, politics on multiple levels have made problematic the implementation of ICPD's Programme of Action, and this will continue to be the case in the coming years. In the area of access to abortion services, ICPD's approach has had at best limited impact and at worst significant, negative ramifications for women's enjoyment of reproductive health. Anti-abortion activism has burgeoned globally in the years since ICPD and can be seen as a proxy for conservative, traditional, and often religious forces whose vision of the family and the nation is one where sex is for procreative purposes within the confines of marriage (between one man and one woman) and where the husband is the economic bread winner (Girard 2004). This backlash, not only against feminism, but also against the realities of most women's lives, has contributed to the hostilities certain governments and non-governmental organizations express internationally. The failure of ICPD to support pregnancy termination as a legitimate exercise of a woman's informed choice about her health has cost women their lives, as well as their health. The politics of abortion, inflected as they are by religious and cultural conservatives, will remain a challenge to the Cairo compromise, no matter what the composition of the U.S. administration.

Politics of a different kind of played out in how the reproductive health and the HIV/AIDS communities have understood each other. ICPD's reticence toward HIV/AIDS prevention and treatment in part can be explained historically. In 1994 HIV was still considered a death sentence; antiretroviral drugs only became publicly available in 1996. In the years since Cairo, HIV/AIDS has come to overshadow attention to reproductive health as a matter of global urgency—even though HIV/AIDS is largely a sexually transmitted infection and has consequences for the enjoyment of reproductive health. Only in the last few years have the reproductive rights of people living with HIV garnered the attention of reproductive health advocates (WHO 2006a). ICPD may not have said enough about prevention, treatment, and care for HIV/AIDS, but with the advent of more widespread access to antiretrovirals, there is a new urgency to bring the two communities together. That HIV has, in some areas of the world, absorbed much of the available health care resources—both human and financial—is another persistent challenge to ICPD, but the rationale for forging common ground goes beyond tapping into financial resources. Rather, it is a larger issue of building functional health systems, pooling scarce human resources, and financially supporting a range of health interventions that meet the goals and aspirations of both communities.

The new, more streamlined global health and development agendas have put ICPD somewhat on the defensive. As important as the MDG indicators are, they miss the profound insights that the years of activism and research leading up to ICPD revealed. Here is where it is critical to keep the core principles of ICPD present while designing and evaluating the strategies needed to achieve the MDGs related to reproductive health. The chapters on population and development in the first section of this volume remind us of the evidence base that must be generated and marshaled, and how this evidence base must be connected to the human rights and empowerment core principles of ICPD.

Overcoming Operational Obstacles

ICPD has weathered recent political assaults and concerns about being omitted from the MDGs with its basic principles remaining intact. However, there are other external factors, as suggested by chapters in this book, that the reproductive health and rights community must be prepared to address. The set of ICPD's operational shortcomings can be organized around a lack of clarity surrounding attitudes toward reproductive and sexual rights (relating to both autonomy in decision making and access to services and information) and an underappreciation of the scope and scale of HIV/AIDS, as well as the importance of global poverty. As some of the chapters argued, policy and programmatic issues such as the MDGs and HIV/AIDS funding mechanisms need not displace ICPD as a concept. However there are a few larger, institutional concerns raised in the final section of the book that could further stymie progress on ICPD.

One of these is the impact of international politics as Francoise Girard's chapter describes the vagaries of the dependence of ICPD on progressive governments and conversely its vulnerability to conservative political challenges. She argues that ICPD's defenders need a long-term strategy as well as conviction in order to successfully institutionalize ICPD through laws, policies, programs and practices. Alaka Basu in her chapter raises another key site for institutionalizing reproductive health—the academy. She argues that it has scarcely embraced reproductive health as defined by ICPD. She makes the case that if ICPD is to have staying power, future professionals must have the knowledge, skills, and experiences that span the range of research, programmatic, and policy issues that constitute reproductive health. Heidi Larson and Michael Reich survey the political landscape at the international institutional level of the United Nations. As much as the implementation of ICPD requires national political will and effort, the UN and its agencies share an important continued responsibility to facilitate the Programme of Action. ICPD, their chapter argues, must be better institutionalized in the current and proposed UN reforms. Finally, Frances Kissling confronts the challenge of religion to institutionalizing ICPD. Resistance to reproductive health, particularly access to information and services related to birth control, pregnancy termination, and sexual health, has emerged from certain religious traditions. Kissling, however, does not dismiss religious convictions but rather views them as opportunities for engagement, and argues that alliances can be built within religious traditions and ultimately help to institutionalize ICPD.

In order to respond to these and other challenges to ICPD raised by the chapters in this book, we offer a few suggestions for advocates, practitioners, and scholars who care about reproductive health and rights. We believe these steps can provide a strategy for the field in the coming years and will permit us to riposte future attacks on ICPD effectively.

1. Improve Measurement and Accountability

Measurement and accountability issues play multifaceted and increasingly important roles in global health. Summary measures of population health are used to document the degree to which a problem requires attention and to mobilize resources to address the problem. Outcome variable measures are used to determine the progress of policies and programs and are increasingly used to hold donors and policy makers accountable for their expenditures. Laura Reichenbach and Joan Kaufman both demonstrate the struggles that the reproductive health field has encountered in seeking to measure the extent of the "problem" of reproductive health as well as the relevant outcomes needed to document progress in the field.

There are three areas related to measurement where reproductive health requires improvement and attention. The first has to do with refining methods for collecting evidence to better document the problem of reproductive health, both in terms of health and more broadly. One approach to building this evidence base is to simply work harder to "get the numbers right" but, as Joan Kaufman describes, this is a challenge for reproductive health because of its unique behavioral, social, cultural, and political nature. As Kaufman argues in her chapter, measuring the contextual factors that impact reproductive health is critical. The causes of poor reproductive health are multi-faceted, as are their implications in terms of health outcomes. We need better conceptual and causal models, and we need to be able to translate these models into operational research that provides us with evidence for advocacy and policy makers. Designing these causal models and collecting the evidence will not be an easy task. Kaufman argues that a multi-level evaluation approach is required to measure the enabling environment for reproductive health—including the social, economic, and political determinants of reproductive health as well as the measurement of intergenerational impacts. The evidence that results from better understandings of the causal relationships between reproductive health and poverty will have an important impact on the future of reproductive health in terms of international donors and institutions.

In a similar vein, reproductive health programs require development of meaningful indicators that measure the value added of human rights to reproductive health outcomes. Generating this evidence will require that the reproductive health and rights field involve development economists and poverty alleviation specialists in the modeling process. A purely technocratic approach will not suffice; the reproductive health and rights community must engage with the broader policy and political environment using conceptual, evidence-based, and political arguments. As Tom Merrick argues in his chapter, better evidence regarding the links between reproductive health and poverty reduction is particularly critical to ensuring that reproductive health stays engaged with the international policy community. Identifying the pathways and the proximate determinants of this linkage is an important area of attention. David Bloom and David Canning's chapter is optimistic that the evidence for these links is stronger than previously believed.

The second area for attention is the improvement of indicators that measure the success of reproductive health policies and programs. Now, more than ever, the reproductive health field must be able to show measurable results of policies and programs to donors and policy makers alike. Achieving this requires differentiation between policy and program indicators. Programmatic indicators communicate improvements in specific reproductive health outcomes as a result of investment in a particular reproductive health program or intervention (i.e., reduction in maternal mortality as a result of investment in emergency obstetric care facilities). Development of programmatic indicators is complicated by the inherent difficulties in measuring reproductive health outcomes (see Kaufman, this volume). More work is still required to improve these types of measures to better reflect reproductive health status (AbouZahr 1999). Policy indicator development requires a different approach, as it goes beyond measuring health outcomes as summary statistical measures to reflect measures of performance or achievement in a particular area. These measures, therefore, are more likely to reflect a broad array of information (both quantitative and qualitative) and to be adapted to the national context. The discussion of policy indicators in the human rights literature can inform and facilitate the development of reproductive health ones (Green 2001).

An important aspect of improvement in indicators that measure the success of reproductive health policies and programs is documenting implementation successes at national and local levels. While this has been done to a large degree, better documentation of how transformative the reproductive health approach can be when it is done effectively is required. Too often, evidence of local success never makes it into policy making discussions. We need to become better equipped at identifying these efforts and to support local partners with documentation and evaluation. Local experience can be used to bolster conceptually sound and well-developed arguments about why investments in reproductive health make a difference. We know that promoting rights and eliminating gender discrimination makes a difference to both health and poverty reduction—but we need to document how, whether through narrative, anecdotal accounts of individuals whose lives have changed, through quantitative aggregate measures, or through a combination of both. Until we collect the proof, ICPD will continue to be vulnerable in today's global health environment.

A third area of measurement is to improve the tracking of resource flows for reproductive health, particularly at the national and subnational levels. This will improve the accountability of both donors and countries receiving development assistance. It will also ultimately strengthen the evidence base related to the cost-effectiveness of reproductive health interventions. This evidence base is necessary for improving the ability of reproductive health and rights advocates to communicate in the language of economists, many of whom are making the financing decisions, when they "sit at the table."

2. Create and Renew Alliances for Strengthened Advocacy

Ensuring that the global reproductive health agenda is on a secure footing requires not just an evidence base but an understanding of how reproductive health is positioned with respect to other agendas and the ability to forge alliances with key partners. Out of a perceived concern that the reproductive health and rights field had become too diffuse and in the interest of maximizing the impact of this book, the MacArthur Foundation asked the editors and producers of this volume to conduct a social network analysis of the reproductive health field to map out the key players and their relationships to one another.[1] The results of this analysis suggest that the field of reproductive health and rights is a loosely knit network rather than hierarchically organized, and encompasses a great diversity of organizations and individuals. Some actors, such as the International Planned Parenthood Federation or the International Women's Health Coalition, were clearly identified as being central to the field. These organizations tended to be thinkers as well as agenda setters. Others organizations, such as the Black Women's Health Initiative or the International Council of AIDS Service Organizations, were identified as potential bridges to adjacent policy domains. The network analysis findings suggest that there is a core locus to the reproductive health field, and there are key actors who have a unique ability to tap into related networks to further the reproductive health and rights agenda. In other words, there are existing and/or potentially easily constructed bridges into allied fields and disciplines ranging from youth advocacy movements to health systems planners that can bolster the Cairo paradigm. An important lesson from this social networking analysis is that reproductive health and rights supporters—particularly those located in the United States—need not feel as alienated or embattled as they might.

The social network analysis and the recommendations of several contributing authors lead us to a series of proposals for how to use the dynamism of our field's structure more strategically. A first step is to engage more actively advocates and practitioners of reproductive health at the domestic and international levels. This calls for better coordination between women's groups at all levels. Regional and national women's groups play the critical role of providing the evidence of reproductive health problems and the effectiveness of their interventions (Vogel 2006). Ensuring that this evidence is heard at the international level and among a range of stakeholders is an important function for national women's groups. Strong advocacy is needed at the national level (Fathalla 2005) and exists in many countries of the world, but regardless of how strong these women's health movements may be, it does not mean they will be heard at the policy making levels. As Tom Merrick argues, women's health advocates at the national level must be "at the table" when health sector priorities are determined. There is clear evidence of the organizing power of ICPD at regional and national levels that must be better acknowledged and celebrated. The success of regional groups in quashing the U.S. attempts to turn back ICPD at the regional reviews of ICPD+10 is a powerful testament to the organizing and catalytic qualities of ICPD and the movements that supported its development.

An additional level of alliance building is to reextend a hand to those from the population field who took part in the original Cairo consensus. Remembering that the concept of reproductive health and rights is the product of the merging of several networks, we must revisit the alliances that built the ICPD. Recent attention to family planning and population issues in both academic (Cleland et al. 2006) and policy circles suggests the need for reproductive health and rights to revisit its relationship with family planning and population (as George Zeidenstein suggests in his chapter). The release of the hearings in the UK Parliament in 2006 as *The Return of the Population Growth Factor: Its Impact on the Millennium Development Goals* is a recent example of how the issue of population stabilization is becoming more important on global policy agendas (APPG 2007). Without revisiting its relationship with family planning and actively engaging those arguing for family planning and population stabilization, the reproductive health field will lose some of the ground it has gained in this area. Family planning programs are an integral and important part of a comprehensive reproductive health approach, and it is important that family planning be maintained as such.

A third level of alliance building is for the reproductive health field to engage more vigorously with the players in related networks close at hand, particularly in HIV/AIDS and in global health policy. The arguments for doing so have been laid out previously in this volume. One key network to tap entails those concerned with strengthening the global health workforce and health systems in general. Clearly everyone in the health sector is better served by supporting functional and appropriately staffed health services; an alliance between safe motherhood advocates and emergency first responders, for example, makes for a creative alignment of bedfellows that is likely to accomplish more than remaining within our own narrowly defined communities.

Finally, we need to reach out to networks where there may be less immediately common ground. The transnational networks that converged to form a sort of skeleton for ICPD need to be knit together anew. The reproductive health field ought to create room for more actors—particularly development planners and those who are actively engaged with the planning and budgeting process (Vogel 2006). These decision makers are central to the ability to make the reproductive health agenda a reality, and we need to be equipped with the data and analysis to make our case. And if the past decade has taught us little else, we must be prepared to engage with faith-based groups and their leaders with the recognition that culture and faith influence individual women's and men's decisions about sexuality and reproduction in profound ways. As Kissling's chapter argues, a discussion of the moral dimensions of reproductive health decision making needs to be had if the ideas of ICPD are to continue to speak to us.

3. Mobilizing Resources: New Strategies

Briefly, the reproductive health community is operating in an increasingly complicated funding and donor assistance world. On the one hand, there is a move toward vertical single-disease global health initiatives. On the other, countries are being encouraged to move toward sector-wide approaches and general budget support. Much of reproductive health is left out of the vertical single disease funding approach, and much gets lost in the basket approach of the World Bank-supported Poverty Reduction Strategy Papers (PRSPs). This suggests the need for a two-pronged approach to tap these complex new funding mechanisms to raise funds for sexual and reproductive health. In this way, those aspects of reproductive health that align with vertical funding streams can be harnessed and incorporated into sector-wide health budgets. It is critical that reproductive health advocates and supporters of women's rights be part of the decision-making process and become savvy about the new funding processes, such as the Global Fund, as well as the sector-wide approaches that are dominating global health.

While there remains much to do, especially in terms of harnessing financial resources, in order to achieve its important goals, ICPD still has great resonance. Recognizing the conceptual strengths of ICPD and celebrating its successful implementation at the national level are important. The field of reproductive health and rights is dynamic, with a landscape that has, and continues to change. Broadening engagement with actors both inside and outside the field will enable networks of reproductive health advocates and practitioners to respond effectively to the unforeseen challenges of the health and development world.

Notes

Chapter 1. Global Reproductive Health and Rights: Reflecting on ICPD

1. The governments assembled at the 1999 ICPD five-year review in New York reendorsed the concepts unanimously in its revised outcome document (UNFPA 1999).

2. Women from the Global South tended to articulate the connection of discrimination against women to macroeconomic systems leading to underdevelopment, corruption, poverty, and human rights abuses in general. Women's movements in the North tended to bracket race/ethnic and class dimensions and focused more on issues of gender.

3. All the nations of the world have ratified at least one human rights treaty that contains one or more human right relevant to reproductive and sexual health.

4. This famous saying came out of the 1974 Bucharest Conference and was attributed to Karan Singh, the Minister representing India at the conference.

5. It is worth noting that the following year, in 1995, women's rights advocates did succeed in having "sexual rights" recognized in the UN Fourth World Conference on Women at Beijing (para. 96) as the ability to control matters related to sexuality.

6. Conversely, the antecedent term "international health" focused on control of epidemics that could cross national boundaries. Others, such as Derek Yach and Douglas Bettcher, insist that global health tracks the transformations understood as "globalization." They argue that the homogenization of culture and diffusion of market values has allowed pathways for ideas and commodities as well as for disease and unhealthy lifestyles to circle the globe at unprecedented rates. From this perspective, international responses to global challenges to public health need multilateral coordination (led by an institution such as WHO) (Brown, Cueto, and Fee 2006).

7. We recognize that not all approaches to global public health take a vertical view. There are champions of addressing underlying social conditions (Farmer 2003), as well as attempts at contextualizing diseases such as tuberculosis, malaria, and HIV as diseases of poverty in the research, design, and implementation of programs (WHO Commission on Social Determinants of Health 2007; WHO Special Programme for Research and Training in Tropical Diseases 2007). There is also emerging insistence on health systems and health infrastructure (see WHO Global Health Workforce Alliance 2007). The latter, however, is slightly redolent of neoverticalization in that it focuses on one piece of the comprehensive approach to health.

8. The MDGs, indeed the greater UN reform processes, might be viewed as a move toward greater verticality in international policy, in the service of greater accountability (see Larson and Reich, this volume). During the 1990s, a series of UN-sponsored conferences were held, ICPD among them. Each conference spawned an outcome document, similar to the ICPD Programme of Action, which called on governments to meet an array of time-bound targets and to implement wide ranging development, health, education, environmental, financial, human rights, and other programs. Whatever might be said of these processes in terms of inefficiency and expense, global civil society participated and helped generate these outcome documents (Petchesky 2003). In other words, these conference processes helped construct the international communities' joint ownership with government of the problems and their solutions. The 2000 Millennium Summit was different. It sought to consolidate the outcome documents and their action points into a simplified and attainable document. The Summit was a process driven from the UN secretary general, tasked to high level bureaucratic appointees, and delivered as the Millennium Development Goals, to be endorsed by the General Assembly. The participants tended to represent finance ministries and donors rather than individual social sectors. While the MDGs were based on already agreed upon international development goals, there were significant omissions with regard to ICPD (see Girard, this volume). What may have arguably been gained by MDG streamlining may have been lost in terms of global ownership. And whether the MDGs endure as the measure for international development policy remains to be seen.

9. As part of his efforts to restructure the U.S. foreign aid system, in 2006 George W. Bush shifted USAID to the State Department rather than allowing it to be a stand-alone agency. The Bush administration also created a variety of new coordinating bodies for global health (Coordinating Office of Global Health at the Centers for Disease Control and Prevention; Office of Global Health Affairs, Department of Health and Human Services; and Office of the U.S. Global AIDS Coordinator). We focus on USAID because of its long history in the field of population.

10. In a similar manner to USAID, the Gates Foundation fashions reproductive health in its own image, while nonetheless acknowledging that "reproductive and maternal health" (defined as "reducing deaths and illness related to pregnancy and prevent unintended pregnancies") (Gates Foundation 2007) is an important priority condition. However, it separates out the ICPD agenda and focuses only on the parts that are amenable to its method of operation, objectives, and values. It funds research and programming related to HIV/AIDS—principally prevention (vaccine/microbicide research)—and some aspects of maternal and neonatal health to the extent that procurement, distribution, and use of vitamins, nutrients, clean water, immunization, and contraception will substantially alleviate the burden of these diseases. Gates contributed substantial financial support to the Averting Maternal Death and Disability Project, which did adopt a broader approach to the delivery of appropriate emergency care; after five years, and a favorable review; however; the foundation chose to not renew its grant (see Roseman, this volume).

Chapter 2. The Global Reproductive Health and Rights Agenda: Opportunities and Challenges for the Future

1. There are many other policy agendas that address reproductive health (national, subnational, and local); this chapter addresses the global policy agenda because of its potential global influence on funding and political support for reproductive health.

2. A large political science literature examines the influences on the agenda setting process. See, for example, Cobb and Ross (1997) and Rochefort and Cobb (1994). In public health, see Reich (1995); Shiffman (2007) and Shiffman, Beer and Wu (2002).

3. See the series of commentaries in *Studies in Family Planning* (June 2005) for different perspectives on the intersections of reproductive health and the MDGs.

4. Reproductive health addresses socially, culturally, and politically charged issues (such as abortion and provision of reproductive health services to adolescents); hence many politicians and policy makers are shying away from the area in this recently politically conservative time.

5. See for example the range of examples on abortion alone presented in *Reproductive Health Matters* 13 (November 2005).

6. The Global Gag Rule refers to the Mexico City Policy, which mandates that no U.S. family planning assistance can be provided to foreign NGOs that perform abortions, provide counseling or referral for abortions, or lobby to make abortion legal or more available in their country. It was reinstated by President George W. Bush on his first day in office in January 2001.

7. See the introduction to this volume for more discussion of the impact of global health on reproductive health.

8. These estimates are slightly lower than the original ICPD estimates but do not include several costs (e.g., facility upgrades, additional health personnel training, community mobilization, HIV/AIDS treatment and care) (Ethelston and Leahy 2006).

9. BOD measures the burden of ill health in a population in disability-adjusted life years (DALYs), which provide a measure of mortality and morbidity related to a particular disease or disability. The BOD and DALYs were the basis for the 1993 World Bank Development Report, *Investing in Health* (World Bank 1993), which has influenced priority setting at the international level as well as the international donor community. Bill Gates read the report more than twice, calling it "a really nice piece of work" and stating that "the DALY concept led Gates and his wife to their first large grant" (Specter 2005: 11).

10. The limitations of the application of BOD and DALYs to reproductive health are well documented (AbouZahr 1999; AbouZahr and Vaughn 2000 among others; Kaufman, this volume) and only briefly mentioned. The well-developed literature critiquing the DALY approach in general is not reviewed here.

Chapter 4. Population, Poverty Reduction, and the Cairo Agenda

1. There is evidence that in the early stages of the transition fertility falls initially among the better-off households, which may widen income gaps and do little for poverty alleviation. However, there is evidence of a cultural spillover effect, with low fertility among elites and highly educated women being echoed

in lower fertility among poorer, less educated women at a much earlier stage than might be expected.

Chapter 5. Mobilizing Resources for Reproductive Health

The views presented here are those of the author and do not represent those of the World Bank or WBI. Many of the points draw on content in WBI's learning program on Poverty, Reproductive Health and Health Sector Reform, as reported in Campbell White, Merrick, and Yazbeck 2006. See also Bernstein and Juul Hansen 2006.

1. That is, available at the time this chapter was initially drafted in 2006.

Chapter 6. Measuring Reproductive Health: From Contraceptive Prevalence to Human Development Indicators

1. They included the following major categories: pregnancy and delivery services including maternal nutrition, quality family planning services, prevention and treatment of reproductive tract infections; sexually transmitted infections and HIV/AIDS; legal abortion services and post-abortion care; adolescent health, prevention of violence against women (female genital cutting, domestic violence, conflict, and emergency situations); voluntarism in childbearing and abortion; sexual rights; reproductive rights.

2. For example, that reduced fertility leads to reduced infant mortality which leads to higher life expectancy, or that reduced fertility leads to higher labor force participation and educational opportunities for women.

3. Ford Foundation Reproductive Health Affinity Group Indicators Committee—Joan Kaufman, Chair, Meiwita Budiharsana, Sarah Costa, Lisa Messersmith, David Winters.

4. Articulated by Amartya Sen in *Development as Freedom* (1999) as the "capabilities approach," it posits that freedom to achieve the fruits of development is as important as the goods and services of development themselves. In this context, agency is a critical index of development, beyond the provision by governments of social development investments and services.

5. Two meetings with external experts were held. A meeting in New York, hosted by IPPF in October 2000, included Rashidah Abdullah, Sajeda Amin, Jane Bertrand, Krishna Bose, Yvette Cuca, Que Dang, Charlotte Ellertson, Lynn Freedman, Alesandra Guedes, Lori Heise, Judith Helzner, Jodi Jacobson, Shireen Jejeebhoy, Pallavi Patel, Rosalind Petchesky, Gita Pillai, Barbara Pillsbury, Geeta Rao Gupta, Iqbal Shah, Melissa Sharer, Margaret (Peg) Sutton, Victoria Ward, Ellen Weiss, and Nancy Yinger. A second meeting was held in Oaxaca, Mexico, in 2001 to which Geeta Rao Gupta was invited to work with the Ford Foundation Indicators Committee to develop the attached conceptual frameworks.

6. The language of the recommended goal is as follows: "Universal access to reproductive health services by 2015 through the primary health system ensuring the same rate of progress or faster amongst the poor and other marginalized groups" (UN 2005a, para. 57(g)).

7. Sexual health issues, as defined by WHO, include the following: HIV/STIs/RTIs, unplanned pregnancy/unsafe abortion, infertility, "sexual well-

being" (sexual satisfaction), gender-based violence, mental health, and female genital mutilation (WHO 2004).

8. Indicators should cover the Enabling Context for Development (such as cultural, secular, and religious legitimacy of women's agency and rights, including laws supportive of women's autonomy and choice); the Pre-requisite Conditions for Sexual and Reproductive Health and Gender Equity (such as gender equitable relationships); Intermediate Outcomes at the Community level for Sexual and Reproductive Health and Gender Equity (such as school-based sex education services); Individual Health Outcomes for women, youth, men (such as healthy use of contraception, abortion, safe pregnancy and delivery, adequate nutrition, prevention and treatment of STIs/RTIs/HIV), prevention and treatment/referral for domestic violence, prevention of other diseases such as malaria, TB, that affect reproductive health; and Intergenerational Outcomes (such as impact of maternal nutrition and infectious disease exposure on children's health).

Chapter 7. Bearing Human Rights: Maternal Health and the Promise of ICPD

1. There has been some serious criticism of the persistent inaccuracies in data surrounding maternal mortality, and the reliance on estimates (Graham and Hussein 2004). It has been suggested, for example, that better data collection may in fact account for the seeming lack of progress (Safe Motherhood Inter-Agency Group 1998). For the purposes of this chapter, we accept for heuristic purposes the global maternal mortality estimates. Additionally, maternal mortality figures are often used as rhetorical place holders or proxies for maternal morbidity—with exponentially more measurement hurdles. It is estimated that there are ten times more injuries than deaths due to pregnancy and childbearing (Hafez 1998).

2. Maternal health is also a useful example of both the challenges and necessity of a rights-based approach to reproductive health. Evidence from these efforts helps define such approaches, which are particularly important as international, national, and nongovernmental agencies look to rights-based approaches as a panacea, not only for reproductive and sexual health, but also for HIV/AIDS, humanitarian crises, and even poverty alleviation.

3. I do not mean to suggest that mothers are irrelevant to their children's survival. Significant correlations exist between the health and education status of women and that of their children (see Jejeebhoy 1996). Nonetheless, this literature participates in instrumentalizing women rather than considering their status as an end in itself.

4. The agencies were UNICEF, UNDP, UNFPA, World Bank, and WHO, along with the International Planned Parenthood Federation and Population Council. Together they formed the Safe-Motherhood Inter-Agency Group after the conference; Family Care International later became the secretariat. Insofar as two international movements called for attention to maternal mortality, a number of women's rights activists would rather have guarded approval of SMI as it principally defined women in terms of motherhood, thereby vilifying any other choice for women (see Berer and Ravindran 1999). Virtually concurrently, a group of women's health and rights activists in 1987 proclaimed its 1988 International Day of Action for Women's Health as focused on "Preventing Maternal Mortality."

5. Many SMI recommendations for action reflect this insight: they were targeted to improve women's status through better education, nutrition, economic independence, and political participation. There were also recommendations, therefore, to improve access to family planning information and services, to develop appropriate technology and management systems, and to secure adequate financing for the recommendations. Finally, NGOs were acknowledged to be an integral element to the success of all interventions.

6. It has to be mentioned that, despite ICPD's potential for connecting reproductive rights with maternal mortality reduction, its Achilles' heel is contained in paragraph 8.25—the compromise that dare not allow abortion to be considered a necessary intervention to terminate unintended pregnancies (see Berer, this volume). In ICPD abortion access was restricted to after-the-fact life saving care and treatment (unless already legal). Where abortion is illegal, there tends to be inadequate access to appropriate family planning services, reflecting discriminatory attitudes toward women. In such contexts it is more likely that women will self abort or seek out abortion services wherever they might be found (Berer 2004). Invariably, many women die of sepsis and hemorrhage, making unsafe abortion a significant direct cause of maternal mortality. In certain respects, the abortion "compromise" reflects the persistent ambivalence in viewing women as individuals rather than vehicles to produce infants (Petchesky 1987). This ambivalence constrains the robust foundation of reproductive agency that the ICPD Programme of Action otherwise articulates.

7. There was a lively, not entirely friendly division of opinion regarding what to do in the name of saving women's lives. See, e.g., Liljestrand and Jerker 2000 (reviewing more broad-based interventions, including TBAs) and Maine and Yamin 1999 (prioritizing emergency obstetric care).

8. As economic, social, and cultural rights obligations are understood to be progressively realized, there is not necessarily a bright line target to which to hold governments accountable. Paul Hunt, UN Special Rapporteur on the Right to the Highest Attainable Standard of Health, uses the following formulation: "Ill health constitutes a human rights violation when it arises, in whole or in part, from the failure of a duty-bearer—typically a State—to respect, protect, or fulfill a human rights obligation. Obstacles stand between individuals and their enjoyment of sexual and reproductive health. From the human rights perspective, a key question is: are human rights duty-bearers doing all in their power to dismantle these barriers?" (UN 2004).

9. One caveat to note is that while indicators such as number of health facilities can show priorities and be used to argue for more resources, it is not at all settled that a failure to meet UN indicators is a human rights violation.

10. The formal international human rights system is based on the Universal Declaration of Human Rights and the eight (and soon to be nine) UN international human rights treaties.

11. For a compilation of relevant treaty body outputs see ACPD 2006.

12. The Center for Reproductive Rights has recently undertaken litigation as part of its strategy to advance women's rights relating to safe pregnancy. It is in the process of filing a petition before the Inter-American Commission due to the death of a pregnant young woman of preventable and treatable causes (pers. communication with Luisa Cabal, Director of International Programs, CRR, November 2007).

13. Research was undertaken using the Office of the High Commissioner for Human Rights treaty body database at www.ohchr.org cross referenced against

the UN Human Rights Treaties database at www.bayefsky.com. Search terms were maternity and pregnancy for the Human Rights Committee and Committee on Economic, Social and Cultural Right (CESCR). Other relevant treaty bodies would include the Committee on Elimination of Discrimination Against Women (CEDAW) and the Committee on the Rights of the Child (CRC).

14. Similarly, CESCR has adopted the human rights analysis relating maternal mortality to the nonfulfillment of the right to health (see UN 1966b, para. 417, 435). The Committee recommends that the state party take measures to reduce child and maternal mortality, and in particular intensify the implementation of its national program on reproductive health, provide further assistance and training to midwives, organize educational campaigns regarding women's sexual and reproductive health, and include such subjects in the school curricula.

15. Both Amnesty International and Human Rights Watch are undertaking fact finding and advocacy strategies in this area. See Amnesty International 2006; Human Rights Watch 2006.

16. The study found that 593 maternal deaths occur for every 100,000 live births and the majority of the maternal deaths (92%) were reported from rural areas. This figure ranks the province of Herat, Afghanistan with the highest rate of maternal mortality outside the African continent. The maternal mortality ratio for Herat Province also exceeds that of all five countries bordering Afghanistan: Pakistan (200/100,000), Iran (60/100,000), Turkmenistan (65/100,000), China (60/100,000), and Tajikistan (120/100,000). In contrast, the United States has an estimated ratio of 12/100,000.

17. Deadly Delays: Maternal Mortality in Peru: a Rights-Based Approach to Safe Motherhood was launched in Spanish in Peru in December 2007 (Physicians for Human Rights, pers. communication 2007).

18. The author of this chapter was involved with this project (as was Sofia Gruskin, a contributor to this collection as well).

19. Its founding members are Averting Maternal Death and Disability Program, Mailman School of Public Health, Columbia University; CARE; Center for Reproductive Rights; Family Care International; Physicians for Human Rights; and UN Special Rapporteur on the Right to the Highest Attainable Standard of Health (Paul Hunt).

20. Such an argument, I believe, does not "reinstrumentalize" motherhood, but rather recognizes and promotes the equal dignity and worth of each individual's life.

Chapter 8. Advocacy Strategies for Young People's Sexual and Reproductive Health: Using UN Processes

1. In official definitions in the UN system, adolescents are ages 10-19, young people are ages 10-24, and youth are ages 15-24. This chapter generally uses "young people" as the most inclusive, but much HIV literature and indicators refer to youth, while ICPD generally refers to "adolescents." The Convention on the Rights of the Child applies to adolescents up to age 18.

2. Calculated from the World Bank Development Data online, in the demographic projections section, total population of 10-24-year-olds taken from 2005 projections.

3. There is copious literature on this subject (see Rivers and Aggleton 1999; WHO 2001b).

4. The most common form of child labor for girls is domestic service, where the risk of sexual harassment from male members of the household is well known.

5. The agreements discussed here include the ICPD Programme of Action, the Beijing Fourth World Conference on Women in 1995, and subsequent consensus agreements in UN conferences, including the 5- and 10-year reviews of ICPD and Beijing, and the UN General Assembly special sessions (UNGASS) on HIV/AIDS in 2001 and Children in 2002.

6. ". . . by 2005, ensure that at least 90 per cent, and by 2010 at least 95 per cent, of young men and women aged 15 to 24 have access to the information, education and services necessary to develop the life skills required to reduce their vulnerability to HIV infection. Services should include access to preventive methods such as female and male condoms, voluntary testing, counselling and follow-up" (UN 1999b: 70).

7. The Center for Reproductive Rights (2002) wrote an account of these negotiations, with a copy of the draft document with all bracketed paragraphs under dispute.

8. Advocates frequently remark that diplomatic memories are short due to turnover in governments and their delegations at the UN, who routinely need education on the content of ICPD and ICPD+5, including the commitments to provide young people with sexual and reproductive health information, education, and services.

9. The United States of America and Somalia have not ratified the Convention.

10. See articles 3, 6, 17, and 24 of the Convention on the Rights of the Child (UN 1989) and article 12 on the right to health of the International Convention on Economic, Social and Cultural Rights (UN 1966b).

11. This seems like useful language for LGBT rights advocates.

12. "Child marriage" is the more precise term, since the UN system defines all individuals under the age of 18 as children, but it is less commonly used.

13. See regional prevalence statistics (Population Reference Bureau 2006). The Population Council website also has several useful resources on child marriage.

14. Shepard and DeJong 2005 contains information on age of marriage laws in the Arab states and Iran in Chapter 2 (Table 2.2, p. 25); Annex Three contains comments by treaty bodies to each country on issues related to young people's sexual and reproductive health, which include comments on early marriage laws and/or practices. For the Latin American and Caribbean Region, Julieta LeMaitre collected pertinent legal data on age of marriage and age of consent, available from the author, or from the regional UNICEF office adolescent program. The Demographic Yearbook 2003, Table 24, has legal marriage data on some countries in the world (UN Department of Economic and Social Affairs 2003a).

15. "Beijing+5" language: "Develop, adopt and fully implement laws and other measures, as appropriate, such as policies and educational programmes, to eradicate harmful customary or traditional practices, including female genital mutilation, early and forced marriage and so-called honour crimes, which are violations of the human rights of women and girls and obstacles to the full enjoyment by women of their human rights and fundamental freedoms" (UN 2000b). Also, "World Fit for Children" reaffirmed this definition, calling for countries to "end harmful traditional or customary practices, such as early and

forced marriage and female genital mutilation, which violate the rights of children and women" (UNICEF 2003: 9).

16. Article 24.3. "States Parties shall take all effective and appropriate measures with a view to abolishing traditional practices prejudicial to the health of children."

17. Article 16.2. "The betrothal and the marriage of a child shall have no legal effect, and all necessary action, including legislation, shall be taken to specify a minimum age for marriage and to make the registration of marriages in an official registry compulsory."

18. In its interpretation of Article 16 (2) of the Convention, para. 36.

19. See note 14.

Chapter 10. Technology, Reproductive Health, and the Cairo Consensus

1. Since this chapter was first drafted, additional microbicide trials have been launched. See http://www.microbicide.org/cs/news_alert_detail?pressrelease .id=53, accessed 30 July 2008.

Chapter 11. The Cairo "Compromise" on Abortion and Its Consequences for Making Abortion Safe and Legal

Thanks to Barbara Crane for helpful comments.

1. In a study in India, for example, 21 of 66 women interviewed considered unwanted pregnancy and abortion a direct consequence of nonconsensual sex, often accompanied by violence when the woman resisted (Ravindran and Balasubramanian 2004).

2. Technical assistance is defined as the transfer of goods and services to another organization. Goods include equipment. Services include organization, facilitation, and participation in workshops, technical meetings, training and program assessments (White House 2001).

3. Although there are no data confirming this, it was widely agreed to be the case among participants at the conference Medical Abortion: An International Forum on Policies, Programmes and Services, Johannesburg, 17-20 October 2004.

4. Whether or not national policy would succeed in doing so was the subject of debate at the conference of the International Society for the Scientific Study of Population, Tours, July 2005.

Chapter 12. Advocacy for Sexuality and Women's Rights: Continuities, Discontinuities, and Strategies Since ICPD

1. For a more detailed discussion about the complexities of global coalition building among the disparate women's rights and health movements, see Garcia-Moreno and Claro 1994 and Correa and Reichmann 1994.

2. Written statements submitted to the Programme of Action, http//www.unfpa.org/icpd/icpd_poa.htm#pt2ch2.

3. In particular, the International Women's Health Coalition, Development Alternatives with Women for a New Era (DAWN), WEDO, and the Center for Women's Global Leadership.

4. The United States of America General Reservation, 17 December 2002, on file with the author.

5. At ICPD+10, no reservations were issued by governments in Asia-Pacific except for the lengthy U.S. "general reservation"; in Latin America and the Caribbean, the U.S. did not join the consensus in the initial meeting in Santiago in March 2004, and therefore had no need to issue a reservation; thinking better of it, the U.S. joined the consensus in the subsequent meeting in Puerto Rico in July 2004, and issued a reservation, along with Costa Rica, Nicaragua, and El Salvador; in Africa, no reservations were entered (the U.S. is not a member of the Economic Commission for Africa).

6. At the Beijing+10 meeting in Mexico, the U.S., El Salvador, and Nicaragua entered reservations.

Chapter 13. Situating Reproductive Health Within the Academy

1. As Gita Sen also highlighted at the IUSSP General Conference in Tours in 2005 (Sen 2005b).

Chapter 14. The Political Limits of the United Nations in Advancing Reproductive Health and Rights

1. The Commission on Population and Development was established in 1946 as the Population Commission, but was renamed following ICPD. It is supported by the UN Population Division.

2. *The State of World Population* 2004 report (UNFPA 2004b) specifically focused on "The Cairo Consensus at Ten: Population, Reproductive Health and the Global Effort to End Poverty."

Chapter 16. Conclusion: Conceptual Successes and Operational Challenges to ICPD: Global Reproductive Health and Rights Moving Forward

1. This study, conducted by Mark Pachucki in June-August 2006, is entitled "Mapping the Field of Global Reproductive Health and Rights; Network Analysis Report" (26 September 2006, on file with editors).

Bibliography

Abernathy M. 2005. *Planning for a Sustainable Supply of Manual Vacuum Aspiration Instruments: A Guide for Program Managers.* Chapel Hill, N.C.: IPAS.

AbouZahr C. 1999. "Disability Adjusted Life Years (DALYs) and Reproductive Health: A Critical Analysis." *Reproductive Health Matters* 7, no. 14: 118–29.

AbouZahr C and Vaughn JP. 2000. "Assessing the Burden of Sexual and Reproductive Ill-Health." *Bulletin of the World Health Organization* 78: 665–76.

Action Canada for Population and Development and International Programme on Reproductive and Sexual Health Law at the University of Toronto. 2006a. *The Application of Human Rights to Reproductive & Sexual Health: A Compilation of the Work of International Human Rights Treaty Bodies.* 3rd ed. Ottawa: Action Canada for Population and Development.

———. 2006b. *Report on the Integration of HIV/AIDS and Sexual and Reproductive Health and Rights.* Ottawa: Action Canada for Population and Development, Ottawa. Accessed 20 April 2007 at http://www.acpd.ca/pdf/Report %20on%20Integration%20of%20HIVAIDS%20and%20SRHR%202006.pdf

African Union. 2003. Protocol to the African Charter on Human and Peoples' Rights on the Rights of Women in Africa. Maputo: African Union. Accessed 1 May 2007 at www.africa-union.org

AIDS Vaccine Advocacy Coalition (AVAC). 2005. *Follow the Money: Money, Development and Research in AIDS Vaccines at the Crossroads.* New York: AVAC.

Aitken IW. 1999. The Implications of Health sector reform for reproductive health and rights. Report of a meeting of the Working Group on Reproductive Health and Family Planning, December 14–15, 1998, Washington, D.C./Tacoma Park, Maryland: Center for Health and Gender Equity [CHANGE]/Population Council: 14–22.

All Party Parliamentary Group on Population, Development and Reproductive Health. 2007. Return of the Population Growth Factor: Its Impact on the MDGs. Report of Hearings by the All Party Parliamentary Group on Population, Development and Reproductive Health, United Kingdom Parliament, London. Accessed 2 August 2007 at http://www.appg-popde vrh.org.uk

Alliance for Microbicide Development. 2007. Alliance for Microbicide Development. Accessed 13 July at http://www.microbicide.org. See http://www.microbicide.org/cs/news_alert_detail?pressrelease.id=53, accessed 30 July 2008.

Allotey P and Reidpath D. 2002. "Objectivity in Priority Setting Tools in Reproductive Health: Context and the DALY." *Reproductive Health Matters* 10, no. 20: 28–46.

Americans for UNFPA. 2006. "Bush Administration Withholds Funds for Global

Women's Health for Fifth Year." Press release, 20 July 2006. Accessed 2 August 2007 at http://www.americansforunfpa.org/NetCommunity/Page.aspx?& pid=345&srcid=253

Amnesty International. 2007. Amnesty International Defends Access to Abortion for Women at Risk. Media release, AI Index: POL 30/012/2007 (Public) News Service 110, 14 June. Accessed 25 July 2007 at http://web.amnesty .org/library/index/ENGPOL300122007

———. 2006. Peru: Poor and Excluded Women: Denial of the Right to Maternal and Child Health. AI Index: AMR 46/004/2006.

Amuchastegui Herrera A and Rivas Zivy M. 2002. "Clandestine Abortion in Mexico: A Question of Mental as Well as Physical Health." *Reproductive Health Matters* 10, no. 19: 95–102.

Anglican Church of Canada. 2002. "Ugandan Priest Infected, Affected by AIDS." 29 November 2002. Accessed 11 July 2007 at http://www.anglican.ca/news/ news.php?newsItem=2002-11-29_xx.news

Annan K. 2006. "In Truman Library Speech, Annan Says UN Remains Best Tool to Achieve Key Goals of International Relations." Speech at Truman Library, 11 December, United Nations, New York. Accessed 13 July 2007 at http://www.un.org/News/ossg/sg/stories/statments_full.asp?statID=40

Ashford LS. 2001. "New Populations Policies: Advancing Women's Health and Rights." *Population Bulletin* 56, no. 1. Washington, D.C.: Population Reference Bureau. Accessed 3 June 2007 at http://www.prb.org/pdf/56.1NewPop PoliciesWomen_Eng.pdf

Askew I and Berer M. 2003. "The Contribution of Sexual and Reproductive Health Services to the Fight Against HIV/AIDS: A Review." *Reproductive Health Matters* 11, no. 22: 51–73.

Averting Maternal Death and Disability Program. 2007. Emergency Obstetric Care, Heilbrunn Department of Population and Family Health, Mailman School of Public Health, Columbia University. Accessed 30 April at http://www.amddprogram.org/index.php?sub=2_1

———. 2006. Report 1999-2005. New York. Accessed 10 September 2007 at http://www.amddprogram.org/resources/1999_2005_report.pdf

Baker B. 2007. *A New Low in the Pharma Drug Wars—Abbott Withdraws Seven Medicines in Thailand.* New York: Health GAP. Accessed 13 July at www.health gap.org/camp/thailand-abbottnewlow.doc

Basu AM. 2005. "The Millennium Development Goals Minus Reproductive Health: An Unfortunate, but Not Disastrous, Omission." *Studies in Family Planning* 36, no. 2: 132–34.

———. 1997. "The New International Population Movement: A Framework for a Constructive Critique." *Health Transition Review* 4, no. 7 (suppl): 7-32.

———. 1996. "The International Conference on Population and Development: What About Men's Rights and Women's Responsibilities?" *Health Transition Review* 6, no. 2: 225–27.

Becker J and Leitman E. n.d. *Introducing Sexuality Within Family Planning: The Experience of the HIV/STD Prevention Projects from Latin America and the Caribbean.* Quality/Calidad/Qualitéseries 8. New York: Population Council. Accessed 20 April 2007 at http://www.popcouncil.org/pdfs/qcq/qcq08.pdf

Becker S. 1999. "Measuring Unmet Need: Wives, Husbands or Couples?" *International Family Planning Perspectives* 25, no. 4: 172–80.

Berer M. 2004. "National Laws and Unsafe Abortion: The Parameters of Change." *Reproductive Health Matters* 12, no. 24: 1–8.

Berer M and Ravindran TKS. 1999. "Preventing Maternal Mortality: Evidence, Resources, Leadership, Action." In M Berer and TKS Ravindran (eds.), *Safe Motherhood Initiatives: Critical Issues.* Oxford: Reproductive Health Matters.

Bernstein S and Juul Hansen C. 2006. *Public Choices, Private Decisions, Sexual and Reproductive Health and the Millennium Development Goals.* New York: UN Millennium Project. Accessed 20 July 2007 at http://www.unfpa.org/publica tions/docs/sexual_health.pdf

Bertrand JT and Escudero G. 2002. *Compendium of Indicators for Evaluating Reproductive Health Programs,* vols. 1, 2. Chapel Hill, N.C.: Evaluation Project.

Bertrand JT, Magnani RJ, and Knowles JC. 1994. *Handbook of Indicators for Family Planning Program Evaluation.* Chapel Hill, N.C.: Evaluation Project.

Bertrand JT and Tsui A. 1995. *Indicators for Reproductive Health Program Evaluation.* Introduction and Final Report of the Subcommittees on Adolescents, STD/HIV, Women's Nutrition, Breastfeeding, Safe Pregnancy. Chapel Hill, N.C.: The Evaluation Project.

Billings DL and Benson J. 2005. "Postabortion Care in Latin America: Policy and Service Recommendations from a Decade of Operations Research." *Health Policy & Planning* 20, no. 3: 158–66.

Billings DL, Moreno C, Ramos C, et al. 2002. "Constructing Access to Legal Abortion in Mexico City." *Reproductive Health Matters* 10, no. 19: 86–94.

Birdsall N and Sinding SW. 1999. "How and Why Population Matters: New Findings, New Issues." In N Birdsall, AC Kelley, and SW Sinding (eds.), *Population Matters: Demographic Change, Economic Growth, and Poverty in the Developing World.* New York: Oxford University Press.

Birn A. 2005. "Gates's Grandest Challenge: Transcending Technology as Public Health Ideology." *The Lancet* 366: 514–19.

Blanc AK and Tsui AO. 2005. "The Dilemma of Past Success: Insiders' Views on the Future of the International Family Planning Movement." *Studies in Family Planning* 36, no. 4: 63–275.

Block J. 2003. "Christian Soldiers on the March." *The Nation,* 3 February, 2. Accessed 25 July 2007 at http://www.thenation.com/doc/20030203/block/2

Bloom DE and Canning D. 2005. "Population, Poverty Reduction, and the Cairo Agenda." In *Report on Seminar on the Relevance of Population Aspects for the Achievement of the Millennium Development Goals.* New York: United Nations.

———. 2003. "How Demographic Change Can Bolster Economic Performance in Developing Countries." *World Economics* 4: 1–14.

Bloom DE, Canning D, Graham B and Sevilla J. 2007. "Global Integration and the Reduction of Poverty." In MR Agosín, DE Bloom, G Chapelier, and J Saigal (eds.), *Solving the Riddle of Globalization and Development.* London: Routledge.

Bloom DE, Canning D, and Malaney P. 2000. "Demographic Change and Economic Growth in Asia." *Population and Development Review* 26, suppl. 1: 257–90.

Bloom DE, Canning D, and Sevilla J. 2003. *The Demographic Dividend: A New Perspective on the Economic Consequences of Population Change.* Population Matters Series. Santa Monica, Calif.: Rand. Accessed 11 July 2007 at http://www.rand.org/pubs/monograph_reports/2007/MR1274.pdf

Bloom DE, Mahal A, Rosenberg L, Sevilla J, et al. 2004. *Asia's Economies and the Challenge of AIDS.* Manila: Asian Development Bank. Accessed 11 July 2007 at http://www.adb.org/Documents/Books/Asia-AIDS/default.asp

Blum R. 2005. "Adolescent Health: Global Issues, Local Challenges." *EJournal*

USA, Growing Up Healthy 10, no. 1. Accessed 18 June 2006 at http://usinfo.state.gov/journals/itgic/0105/ijge/blum.htm

Bogecho D and Upreti M. 2006. "The Global Gag Rule—An Antithesis to the Rights Based Approach to Health." *Health and Human Rights* 9, no. 1: 17–32.

Bok S. 1994. "Population and Ethics: Expanding the Moral Space." In G Sen, A Germain, and L Chen (eds.), *Population Policies Reconsidered: Health, Empowerment, and Rights*. Cambridge, Mass.: Harvard University Press.

Boland R, Rao S and Zeidenstein G. 1994. "Honoring Human Rights in Population Policies: From Declaration to Action." In G Sen, A Germain, and L Chen (eds.), *Population Policies Reconsidered: Health, Empowerment, and Rights*. Cambridge, Mass.: Harvard University Press.

Bongaarts J. 1978. "A Framework for Analyzing the Proximate Determinants of Fertility." *Population and Development Review* 4, no. 1: 105–32.

Bongaarts J, Mauldin WP, and Phillips JF. 1990. "The Demographic Impact of Family Planning Programs." *Studies in Family Planning* 21, no. 6: 299–310.

Borghi J, Ensor T, Somanthian A, et al. on behalf of The Lancet Maternal Survival Series Steering Group. 2006. "Mobilising Financial Resources for Maternal Health." *The Lancet* 368, no. 9545: 1457–65.

Bose A. 1995. "The Family Welfare Programme in India: Changing Paradigm." In H Mohan Mathur (ed.), *The Family Welfare Programme in India*. Delhi: Vikasi.

Boseley S. 2006. "Gates Breaks Ranks with Attack on US Aids Policy." *The Guardian*, 15 August. Accessed 24 July 2007 at http://www.guardian.co.uk/aids/story/0,1844772,00.html

Boserup M. 1978. "Fear of Doomsday: Past and Present." *Population and Development Review* 4, no. 1: 133-43.

"Brazil to Ease Abortions for Pregnant Rape Victims." 2005. *Reproductive Health Matters* 13, no. 26: 186.

Brown TM, Cueto M, and Fee E. 2006. "The World Health Organization and the Transition from "International" to "Global" Public Health." *American Journal of Public Health* 96, no. 1: 62–72.

Brown W. 1997. "The Impossibility of Women's Studies." *Differences* 9, no. 3: 79–101.

Bruce J. 1994, "Population Policy Must Encompass More than Family Planning Services." in LA Mazur (ed.), *Beyond the Numbers: A Reader on Population, Consumption and the Environment*. Washington, D.C.: Island Press.

Bruce J and Clark S. 2004. *The Implications of Early Marriage for HIV/AIDS Policy*. New York: Population Council. Accessed 30 April 2007 at www.popcouncil.org/pdfs/EMBfinalENG.pdf

———. 2003. "Including Married Adolescents in Adolescent Reproductive Health and HIV/AIDS Policy." Paper prepared for WHO/UNFPA/Population Council Technical Consultation on Married Adolescents, 9–12 December. Accessed 5 March 2006 at http://www.popcouncil.org/pdfs/CMImplications.pdf

de Bruyn M. 2002. *Reproductive Choice and Women Living with HIV*. Chapel Hill, N.C.: Ipas.

Bulatao RA. 1998. *The Value of Family Planning Programs in Developing Countries*. Los Angeles: RAND.

Bunch C. 1995. "Transforming Human Rights from a Feminist Perspective." In J Peters and A Wolper (eds.), *Women's Rights, Human Rights*. New York: Routledge.

Campbell White A, Merrick TW, and Yazbeck AS. 2006. *Reproductive Health: The Missing Millennium Development Goal.* Washington, D.C.: World Bank.

Canadian International Development Agency. 2007. Canada's New Government Announces Funding to Help Women and Reconstruction in Kandahar. Media release, 8 January. Accessed 30 April at http://www.acdicida.gc.ca/CIDAWEB/acdicida.nsf/En/MIC-181047-KP6

Caro DA, Murray SF, and Putney P. 2004. Evaluation of the Averting Maternal Death and Disability Program. Columbia University, New York. Accessed 30 April 2007 at http://www.amddprogram.org/resources/2004%20AMDD%20EVALUATION%20REPORT.pdf

Casterline JB and Sinding SW. 2000. "Unmet Need for Family Planning in Developing Countries and Implications for Population Policy." *Population and Development Review* 26, no. 4: 691–723.

Catholic World News. 2004. Doctors Seek Legalization of Anencephaly Abortion in Peru. Accessed 1 May 2007 at http://www.cwnews.com/news/viewstory.cfm?recnum=33647.

Center for Communication Programs. 2007. Resources for HIV/AIDS and Sexual and Reproductive Health Integration. Accessed 13 July at http://hivandsrh.org

Center for Reproductive Law and Policy. 2002. *Abortion in Nepal: Women Imprisoned.* New York: Forum for Women, Law and Development, Center for Reproductive Law and Policy.

———. 1999. *Reproductive Rights of Young Girls and Adolescents in Mali: Shadow Report.* New York: Center for Reproductive Law and Policy. Accessed 1 August 2007 at http://www.reproductiverights.org/pdf/sr_mali_0999_eng.pdf

Center for Reproductive Rights. 2007. *The World's Abortion Laws.* New York: Center for Reproductive Rights.

———. 2005. UN Human Rights Committee Makes Landmark Decision Establishing Women's Right to Access to Legal Abortion. Accessed 17 November at www.reproductiverights.org/pr_05_1117KarenPeru.html

———. 2003. *The Bush Global Gag Rule: Endangering Women's Health, Free Speech and Democracy. International Fact Sheet.* New York: Center for Reproductive Rights.

———. 2002. *Background on the Negotiations for the United Nations Special Session on Children.* New York: Center for Reproductive Rights. Accessed 20 February 2006 at http://www.crlp.org/ww_adv_child_neg.html

Center for Reproductive Rights and Association des Juristes Maliennes. 2003. *Claiming Our Rights: Surviving Pregnancy and Childbirth in Mali.* New York: Center for Reproductive Rights.

Cervical Barrier Advancement Society. 2007. The Cervical Barrier Advancement Society. Accessed 13 July at http://www.cervicalbarriers.org

Chapman A. 1996. "A 'Violations Approach' for Monitoring the International Covenant on Economic, Social and Cultural Rights." *Human Rights Quarterly* 18, no. 1: 23–66.

Chatterjee P. 2005. "Doctors' Group Proposes One-Child Policy for India." *The Lancet* 365, no. 9471: 1609.

Chesler E. 1992. *Woman of Valor: Margaret Sanger and the Birth Control Movement in America.* New York: Simon and Schuster.

Clark S. 2004. "Early Marriage and HIV Risks in Sub-Saharan Africa." *Studies in Family Planning* 35, no. 3: 149–60.

Cleland J, Bernstein S, Ezeh A, Faundes A, Glasier A, and Innis J. 2006. "Family

Planning: The Unfinished Agenda." The Lancet Sexual and Reproductive Health Series. *The Lancet* 368, no. 9549: 1810–27.

Coalition on Abortion/Breast Cancer. 2006. Coalition on Abortion/Breast Cancer website. Accessed 28 July 2007 at http://www.abortionbreastcancer.com/start/

Cobb R and Ross M. 1997. *Cultural Strategies of Agenda Denial: Avoidance, Attack, and Redefinition.* Lawrence: University of Kansas Press.

Condorcet J. 1976. *Condorcet: Selected Writings*, KM Baker (ed.). Indianapolis: Bobbs-Merrill.

Cook RJ. 1999. "Advancing Safe Motherhood Through Human Rights." *Journal of the Society of Gynecology and Obstetrics of Canada* 21: 363–71.

_____. 1998. "Human Rights Law and Safe Motherhood." *European Journal of Health Law* 5, no. 4: 357–75.

_____. 1997. "Reproductive Health Law: Where Next After Cairo and Beijing?" *Med Law* 16, no. 1: 169–78.

_____. 1994. *Women's Health and Human Rights: The Promotion and Protection of Women's Health Through International Human Rights Law.* Geneva: WHO.

_____. 1989. "Reducing Maternal Mortality: A Priority for Human Rights Law." In SAM McLean (ed.), *Issues in Human Reproduction.* Aldershot: Gower.

Cook RJ and Bevilacqua MBG. 2004. "Invoking Human Rights to Reduce Maternal Deaths." *The Lancet* 363: 73.

Cook RJ and Dickens BM. 2001. *Advancing Safe Motherhood Through Human Rights.* WHO/RHR/01.5. Geneva: WHO.

Cook RJ, Dickens BM, and Fathalla MF. 2003. *Reproductive Health and Human Rights: Integrating Medicine, Ethics and Law.* Oxford: Oxford University Press.

Cook RJ and Fathalla M. 1996. "Advancing Reproductive Rights Beyond Cairo and Beijing." *International Family Planning Perspectives* 22, no. 3: 115–121.

Cornu C. 2002. *Towards a More Meaningful Involvement of People Living with HIV/AIDS.* Brighton: International HIV/AIDS Alliance.

Correa S. 1997. "From Reproductive Health to Sexual Rights: Achievements and Future Challenges." *Reproductive Health Matters* 5, no. 10: 107–16.

Correa S et al. 2005. "Thinking Beyond ICPD+10: Where Should Our Movement Be Going?" *Reproductive Health Matters* 13, no. 25: 109–19.

Correa S and Petchesky R. 1994. "Reproductive and Sexual Rights: A Feminist Perspective." In G Sen, A Germain and L Chen (eds.), *Population Policies Reconsidered: Health, Empowerment and Rights.* Cambridge, Mass.: Harvard University Press.

Correa S and Reichmann R. 1994. *Population and Reproductive Rights: Feminist Perspectives from the South.* London: Zed Books.

Costello A, Azad K, and Barnett S. 2006, "Comment: An Alternative Strategy to Reduce Maternal Mortality." *The Lancet* 368: 1477–99.

Costello A and Osrin D. 2005. "The Case for a New Global Fund for Maternal, Neonatal, and Child Survival." *The Lancet* 366: 603–5.

Countdown 2015. 2007. Countdown 2015: Sexual and Reproductive Health and Rights for All website. Accessed 2 June at http://www.countdown2015.org/home.aspx

Coyaji K, Elul B, Krishna U, et al. 2001. "Mifepristone Abortion Outside the Urban Research Hospital Setting in India." *The Lancet* 357: 120–22.

Crane BB and Dusenberry J. 2004. "Power and Politics in International Funding for Reproductive Health: The U.S. Global Gag Rule." *Reproductive Health Matters* 12, no. 24: 128–37.

Crossette B. 2005. "Reproductive Health and the Millennium Development Goals: The Missing Link." *Studies in Family Planning* 36, no. 1.

De Pinho H. 2005. "Towards the Right Reforms: The Impact of Health Sector Reforms on Sexual and Reproductive Health." *Development* 48, no. 4: 61–68.

Deen T. 2008. "Family Planning Gets Mere Sliver of Aid Pie." Inter Press Service News Agency, 11 April.

———. 2006. "UN Bodies Survive U.S. Funding Threats." Inter Press Service News Agency (IPS), 10 September.

Dehne KL and Riedner G. 2005. *Sexually Transmitted Infections Among Adolescents: The Need for Adequate Health Services.* Geneva: WHO, Department of Child and Adolescent Health. Accessed 5 March 2006 at http://www.who.int/child-adolescent-health/publications/ADH/ISBN_92_4_156288_9.htm

DeJong J. 2000. "The Role and Limitations of the Cairo International Conference on Population and Development." *Social Science and Medicine* 51, no. 6: 941–53.

DeLay P, Greener R, and Izazola JA. 2007, "Are We Spending Too Much on HIV/AIDS?" *BMJ* 334: 345.

Demeny P. 2003. *Population Policy: A Concise Summary.* Policy Research Division Working Paper 173. New York: Population Council. Accessed 30 April 2007 at http://www.popcouncil.org/pdfs/wp/173.pdf

Department for International Development, UK. 2004. *Sexual and Reproductive Health and Rights: A Position Paper.* London: DFID.

Dixon-Mueller R. 1993. *Population Policy and Women's Rights: Transforming Reproductive Choice.* Westport, Conn.: Praeger.

Dixon-Mueller R and Germain A. 2006. "Fertility Regulation and Reproductive Health in the Millennium Development Goals: The Search for a Perfect Indicator?" *American Journal of Public Health* 10.

Dollar D and Kraay A. 2002. "Spreading the Wealth." *Foreign Affairs* 81, no. 1.

Donaldson PJ and Tsui AO. 1994. "The International Family Planning Movement." In LA Mazur (ed.), *Beyond the Numbers: A Reader on Population, Consumption and the Environment.* Washington, D.C.: Island Press.

Doyal L. 1995. *What Makes Women Sick: Gender and the Political Economy of Health.* New Brunswick, N.J.: Rutgers University Press.

Druce D, Dickinson C, et al. 2006. Strengthening Linkages for Sexual and Reproductive Health, HIV and AIDS: Progress, Barriers and Opportunities for Scaling Up. Final report, August. DFID Health Resource Centre. Accessed 20 April 2007 at http://www.dfidhealthrc.org/publications/HIV_SRH_strengthening_responses_06.pdf

Ecks, S and Sax WS (eds.). 2005 *The Ills of Marginality: New Perspectives on Subaltern Health. Special Issue of Anthropology and Medicine* 12, no. 3.

Ehrlich PR. 1968. *The Population Bomb.* New York: Ballantine.

El Feki S. 2004. "The Birth of Reproductive Health: A Difficult Delivery." *PLOS Medicine* 1, no. 1: 6–9.

Ellertson C, Elul B, Ambardekar S, et al. 2000. "Accuracy of Assessments of Pregnancy Duration by Women Seeking Early Abortion." *The Lancet* 355, no. 9207: 877–81.

Engelman R. 1998. *Plan and Conserve: A Source Book on Linking Population and Environmental Services in Communities.* Washington, D.C.: Population Action International.

England R. 2007. "Are We Spending Too Much on HIV?" *BMJ* 334: 344.

Ethelston S. 2004a. "Aid Is Back! Sexual and Reproductive Health Faces a Fight for Resources in the New Landscape of Development Assistance." *ICPD at 10: Countdown 2015* special issue. London: International Planned Parenthood Federation.

_____. 2004b. *Progress and Promises: Trends in International Assistance for Population and Reproductive Health.* Washington, D.C.: Population Action International.

Ethelston S and Leahy E. 2006. *Reproductive Health: Who Pays? How Much?* Washington, D.C.: Population Action International.

European Court of Human Rights. 2007. *Tysiac v. Poland* (Application no. 5410/03). 20 March, final 24 September.

Farmer P. 2003. *Pathologies of Power: Health, Human Rights, and the New War on the Poor.* Berkeley: University of California Press.

Fathalla MF. 2005. "The Reproductive Health Community: A Valuable Asset for Achieving the MDGs." *Studies in Family Planning* 36, no. 2: 135–37.

_____. 1988. "Promotion of Research in Human Reproduction: Global Needs and Perspectives." *Human Reproduction* 3: 7–10.

Fedele L, Bianchi S, Raffaelli R, et al. 1997. "Treatment of Adenomyosis-Associated Menorrhagia with a Levonorgestrel-Releasing Intrauterine Device." *Fertility and Sterility* 68: 426–29.

Ferreira da Costa LL, Hardy E, Duarte Osis MJ, and Faúndes A. 2005. "Termination of Pregnancy for Fetal Abnormality Incompatible with Life." *Reproductive Health Matters* 13, no. 26: 139–46.

Finkle JL and Crane BB. 1985. "Ideology and Politics at Mexico City: The United States at the 1984 International Conference on Population." *Population and Development Review* 11, no. 1: 1–28.

_____. 1975. "The Politics of Bucharest: Population, Development, and the New International Economic Order." *Population and Development Review* 1, no. 1: 87–114.

Finkle JL and MacIntosh A. 2002. "United Nations Population Conferences: Shaping the Policy Agenda for the Twenty-First Century." *Studies in Family Planning* 33, no. 1: 11–23.

Forbes A. 2006. "Moving Toward Assured Access to Treatment in Microbicide Trials." *PLoS Medicine* 3, no. 7: e153. Accessed 13 July 2007 at http://doi:10.1371/journal.pmed.0030153

Ford Foundation and IPPF/WHR. 2002. *Sexual and Reproductive Health Indicator Development: An Annotated Bibliography.* New York: Ford Foundation.

Fortney J. 1995. *Reproductive Morbidity: A Conceptual Framework.* Family Health International Working Paper WP95-02. Research Triangle Park, N.C.: Family Health International.

Freedman LP. 2005. "Human Rights and the Politics of Risk and Blame." In Gruskin S, Grodin M, Annas G, and Marks SP (eds.), *Perspectives in Health and Human Rights.* New York: Routledge.

_____. 2002. "Shifting Visions: 'Delegation' Policies and the Building of a 'Rights-Based' Approach to Maternal Mortality." *Journal of the American Medical Women's Association* 57, no. 3: 154–58.

_____. 2001. "Using Human Rights in Maternal Mortality Programs: From Analysis to Strategy." *International Journal of Gynecology and Obstetrics* 75: 51-60.

Freedman LP and Isaacs SL. 1993. "Human Rights and Reproductive Choice." *Studies in Family Planning* 24, no. 1: 18–30.

Freedman LP, Waldman RJ, de Pinho H, et al. 2005a. *Who's Got the Power? Transforming Health Systems for Women and Children,* UN Millennium Project Task Force on Child Health and Maternal Health. New York: UN Millennium

Project. Accessed 20 July 20 2007 at http://www.unmillenniumproject.org/documents/maternalchild-complete.pdf

Freedman LP, Waldman RJ, de Pinho H, et al. 2005b. "Transforming Health Systems to Improve the Lives of Women and Children." *The Lancet* 365: 997–1000.

Freedman R. 1997. "Do Family Planning Programs Affect Fertility Preferences? A Literature Review." *Studies in Family Planning* 28, no. 1: 1–13.

Garcia-Lerma J et al. 2006, "Prevention of Rectal SHIV Transmission in Macaques by Tenofovir/FTC Combination." Abstract 32LB, Thirteenth Conference on Retroviruses and Opportunistic Infections, Denver.

Garcia-Moreno C and Claro A. 1994, "Challenges from the Women's Health Movement: Women's Rights versus Population Control." In G Sen, A Germain and L Chen (eds.), *Population Policies Reconsidered: Health, Empowerment and Rights.* Cambridge, Mass.: Harvard University Press.

Gardiner N. 2006. Kofi Annan's Legacy of Failure. WebMemo 1283. Washington, D.C.: Heritage Foundation.

Garrett L. 2007."The Challenge of Global Health." *Foreign Affairs* 86, no. 1. Accessed 1 August at http://www.foreignaffairs.org/20070101faessay 86103/laurie-garrett/the-challenge-of-global-health.html

Gates Foundation. 2007. Global Health—Priority Diseases and Conditions Website. Accessed 2 June at http://www.gatesfoundation.org/GlobalHealth /Pri_Diseases

Gender and Health Equity Network. n.d. Gender and Health Equity Network Website. Accessed 22 July 2007 at http://www.ids.ac.uk/ghen

Germain A. 2000. "Population and Reproductive Health: Where Do We Go Next?" *American Journal of Public Health* 90, no. 12: 1845–47.

Germain A and Dixon-Mueller R. 2005. "Reproductive Health and the MDGs: Is the Glass Half Full or Half Empty?" *Studies in Family Planning* 36, no. 2: 137–40.

Germain A and Kidwell J. 2005. "The Unfinished Agenda for Reproductive Health: Priorities for the Next 10 Years." *International Family Planning Perspectives* 31, no. 2: 90–93.

Gillespie DG. 2004a. "Whatever Happened to Family Planning and, for That Matter, Reproductive Health?" *International Family Planning Perspectives* 30: 34–38.

_____. 2004b. "The Meeting That Did Not Happen: Cairo, 10 Years On." *The Lancet* 364: 1566–67.

Girard F. 2004. *Global Implications of U.S. Domestic Policy and International Policies on Sexuality.* IWGSSP Working Paper 1, June. New York: International Working Group for Sexuality and Social Policy, Columbia University Mailman School of Public Health. Accessed 2 August 2007 at http://www.mail man.hs.columbia.edu/cgsh/IWGSSPWorkingPaper1English.pdf

_____. 2002. "UN Special Session on Children: Bush Administration Continues Its Attacks on Sexual and Reproductive Health." *Reproductive Health Matters* 10, no. 20: 141–43.

_____. 2001a. *Reflections on the Declaration of Commitment on HIV/AIDS Adopted by the UN's General Assembly Special Session on HIV/AIDS.* International Women's Health Coalition website. Accessed 20 February 2006 at http://www.iwhc .org/global/un/unhistory/hivaidsreflections.cfm

_____. 2001b. "Reproductive Health Under Attack at the United Nations." *Reproductive Health Matters* 9, no. 18: 68.

Glasier A and Gulmezoglu AM. 2006. "Putting Sexual and Reproductive Health on the Agenda." *The Lancet* 368: 1550–51.

Global Gag Rule Impact Project. 2003. Access Denied: U.S. Restrictions on International Family Planning. Washington, D.C. Accessed 5 February 2006 at Global Gag Rule Impact Project www.globalgagrule.org

Graham W and Hussein J. 2004. "The Right to Count." *The Lancet* 363, no. 9402: 67–68.

Greco G., Powell-Jackson T, Borghi, J, and Mills A. 2008. "Countdown to 2015: Assessment of Donor Assistance to Maternal, Newborn, and Child Health Between 2003 and 2006." *The Lancet.* 371: 1268–75.

Greene ME and Merrick TW. 2005. *Poverty Reduction: Does Reproductive Health Matter?* World Bank HNP Discussion Paper Series. Washington, D.C.: World Bank.

Grimes DA. 1998. "Worldwide Perspective on IUD Use." *Contraception Report* 9, no. 4: 4–8.

Grown C, Gupta GR, and Kes A. 2005. *Taking Action: Achieving Gender Equality and Empowering Women.* Report of UN Millennium Project Task Force on Education and Gender Equality. London: Earthscan and Millennium Project.

Gruskin S. 2004. "Stalled on the Road to Reproductive Health." *American Journal of Public Health* 94, no. 8.

Gruskin S, Cottingham J, Roseman MJ et al. 2006. "Maternal and Neonatal Health: Using a Human Rights Approach." Presentation at American Public Health Association 134th Annual Meeting and Exposition, Boston, 5 November.

Gruskin S, Ferguson L, and Bogecho D. 2007. "Beyond the Numbers: Using Rights-Based Perspectives to Enhance ARV Scale-Up." *AIDS* 21 (suppl 5): S13–S19.

Gruskin S, Ferguson. L, and O'Malley J. 2007. "Ensuring Sexual and Reproductive Health for People Living with HIV: An Overview of Key Human Rights, Policy and Health Systems Issues." *Reproductive Health Matters* 15, no. 29 (supplement).

Gruskin S, Roseman MJ, and Ferguson L. 2007. "Reproductive Health and HIV/AIDS: Using International Human Rights and Policies to Frame Appropriate Responses." *McGill International Journal of Sustainable Development Law and Policy* 3, no. 1.

The Guardian. 2007. "Mexico City Faces Court Challenge After Legalising Abortions." Guardian UK Unlimited (online), 25 April. Accessed 1 August at http://www.guardian.co.uk/international/story/0,2065182,00.html

Guay LA, Musoke P, Fleming T, et al. 1999, "Intrapartum and Neonatal Single-Dose Nevirapine Compared with Zidovudine for Prevention of Mother-to-Child Transmission of HIV-1 in Kampala, Uganda: HIVNET 012 Randomized Trial." *The Lancet* 354, no. 9181: 795–802.

Gwatkin DR. 2000. "Health Inequalities and the Health of the Poor: What Do We Know? What Can We Do?" *Bulletin of the World Health Organization* 78: 3-17.

Gwatkin DR et al. 2004. *Initial Country Level Information about Socio-Economic Differences in Health, Nutrition and Population.* 2nd ed. Washington, D.C.: World Bank.

Gynuity Health Projects. 2005. *Global Maps of the Availability of Mifepristone and Misoprostol.* New York: Gynuity Health Projects.

Haberland N and Measham D. 2002. *Responding to Cairo: Case Studies of Changing Practice in Reproductive Health and Family Planning.* New York: Population Council.

Hafez G. 1998. "Maternal Mortality: A Neglected and Socially Unjustifiable Tragedy: Why WHO Selected 'Safe Motherhood' as the Slogan for World Health Day." *Eastern Mediterranean Health Journal* 4, no. 1: 7–10.

Hardee K, Agarwal K, Luke N, Wilson E, Pendzich M, Farrell M, and Cross H. 1999. "Post-Cairo Reproductive Health Policies: A Comparative Study of Eight Countries." *International Family Planning Perspectives* 25 (Suppl.): S2–S9.

Harkavy O. 1995. *Curbing Population Growth: An Insider's Perspective on the Population Movement.* New York: Plenum Press.

Hartmann B. 2005. "Refuting Security Demographics: In Dialogue with Betsy Hartmann." *Development* 48, no. 4: 16–20.

_____. 1998. "Population, Environment and Security: A New Trinity." *Environment and Urbanization* 10, no. 2: 113–28.

_____. 1995. *Reproductive Rights and Wrongs: The Global Politics of Population Control.* Boston: South End Press.

Haslegrave M. 2004. "Implementing the ICPD Programme of Action: What a Difference a Decade Makes." *Reproductive Health Matters* 12. no. 23: 12–18.

Haslegrave M and Bernstein S. 2005. "ICPD Goals: Essential to the Millennium Development Goals." *Reproductive Health Matters* 13, no. 25: 106-8.

Haslegrave M and Olatunbosun O. 2003. "Incorporating sexual and reproductive health care in the medical curriculum in developing countries." *Reproductive Health Matters* 11, no. 21: 49–58.

Hassan R. 2007. *Are Human Rights Compatible with Islam? The Issue of the Rights of Women in Muslim Communities.* Milwaukee: Religious Consultation on Population, Reproductive Health and Ethics. Accessed 11 July at http://www.religiousconsultation.org/hassan2.htm

Hatcher RA et al. 1998. *Contraceptive Technology.* 17th ed. New York: Ardent Media.

Hausmann R and Szekely M. 2001. "Inequality and the Family in Latin America." In N Birdsall, AC Kelley and SW Sinding (eds.), *Population Matters: Demographic Change, Economic Growth, and Poverty in the Developing World.* New York: Oxford University Press.

Hawkins K, Newman K, Thomas D, and Carlson C. 2005. "Developing a Human Rights-Based Approach to Addressing Maternal Mortality: Desk Review." London: DFID Health Resource Centre.

Hessini L. 2005, "Global Progress in Abortion Advocacy and Policy: An Assessment of the Decade Since ICPD." *Reproductive Health Matters* 13. no. 25: 88–100.

Hierro López LA. 2004. *Uruguay y la ley sobre el aborto avances y parálisis.* Summary by L Abracinskas. Accessed 13 September from Latin American and Caribbean Committee for the Defense of Women's Rights Website http://www.cladem.org/espanol/nacionales/uruguay/uyarticuloavances1.asp

Hirve S. 2004. "Abortion Law, Policy and Services in India: A Critical Review." *Reproductive Health Matters* 12, no. 24: 114–21.

Hogerzeil H., Sansom M, et al. 2006. "Is Access to Essential Medicines as Part of the Fulfilment of the Right to Health Enforceable Through the Courts?" *The Lancet* 368, no. 9532: 305–11.

hooks b. 1981, *Ain't I a Woman: Black Women and Feminism.* Boston: South End Press.

Horton R. 2006. "Reviving Reproductive Health." *The Lancet* 368, no. 9547: 1549.

Human Rights Committee. 2005. *Karen Noelia Llantoy Huamán v. Peru, Communication No. 1153/2003.* Document CCPR/C/85/D/1153/2003,

Human Rights Committee 85th session, 17 October–3 November. Accessed 1 August 2007 at http://www1.umn.edu/humanrts/undocs/1153-2003.html

_____. 2003. *Concluding Observations of the Human Rights Committee, Mali.* Document CCPR/CO/77/MLI. Accessed 1 August 2007 at http://www1.umn.edu/humanrts/hrcommittee/mali2003.html

Human Rights Watch. 2006. A High Price to Pay: Detention of Poor Patients in Burundian Hospitals (September). http://hrw.org/reports/2006/burundi0906/index.htm

_____. 2002. "Ignorance Only: HIV/AIDS, Human Rights and Federally Funded Abstinence-Only Programs in the U.S.: Texas: A Case Study." HRW 14, no. 5 (G). New York: Human Rights Watch. Accessed 2 June 2007 at http://hrw.org/reports/2002/usa0902/USA0902.pdf

Inhorn MC. 2004. Presentation at Reproductive Health in the Twenty-First Century Conference, 14-15 October, Radcliffe Institute for Advanced Studies, Harvard University.

Inter-American Commission on Human Rights. 2007. Annual Report, Mexico, *Paulina Ramírez v. Mexico*, No. 21/07, Petition 161-02 Friendly Settlement. Accessed 30 April at http://www.cidh.oas.org/annualrep/2007eng/Mexico16102eng.htm

International Planned Parenthood Federation. 2007. Global Gag Rule. Accessed 20 July at http://www.ippf.org/en/What-we-do/Advocacy/Global+gag+rule.htm

_____. 2006. "United Nations General Assembly Adopts Universal Access Target for Reproductive Health." Press release, 5 October. Accessed 20 April 2007 at http://www.ippf.org/en/News/Press-releases/UN+General+Assembly+adopts+target.htm

_____. 2002. *Manual to Evaluate Quality of Care from a Gender Perspective.* New York: IPPF Western Hemisphere Region.

International Women's Health Coalition. 2005. *IWHC Factsheet: Child Marriage.* New York: IWHC. Accessed 6 June 2007 at http://www.iwhc.org/resources/childmarriagefacts.cfm

_____. 1994. *Challenging the Culture of Silence: Building Alliances to End Reproductive Track Infections.* Rapporteurs Antrobus P, Germain A, and Nowrojee. New York: IWHC.

Isaacs SL. 1995. "Incentives, Population Policy, and Reproductive Rights: Ethical Issues." *Studies in Family Planning* 26, no. 6: 363–67.

Jackson JB, Musoke P, Fleming T et al. 2003. "Intrapartum and Neonatal Single-Dose Nevirapine Compared with Zidovudine for Prevention of Mother-to-Child Transmission of HIV-1 in Kampala, Uganda: 18-Month Follow-Up to the HIVNET 012 Randomised Trial." *The Lancet* 362, no. 9387: 859–68.

Jahan R and Germain A. 2004. "Mobilising Support to Sustain Political Will Is the Key to Progress in Reproductive Health." *The Lancet* 364: 742–44.

Jain A. 1998. "Population Policies That Matter." In A Jain (ed.), *Do Population Policies Matter? Fertility and Politics in Egypt, India, Kenya and Mexico.* New York: Population Council.

Jain A and Bruce J. 1994. "A Reproductive Health Approach to the Objectives and Assessment of Family Planning Programmes." In G Sen, A Germain and L Chen (eds.), *Population Policies Reconsidered: Health, Empowerment, and Rights.* Cambridge, Mass.: Harvard University Press.

Jejeebhoy SJ. 1996. *Women's Education, Autonomy, and Reproductive Behaviour: experience from developing countries.* Oxford: Clarendon Press.

Jimenez EY and Murthi M. 2006. "Investing in the Youth Bulge." *Finance & Development* 43, no. 3.

Johnson HB. 2004. "Is Reproductive Health Care Cost-Efficient? The Case of Abortion and Post-Abortion Care." Report, Ipas, Chapel Hill, N.C.

Kantner J and Kantner A. 2006. *The Struggle for International Consensus on Population and Development.* New York: Palgrave Macmillan.

Kates J, Morison JS and Lief E. 2006. "Global Health Funding: A glass half full?" *The Lancet* 368, no. 9531: 187–88.

Katz A. 2005. "The Sachs Report: Investing in Health for Economic Development—Or Increasing the Size of the Crumbs from the Rich Man's Table? Part II." *International Journal of Health Services* 35, no. 1: 171–88.

Kaufman J and Jing F. 2002. "Privatisation of Health Services and the Reproductive Health of Rural Chinese Women." *Reproductive Health Matters* 10, no. 20: 108–16.

Kaufman J and Messersmith L. 2006. "Integrating the Fields of Sexual and Reproductive Health and HIV/AIDS." Paper presented at the 2006 Population Association of America conference, Los Angeles.

Keck M and K. Sikkink K. 1998. *Activists Beyond Borders: Advocacy Networks in International Politics.* Ithaca, N.Y.: Cornell University Press.

Kestler E, Valencia L, Del Valle V, et al. 2006. "Scaling Up Post-Abortion Care in Guatemala." *Reproductive Health Matters* 14, no. 27: 138–47.

Kim J and Motsei M. 2002, "Women Enjoy Punishment: Attitudes and Experiences of Gender Based Violence Among PHC Nurses in Rural South Africa." *Social Science and Medicine* 54: 1243–54.

Kingdon J. 1984. *Agendas, Alternatives, and Public Policies.* Boston: Little, Brown.

Kissling F. 2004. "Is There Life After Roe? How to Think About the Fetus." *Conscience* (Winter). Accessed 1 April 2007 at Catholics for Choice Website, http://www.catholicsforchoice.org/conscience/archives/c2004win_lifeafter roe.asp

———. 1999. "The Vatican at the United Nations: Cairo+5." *Conscience* 20, no. 2: 15–16.

Kitts J and Lal S. 2006. *Toward Greater Integration of HIV/AIDS and Sexual and Reproductive Health and Rights.* Ottawa: Action Canada for Population and Development.

Klugman B. 2005. "Sexual Rights in Southern Africa." In Gruskin S, Grodin M, Annas G, and Marks SP (eds.), *Perspectives in Health and Human Rights.* New York: Routledge.

Klugman J (ed.). 2002. *A Sourcebook for Poverty Reduction Strategies.* 2 vols. Washington, D.C.: World Bank.

Kresge KJ. 2005. "New Strides in Protecting Infants from HIV." *International AIDS Vaccine Initiative Report* 9, no. 2. Accessed 1 April 2007 at http://www.iavire port.org/Issues/Issue92/NewStridesInProtectingInfantsFromHIV.asp

Lakha F, Henderson C, and Glasier A. 2005. "The Acceptability of Self-Administration of Subcutaneous Depo-Provera." *Contraception* 72: 1, 1 4–18.

Langer A. 2006. "Cairo After 12 years: Successes, Setbacks, and Challenges." *The Lancet* 368: 1552–54.

Lapham RJ and Mauldin WP. 1985. "Contraceptive Prevalence: The Influence of Organized Family Planning Programs." *Studies in Family Planning* 16, no. 3: 117-37.

Lee K and Walt G. 1995. "Linking National and Global Population Agendas:

Case Studies from Eight Developing Countries." *Third World Quarterly* 16, no. 2: 257-72.

Liljestrand J. 2000. "Strategies to Reduce Maternal Mortality Worldwide." *Current Opinion in Obstetrics and Gynecology* 12, no. 6: 513-17.

Liu PY, Swerdloff RS, Christenson PD, et al. 2006. "Rate, Extent, and Modifiers of Spermatogenic Recovery After Hormonal Male Contraception: An Integrated Analysis." *The Lancet* 367, no. 9520: 1412-20.

Løkeland M. 2004. "Abortion: The Legal Right Has Been Won, But Not the Moral Right." *Reproductive Health Matters* 12, no. 24: 167–73.

Lopez A et al. 2002. "Global and Regional Burden of Disease and Risk Factors, 2001: Systematic Analysis of Population Health Data." *The Lancet* 36, no. 9524: 1747–57.

Loudon I. 1992. *Death in Childbirth: An International Study of Maternal Care and Maternal Mortality, 1880-1950.* Oxford: Oxford University Press.

Lush L. 2002. "Service Integration: An Overview of Policy Developments." *International Family Planning Perspectives* 28, no. 2: 71–76.

MacKellar L. 2005. "Priorities in Global Assistance for Health, AIDS, and Population." *Population and Development Review* 31, no. 2: 293–312.

Maine D and Yamin AE. 1999. "Maternal Mortality as a Human Rights Issue: Measuring Compliance with International Treaty." *Human Rights Quarterly* 21, no. 3: 563–607.

Malthus TR. 1986. *An Essay on the Principle of Population.* 6th ed. (1826) with variant readings from the 2nd edition (1803). EA Wrigley and D Souden (eds.). London: W. Pickering.

Mamdani M. 1972. *The Myth of Population Control: Family, Caste, and Class in an Indian Village.* New York: Monthly Review Press.

Markham I. 2007. "Episcopalians, Homosexuality and the General Convention 2006." *Reviews in Religion and Theology* 4, no. 1: 1–5.

Mason A and Lee SH. 2004. "The Demographic Dividend and Poverty Reduction." Paper prepared for Seminar on the Relevance of Population Aspects for the Achievement of the Millennium Development Goals, 17-19 November, UN Population Division, Department of Economic and Social Affairs, New York. Accessed 30 April 2007 at http://www.un.org/esa/popula tion/publications/PopAspectsMDG/19_MASONA.pdf

Matthews J. 1992. "Politically Correct Environmentalists." *Washington Post,* 12 April, C-7.

Mayhew S. 1996, "Integrating MCH/FP and STD/HIV Services: Current Debates and Future Directions." *Health Policy Planning* 11, no. 4: 339–53.

Mayhew S, Lush L, Cleland J, and Walt G. 2000. "Implementing the Integration of Component Services for Reproductive Health." *Studies in Family Planning* 31, no. 2: 151–62.

McCafferty C, Leigh E, and Lamb N. 2002. *China Mission Report by UK MPs,* 1-9 April. Accessed 28 May 2007 at http://www.planetwire.org/wrap/files.fcgi/ 2955_UK_report.htm

McFeely T. 2007. "No Amnesty for the Unborn." *National Catholic Register,* 17-23 June. Accessed 25 July at http://ncregister.com/site/article/2904

McNicoll G. 2003. *Population and Development: An Introductory View.* Policy Research Division Working Paper 174. New York: Population Council. Accessed 30 April 2007 at http://www.popcouncil.org/pdfs/wp/174.pdf.

Meadows DH, Meadows DL, Randers J, and Behrens WW. 1972. *The Limits to Growth.* New York: University Books.

Meriggiola MC, Cerpolini S, Bremner WJ, et al. 2006. "Acceptability of an Injectable Male Contraceptive Regimen of Norethisterone Enanthate and Testosterone Undecanoate for Men." *Human Reproduction* 21, no. 8: 2033–40.

Merrick T. 2005. "Mobilizing Resources for Reproductive Health." Prepared for the David and Lucile Packard Foundation, Population Program Review Task Force, August.

Mertens W. 1994. *The Context of IUSSP Contribution to the International Conference on Population and Development*. Policy and Research Paper 1. Paris: International Union for the Scientific Study of Population. http://www.iussp.org/Publications_on_site/PRP/prp1.php

Microbicide Trials Halted in Africa, India Because of Possible Increased Risk of HIV Transmission. 2007. 5 February. Accessed 13 July at http://www.medical newstoday.com/medicalnews.php?newsid=62119

Miller A. 2000. "Sexual But Not Reproductive: Exploring the Junction and Disjunction of Sexual and Reproductive Rights." *Health and Human Rights* 4, no. 2: 69–109.

Miller G. 2005. *Contraception as Development? New Evidence from Family Planning in Colombia.* NBER Working Paper W11704. Cambridge, Mass.: NBER.

Miller K, Shortridge E, and Martin S. 2006. "Is Low Maternal Mortality Possible Where Abortion Is Illegal? A Global Ecological Study." Manuscript, Ibis Reproductive Health, Cambridge, Mass.

Moench T, Chipato T, and Padian N. 2001. "Preventing Disease by Protecting the Cervix: The Unexplored Promise of Internal Vaginal Barrier Devices." *AIDS* 15: 1595–1602.

Mohanty CT. 2002. "'Under Western Eyes': Revisited: Feminist Solidarity Through Anticapitalist Struggles." *Signs: Journal of Women in Culture and Society* 28, no. 2: 499–535.

_____. 1988. "Under Western Eyes: Feminist Scholarship and Colonial Discourses." *Feminist Review* 30: 61–88.

Mosley WH and Chen LC. 1984. "An Analytical Framework for the Study of Child Survival in Developing Countries." *Population and Development Review*, Supplement: *Child Survival: Strategies for Research* 10: 25–45.

Mueller D and Germaine A. 2005. "Fertility Regulation and Reproductive Health in the Millennium Development Goals: The Search for the Perfect Indicator?" *American Journal of Public Health* 10.

Mumford SD. 1986. *The Pope and the New Apocalypse: The Holy War Against Family Planning.* Research Triangle, N.C.: Center for Research on Population and Security.

Murray CJ and Lopez AD. 1998. *Health Dimensions of Sex and Reproduction.* Geneva: WHO.

_____ (eds.). 1996a. *The Global Burden of Disease: A Comprehensive Assessment of Mortality and Disability from Diseases, Injuries, and Risk Factors in 1990 and Projected to 2020.* Geneva: WHO.

_____ (eds.). 1996b. *Global Health Statistics: A Compendium of Incidence, Prevalence, and Mortality Estimates for over 200 Conditions.* Boston: Harvard School of Public Health for WHO and World Bank.

Murray CJ, Salomon JA, Mathers CD, and Lopez AD. 2002. *Summary Measures of Population Health: Concepts, Ethics, Measurement and Applications.* Geneva: WHO.

Myer L, Rabkin M, Abrams EJ, et al. 2005. "Focus on Women: Linking HIV Care and Treatment with Reproductive Health Services in the MTCT-Plus Initiative." *Reproductive Health Matters* 13, no. 25: 136–46.

National Center for Health Statistics. 2004. NCHS Health Definitions. Hyattville, Md. Accessed 1 February 2006 at http://www.cdc.gov/nchs/datawh/nchs defs/tfr.htm

National Research Council. 1997. *Reproductive Health in Developing Countries: Expanding Dimensions, Building Solutions.* Washington, D.C.: National Academy Press.

———. 1986. *Population Growth and Economic Development: Policy Questions.* Washington, D.C.: National Academy Press.

Ngai SW, Fan S, Li S, et al. 2005. "A Randomized Trial to Compare 24 h Versus 12 h Double Dose Regimen of Levonorgestrel for Emergency Contraception." *Human Reproduction* 20, no. 1: 307–11.

Nowels L. 2003. "Population Assistance and Family Planning Programs: Issues for Congress." *Issue Brief for Congress,* updated 13 February. Order Code IB96026.

Nundy SM, Chir M, and Gulhati C. 2005. "A New Colonialism? Conducting Clinical Trials in India." *New England Journal of Medicine* 352, no.16: 1633–36.

Nussbaum M. 1999. "The Professor of Parody." *New Republic,* 22 February.

Obermeyer C. 1999. "The Cultural Context of Reproductive Health: Implications for Monitoring the Cairo Agenda." *International Family Planning Perspectives* 25 (Suppl): 50–55.

Office of Population Research, Princeton University and the Association of Reproductive Health Professionals. 2007. Emergency Contraception Website. Accessed July 13, 2007 at http://ec.princeton.edu.

Okie S. 2006. "Global Health: The Gates-Buffett Effect." *New England Journal of Medicine* 355, no. 11: 1084–88.

Olatunbosun OA and Edouard L. 1997. "The Teaching of Evidence-Based Reproductive Health in Developing Countries." *International Journal of Gynecology and Obstetrics* 56: 171–76.

O'Malley J. 2007. "Sexual & Reproductive Health Needs & Aspirations of Vulnerable Populations." Plenary presentation, International Conference on Actions to Strengthen Linkages Between SRH and HIV/AIDS, Mumbai, 4–8 February.

———. 2004. *SRH HIV: Can This Marriage Work? Countdown 2015 ICPD at 10.* London: International Planned Parenthood Federation.

Ooms G and Schrecker T. 2005. "Expenditure Ceilings, Multilateral Financial Institutions, and the Health of Poor Populations." *The Lancet* 365: 1821-23.

Organon. 2007. Nuvaring Website. Accessed 13 July at http://www.nuvaring.com

Ortho. 2007. Ortho Evra Website. Accessed 13 July 1at http://www.orthoevra.com

Oye-Adeniran BA, Umoh AV, and Nnatu SNN. 2002. "Complications of Unsafe Abortion: A Case Study and the Need for Abortion Law Reform in Nigeria." *Reproductive Health Matters* 10, no. 19: 18–21.

Pachucki M. 2006. Mapping the Field of Global Reproductive Health and Rights; Network Analysis Report (unpublished, on file with editors).

Pakarinen P, Toivonen J, and Luukkainen T. 2001. "Therapeutic Use of the LNG IUS, and Counseling." *Seminars in Reproductive Medicine* 19, no. 19: 365–72.

PEPFAR Watch. 2007. Center for Health and Gender Equity, Takoma Park, Md. Accessed 11 July at http://www.pepfarwatch.org

Petchesky RP. 2003. *Global Prescriptions: Gendering Health and Human Rights*. London: Zed Books.

_____. 1987. "Fetal Images: The Power of Visual Culture in the Politics of Reproduction." *Feminist Studies* 13, no. 2: 263–92.

Pfizer. 2005. Depo-Subq Provera 104. Accessed 13 July 2007 at http://www.depo-subqprovera104.com

Pharmacy Access Partnership. 2007. Pharmacy Access Partnership: Promoting Community Health Through Pharmacies. Accessed 13 July at http://www.pharmacyaccess.org

Physicians for Human Rights. 2007. *Deadly Delays: Maternal Mortality in Peru: a Rights-Based Approach to Safe Motherhood*. Cambridge: Physicians for Human Rights. Accessed 28 July 2008 from http://physiciansforhumanrights.org/library/report-2007-11-28.html

Physicians for Human Rights. 2002. *Maternal Mortality in Herat Province: The Need to Protect Women's Rights*. Boston: Physicians for Human Rights. Accessed 30 April 2007 from http://physiciansforhumanrights.org/library/2002-09-10.html

Polish Federation for Women and Family Planning. 2005. *Contemporary Women's Hell: Polish Women's Stories*. Warsaw: Polish Federation for Women and Family Planning.

Population Action International. 2004a. What Is U.S. International Population Assistance? FACT Sheet. Washington, D.C.: Population Action International. Accessed 24 July 2007 at http://www.populationaction.org/Publications/Fact_Sheets/FS20/Intl_Pop_Assist.pdf

_____. 2004b. *Progress & Promises: Trends in International Assistance for Reproductive Health and Population*. Washington, D.C.: Population Action International.

Population Council. 2007. Population Council Website. Accessed 25 July at http://www.popcouncil.org/ta/mar.html

_____. 2004. *Forced Sexual Relations Among Married Young Women in Developing Countries*. New Delhi: Population Council. Accessed 5 March 2006 at http://www.who.int/reproductivehealth/adolescent/docs/population_syntheis1.pdf

Population Reference Bureau. 2006. World's Youth 2006 Data Sheet. Washington, D.C.; Population Reference Bureau. Accessed 4 March at http://www.prb.org/pdf06/WorldsYouth2006DataSheet.pdf

Powell-Jackson T, Borghi J, et al. 2006. "Countdown to 2015: Tracking Donor Assistance to Maternal, Newborn, and Child Health." *The Lancet* 368: 1077–87.

Presser H and Sen G. 2000. *Women's Empowerment and Demographic Processes: Moving Beyond Cairo*. Oxford: Oxford University Press.

Ravindran S and de Pinho H. 2005. "*The Right Reforms? Health Sector Reforms and Sexual and Reproductive Health*." South. Africa: Women's Health Project, School of Public Health, University of the Witwatersrand.

Ravindran TKS and Balasubramanian P. 2004. "'Yes' to Abortion But 'No' to Sexual Rights: The Paradoxical Reality of Married Women in Rural Tamil Nadu, India." *Reproductive Health Matters* 12, no. 23: 88–99.

Reich MRR. 1995. "The Politics of Agenda Setting in International Health: Child Health Versus Adult Health in Developing Countries." *Journal of International Development* 7, no. 3: 489–502.

Reichenbach L. 2002. "The Politics of Priority Setting for Reproductive Health: Breast and Cervical Cancer in Ghana." *Reproductive Health Matters* 10, no. 20: 47–58.

Religion Counts. 2002. *Religion and Public Policy at the UN.* Washington: Religion Counts. Accessed 11 July 2007 at http://www.catholicsforchoice.org/top ics/politics/documents/2000religionandpublicpolicyatheun.pdf

Richey LA. 2003. *Rethinking Uganda: The Impact of AIDS on Reproductive Health and Rights Reforms in Sub-Saharan Africa.* IIS/GI Keongevej Working Paper 03.8. Copenhagen: Institute for International Studies.

Rivers K and Aggleton P. 1999. *Adolescent Sexuality, Gender, and the HIV Epidemic.* New York: UNDP HIV and Development Programme.

Robinson NJ, Mulder DW, Auvert B, et al. 1997. "Proportion of HIV Infections Attributable to Other Sexually Transmitted Diseases in a Rural Ugandan Population: Simulation Model Estimates." *International Journal of Epidemiology* 26, no. 1: 180–89.

Rochefort D and Cobb R. 1994. *The Politics of Problem Definition: Shaping the Policy Agenda.* Lawrence: University of Kansas Press.

Roddy RE, Zekeng L, Ryan KA, et al. 1998. "A Controlled Trial of Nonoxynol-9 Film to Reduce Male-to-Female Transmission of Sexually Transmitted Diseases." *New England Journal of Medicine* 339, no. 8: 504–10.

Ronsmans C and Graham W, on behalf of Maternal Survival Series Steering Group. 2006. "Maternal Mortality: Who, When, Where, and Why." *The Lancet* 368: 1189–2000.

Roseman M. 1999. "Birthing the Republic: Midwives, Medicine and Morality in France." PhD dissertation, Columbia University.

Rosenfield A and Maine D. 1985. "Maternal Mortality—A Neglected Tragedy: Where Is the M in MCH?" *The Lancet* 2: 83–85.

Russett B. 1996. "Ten Balances for Weighing UN Reform Proposals." *Political Science Quarterly* 111, no. 2: 259–69.

Sachs JD. 2001. *Macroeconomics and Health: Investment in Health for Economic Development.* Report of the Commission on Macroeconomics and Health. Geneva: WHO.

Safe Motherhood Inter-Agency Group, Family Care International. 1998. Safe Motherhood Fact Sheets. New York: Family Care International.

Sahil F. 2007. "UNICEF and Partners Come Together to Help Reduce Maternal Mortality in Afghanistan." Media release, UNICEF, 2 April. Accessed 30 April at http://www.unicef.org/infobycountry/afghanistan_39281.html

Sai F. 2005. *Time to Move On: Countdown 2015 ICPD at 10.* New York: International Planned Parenthood Federation.

Sawires SR et al. 2007. "Male Circumcision and HIV/AIDS: Challenges and Opportunities." *The Lancet* 369: 708-13.

Schaff EA, Eisinger SH, Stadalius LS, et al. 1999. "Low-Dose Mifepristone 200 mg and Vaginal Misoprostol for Abortion." *Contraception* 59, no. 1: 1–6.

Schaff EA, Stadalius LS, Eisinger SH and Franks P. 1997. "Vaginal Misoprostol Administered at Home After Mifepristone (RU486) for Abortion." *Journal of Family Practice* 44: 353–60.

Schindlmayr T. 2004. "Explicating Donor Trends for Population Assistance." *Population Research and Policy Review* 23, no. 1: 25–54.

Seltzer JR. 2002. *The Origins and Evolution of Family Planning Programs in Developing Countries.* Los Angeles: Rand Corporation.

Sen A. 1999. *Development as Freedom.* New York: Random House Anchor Books.

Sen G. 2005a. *Neolibs, Neocons, and Gender Justice: Lessons from Global Negotiations.* UNRISD Occasional Paper 9. Geneva: UN Research Institute for Social Development.

_____. 2005b. "Gender Equality and Human Rights: ICPD as a Catalyst?" In *The ICPD Vision: How Far Has the 11-Year Journey Taken Us?* Report from UNFPA Panel Discussion at IUSSP 25th International Population Conference, 19 July. Tours: UNFPA.

_____. 1994. "Women's Status, Empowerment and Reproductive Outcomes." In G Sen, A Germain, and L Chen (eds.), *Population Policies Reconsidered: Health, Empowerment, and Rights.* Cambridge, Mass.: Harvard University Press.

Sen G and Correa S. 1999. "Gender Justice and Economic Justice: Reflections on the Five-Year Reviews of the UN Conferences of the 1990s." Paper prepared for the UN Development Fund for Women.

Sen G, George A, and Östlin P. 2002. *Engendering International Health: The Challenge of Equity.* Cambridge, Mass.: MIT Press.

Sen G, Germain A, and Chen L. 1994, "Reconsidering Population Policies: Ethics, Development and Strategies for Change." In G Sen, A Germain, and L Chen (eds.), *Population Policies Reconsidered: Health, Empowerment and Rights.* Cambridge, Mass.: Harvard University Press.

Sen G, Govender V, and Cottingham J. 2006. *Maternal and Neonatal Health: Surviving the Roller-Coaster of International Policy.* Geneva: Maternal-Newborn Health and Poverty Project, WHO. Accessed 30 April 2007 at http://www.ids.ac.uk/ghen/resources/papers/MaternalMortality2006.pdf

Serour GI, Ragab AR, and Hassanein M. 1996. "The Position of Muslim Culture Towards Abortion." *Population Sciences* 16: 1–17.

Shakya G, Kishore S, Bird C, and Barak J. 2004. "Abortion Law Reform in Nepal: Women's Right to Life and Health." *Reproductive Health Matters* 12, no. 24: 75–84.

Shell-Duncan B. 2001. "The Medicalization of Female Circumcision: Harm Reduction of Promotion or Promotion of a Dangerous Practice?" *Social Science and Medicine* 52: 1013–28.

Shepard BL and DeJong JL. 2005. *Breaking the Silence and Saving Lives: Young People's Sexual and Reproductive Health in the Arab States and Iran.* Boston: François-Xavier Bagnoud Center for Health and Human Rights.

Shiffman, J. 2008. "Has Donor Prioritization of HIV/AIDS Displaced Aid for Other Health Issues?" *Health Policy and Planning* 23: 95–100.

_____. 2007. *Generating Political Priority for Public Health Causes in Developing Countries: Implications from a Study on Maternal Mortality.* Brief. Washington, D.C.: Center for Global Development.

_____. 2006. "HIV/AIDS and the Rest of the Global Health Agenda." *Bulletin of the World Health Organization* 84, no. 12: 923.

Shiffman J, Beer T, and Wu Y. 2002. "The Emergence of Global Disease Control Priorities." *Health Policy and Planning* 17, no. 3: 225-34.

Simmons GB and Lapham RJ. 1987. "Overview and Framework." In RJ Lapham and GB Simmons (eds.), *Organizing for Effective Family Planning Programs.* Washington, D.C.: National Academy Press.

Sinding S. 2006. "Population and Sexual and Reproductive Health and Rights: State of the Field and Some Suggestions for Future Program Actions." Prepared for David and Lucile Packard Foundation Population Program Review Task Force, January.

_____. 2005a. "Keeping Sexual and Reproductive Health at the Forefront of Global Efforts to Reduce Poverty." *Studies in Family Planning* 36, no. 2: 140–43.

_____. 2005b. "Why Is Funding for Population Activities Declining?" *Asia-Pacific Population Journal* 20, no. 2: 3–9.

_____. 2000. "The Great Population Debates: How Relevant Are They for the 21st Century." *American Journal of Public Health* 90, no. 12: 1841–44.

Singh S. 2006. "Hospital Admissions Resulting from Unsafe Abortion: Estimates from 13 Developing Countries." *The Lancet* 368: 1887–92.

Singh S, Darroch JE, Vlassof M, and Nadeau J. 2003. *Adding It Up: The Benefits of Investing in Sexual and Reproductive Health Care.* New York: Alan Guttmacher Institute.

Snow RC. 2001. "Female Genital Cutting: Distinguishing the Rights from the Health Agenda (editorial). *Tropical Medicine and International Health* 6: 89–91.

Sonfeld, Alan. 2002. "Looking at Men's Sexual and Reproductive Health Needs." *Guttmacher Report on Public Policy* 5, no. 2.

Specter M. 2005. "What Money Can Buy." *New Yorker* 81, no. 33: 56–71.

Speidel JJ. 2005. "Population Donor Landscape Analysis." For review of Packard Foundation International Grantmaking in Population, Sexual and Reproductive Health and Rights, 6 September. Accessed 29 November 2006 at http://www.packard.org/assets/files/population/program%20review /pop_rev_speidel_030606.pdf

Starrs A. 1987. *Preventing the Tragedy of Maternal Deaths: A Report on the International Safe Motherhood Conference, Nairobi, Kenya, February 1987.* Washington, D.C.: World Bank.

Stillwaggon E. 2006. *AIDS and the Ecology of Poverty.* London: Oxford University Press.

Sundari TK. 1992. "The Untold Story: How the Health Care Systems in Developing Countries Contribute to Maternal Mortality." *International Journal of Health Services* 22, no. 3: 513–28.

Swedish International Development Cooperation Agency. 2006. *Sweden's International Policy on Sexual and Reproductive Health and Rights.* Stockholm: Ministry for Foreign Affairs.

Thaddeus S and Maine D. 1994. "Too Far to Walk: Maternal Mortality in Context." *Social Science and Medicine* 38: 1091–10.

Thapa S. 2004. "Abortion Law in Nepal: The Road to Reform." *Reproductive Health Matters* 12, no. 24: 85–94.

Tinker A., Finn K, and Epp J. 2000. *Improving Women's Health: Issues and Interventions.* Washington, D.C.: World Bank, Health, Nutrition, and Population.

Trussell J. 2004. "Contraceptive Efficacy." In RA Hatcher, J Trussell, and F Stewart, et al. (eds), *Contraceptive Technology.* 18th rev. ed. New York: Ardent Media.

Tsui AO. 2001. "Population Policies, Family Planning Programs, and Fertility." In *Global Fertility Transition. Population and Development Review* 27 (suppl).

United Nations. 2007. *Recommendations Contained in the Report of the High-Level Panel on United Nations System-Wide Coherence in the Areas of Development, Humanitarian Assistance, and the Environment.* Document A/61/836, UN General Assembly, New York. Accessed 1 August at www.undg.org /docs/7136/A-61-836%20(SG%20Ban%20Note%20on%20HLP).doc

_____. 2006a. *Report of the Secretary General on the Work of the Organization.* Document A/61/1, United Nations, New York. Accessed 20 July 2007 at http://www.un.org/Docs/journal/asp/ws.asp?m=A/61/1(SUPP)

_____. 2006b. *Delivering as One: Report of the Secretary General's High Level Panel on UN System-Wide Coherence in the Areas of Development, Humanitarian Assistance, and the Environment.* Document A/61/583, 20 November, United Nations, New York.

_____. 2005a. *World Summit Outcome,* Document A/Res/60/1, 24 October 2005, United Nations, New York. Accessed 20 July 2007 at http://www.un.org/ Docs/journal/asp/ws.asp?m=A/RES/60/1

_____. 2005b. *In Larger Freedom: Towards Development, Security, and Human Rights for All. Report of the Secretary-General.* Document A/59/2005, 21 March, United Nations, New York. Accessed 27 July 2007 at http://www.un.org/largerfree dom

_____. 2004. *The Right of Everyone to the Enjoyment of the Highest Attainable Standard of Physical and Mental Health: Report of the Special Rapporteur, Paul Hunt.* Document E/CN.4/2004/49, Commission on Human Rights, Geneva. Accessed 2 June 2007 at http://daccessdds.un.org/doc/UNDOC/ GEN/G04/109/33/PDF/G0410933.pdf?OpenElement

_____. 2001a. *Follow-Up to the Outcome of the Millennium Summit. Road Map Towards the Implementation of the United Nations Millennium Declaration, Report of the Secretary-General.* Document A/56/326, UN General Assembly, 6 September, United Nations, New York. Accessed 16 February 2007 at http://www.un .org/millenniumgoals/sgreport2001.pdf?OpenElement

_____. 2001b. United Nations General Assembly Special Session (UNGASS) on HIV/AIDS, *Declaration of Commitment on HIV/AIDS: "Global Crisis—Global Action."* Document A/RES/S-26/2, UN General Assembly Special Session on HIV/AIDS, 2 August. Accessed 20 April 2007 at http://www.un.org/ga/aids/ coverage/FinalDeclarationHIVAIDS.html

_____. 2000a. *United Nations Millennium Declaration,* Document A/RES/55/2. September 2000, United Nations, New York. Accessed 20 July 2007 at http://www.un.org/millennium/declaration/ares552e.pdf

_____. 2000b. *Further Actions and Initiatives to Implement the Beijing Declaration and Platform for Action* ("Beijing + Five Document"). Document A/RES/S-23/3, June. United Nations, New York. Accessed 20 July 2007 at http://www.un.org/womenwatch/daw/followup/ress233e.pdf

_____. 1999a. *Report of the Ad Hoc Committee of the Whole of the Twenty-first Special Session of the General Assembly* ("ICPD + Five Document"). Document A/S-21/5/Add.1, July. United Nations, New York. Accessed 20 July 2007 at http://www.un.org/popin/unpopcom/32ndsess/gass/215e.pdf

_____. 1999b. *Key Actions for the Further Implementation of the Programme of Action of the International Conference on Population and Development.* Document A/RES/S-21/2, 30 June-2 July, United Nations, New York. Accessed 20 July 2007 at http://www.un.org/documents/ga/res/21sp/a21spr02.htm

_____. 1995. *Programme of Action, adopted at the International Conference on Population and Development, Cairo, 5–13 September 1994.* Document ST/ESA/SER.A/149, United Nations, New York. Accessed 4 November 2005 at http://www.unfpa.org/icpd/docs/icpd/icpd-poa-04reprint_eng.pdf

_____. 1989. Convention on the Rights of the Child. Document A/RES/44/25, 20 November, United Nations, New York. Accessed 25 July 2007 at http://www.un.org/documents/ga/res/44/a44r025.htm

_____. 1984. *Report of the International Conference on Population.* Document E.84.XIII.84/PC/9, Mexico City, 6–14 August, United Nations, New York. Accessed 29 July 2007 at http://www.un.org/popin/icpd/recommenda tions/expert/10.html

_____. 1979. Convention on the Elimination of All Forms of Discrimination against Women. Document A/34/46, 18 December. United Nations, New York.

_____. 1968. Proclamation of the International Conference on Human Rights at Teheran. Document A/CONF. 32/41 at 3, 14 May. United Nations, New York.

_____. 1966a. International Covenant on Civil and Political Rights. Document A/6316, 16 December, United Nations, New York.

_____. 1966b. International Covenant on Economic, Social and Cultural Rights. Document A/6316, 16 December, United Nations, New York.

UNAIDS. 2006a. *Report on the Global AIDS Epidemic 2006.* Geneva: UNAIDS. Accessed 20 July 2007 at http://data.unaids.org/pub/GlobalReport/2006/GR06_en.zip

_____. 2006b. *Meeting the Sexual and Reproductive Health Needs of People Living with HIV.* Brief Series, Guttmacher Institute and the Joint United Nations Programme on HIV/AIDS 6.

_____. 2000. *Enhancing the Greater Involvement of People Living with or Affected by HIV/AIDS (GIPA) in Sub-Saharan Africa: A UN Response: How Far Have We Gone?* Key Material, UNAIDS Best Practice Collection, October, United Nations, New York. Accessed 29 July 2007 at http://data.unaids.org/Publications/IRC-pub01/JC274-GIPA-ii_en.pdf

UNAIDS/WHO. 2005. *AIDS Epidemic Update.* Geneva: UNAIDS/WHO. Accessed 4 March 2006 at http://www.unaids.org/epi/2005/doc/report _pdf.asp

United Nations Children's Fund. 2003. *Building a World Fit for Children.* UN General Assembly Special Session on Children, Document A/S-27/19/Rev.1, 8-10 May 2002, United Nations, New York. Accessed 20 July 2007 at http://www.unicef.org/specialsession/docs_new/documents/A-RES-S27-2E.pdf

_____. 2002. *Adolescence: A Time That Matters.* New York: United Nations Children's Fund. Accessed 6 March 2004 at http://www.unicef.org/publica tions/files/pub_adolescence_en.pdf

_____. 2001. "Early Marriage." *Innocenti Digest* 7. Florence: Innocenti Research Centre, United Nations Children's Fund. Accessed 6 June 2007 at http://www.unicef-icdc.org/publications/pdf/digest7e.pdf

_____. 1998. *Report on UNICEF Activities as Follow-Up to the International Conference on Population and Development.* Document E/ICEF/1998/9. Executive Board Progress Report, UNICEF, New York.

United Nations Commission on Population and Development. 2005a. *Report on the Thirty-Eighth Session.* Document E/CN.9/2005/10, Resolution 2005/2, 4–8, 14 April. United Nations, New York. Accessed 20 July 2007 at http://www.un.org/esa/population/cpd/cpd2005/comm2005.htm

_____. 2005b. *The Flow of Financial Resources for Assisting in the Implementation of the Programme of Action of the International Conference on Population and Development.* Document E/CN.9/2005/5, United Nations Economic and Social Council, New York. Accessed 29 July 2007 at http://www.un.org/esa/population /cpd/cpd2005/comm2005.htm

_____. 2004. *Report on the Thirty-Seventh Session.* Document E/CN.9/2004/9, 22–26 March and 6 May, United Nations, New York. Accessed 20 July 2007 at http://www.un.org/esa/population/cpd/cpd2004/comm2004.htm

_____. 2003. *Population, Education, and Development.* Document E/CN.9/

2003/L.5, 31 March-4 April. Accessed 20 July 2007 at http://www.un.org/esa/population/cpd/cpd2003/comm2003.htm

UN Commission on the Status of Women. 2005. *Report on the Forty-Ninth Session.* Document E/CN.6/2005/11, 28 February, 22 March, United Nations, New York. Accessed 20 July 2007 at http://www.daccess-ods.un.org/TMP/7657073.html

UN Committee Against Torture. 2004. *Conclusions and Recommendations of the Committee Against Torture: Chile.* 14/06/2004. Document. CAT/C/CR/32/5, 14 June, Office of the UN High Commissioner for Human Rights, Geneva. Accessed 1 August 2007 at http://www.unhchr.ch/tbs/doc.nsf/(Symbol)/CAT.C.CR.32.5.En?Opendocument

UN Committee on Economic, Social and Cultural Rights. 2000. *The Right to the Highest Attainable Standard of Health.* General Comment 14 (8), Document E/C.12/2000/4, 11 August. Office of the UN High Commissioner for Human Rights, Geneva. Accessed 25 July 2007 at http://www.unhchr.ch/tbs/doc.nsf/(symbol)/E.C.12.2000.4.En

UN Committee on the Elimination of Discrimination Against Women. 1995. *Procedural Decisions of the Committee on the Elimination of Discrimination Against Women,* 14th Session, Document A/50/38, 2 March 2005, United Nations, New York. Accessed 25 July 2007 at http://www1.umn.edu/humanrts/cedaw/decisions/session14-1995.html

_____. 1994. *Equality in Marriage and Family Relations.* General Comment 21, 2 April, Office of the UN High Commissioner for Human Rights, Geneva. Accessed 25 July 2007at http://www.unhchr.ch/tbs/doc.nsf/0/7030ccb 2de3baae5c12563ee00648f1f?Opendocument

UN Committee on the Rights of the Child. 2003a. *HIV/AIDS and the Rights of the Child.* General Comment 3, Document CRC/GC/2003/1, 17 March, Office of the UN High Commissioner for Human Rights, Geneva. Accessed 6 June 2007 at http://www.unhchr.ch/tbs/doc.nsf/(symbol)/CRC.GC.2003.3.En? OpenDocument

_____. 2003b. *Adolescent Health and Development in the Context of the Convention on the Rights of the Child.* General Comment. 4 (21), Document CRC/GC/2003/4, 17 March, Office of the UN High Commissioner for Human Rights, Geneva. Accessed 6 June 2007 at http://www.unhchr.ch/tbs/doc.nsf/(symbol)/CRC.GC.2003.4.En

_____. 1999. *Concluding Observations of the Committee on the Rights of the Child: Mali.* 02/11/99, Document CRC/C/15/Add.113 2 November, Office of the UN High Commissioner for Human Rights, Geneva. Accessed 1 August 2007 at http://www.unhchr.ch/tbs/doc.nsf/(Symbol)/08f88d9b4806b60580256810 0056a532?Opendocument

UN Department of Economic and Social Affairs, Population Division. 2003a. *Demographic Yearbook 2003.* United Nations, New York. Accessed 25 July 2007 at http://unstats.un.org/unsd/Demographic/products/dyb/DYB2003/NotesTab24.pdf

_____. 2003b. *World Contraceptive Use.* United Nations, New York. Accessed 29 July 2007 at http://www.un.org/esa/population/publications/contraceptive 2003/wcu2003.htm

_____, Division for the Advancement of Women. 1995. Fourth World Conference on Women, September, Beijing, China. Accessed 25 July 2007 at http://www.un.org/womenwatch/daw/beijing/platform

UN Economic Commission for Africa. 2004. *Report of the Seventh African Regional Conference on Women, Outcome and the Way Forward*, United Nations, New York. Accessed 20 July 2007 at http://www.uneca.org/eca_programmes/acgd/de fault.htm

UN Economic and Social Commission for Asia and the Pacific. 2004. *Report of the High-Level Intergovernmental Meeting to Review Regional Implementation of the Beijing Platform for Action and Its Regional and Global Outcomes.* Document E/ESCAP/BPA/Rep, September, United Nations, New York. Accessed 20 July 2007 at http://www.unescap.org/EDC/English/IntergovMeetings/BPA/ BPA_Rep.pdf

———. 2003. *Report of the Fifth Asia and Pacific Population Conference.* Document E/ESCAP/1271, 17 March, United Nations, New York. Accessed 20 July 2007 at http://ww.unescap.org/59/e/E1271e.pdf

UN Economic Commission for Latin America and the Caribbean. 2004a. *Report of the Open-Ended Meeting of the Presiding Officers of the Sessional Ad Hoc Committee on Population and Development,* Document LC/L.2141, 11 March 2004. Accessed 20 July 2007 at http://www.cepal.org.ar/publicaciones/xml/4/ 15014/LCL2141i.pdf

———. 2004b. *Report of the Ninth Regional Conference on Women in Latin America and the Caribbean.* Document LC/G.2256 (CRM.9/6), June, United Nations, New York. Accessed 20 July 2007 at http://www.peacewomen.org/un/Beijing 10%20/ECLACResDoc.pdf

UN Millennium Project. 2005. *Investing in Development.* New York: United Nations. Accessed 20 July 2007 at http://www.unmillenniumproject.org/re-ports/fullreport.htm

UN Population Fund (UNFPA). 2007. *Using Culturally Sensitive Approaches to Achieve Universal Goals.* New York: United Nations Population Fund. Accessed 11 July at http://www.unfpa.org/culture/overview.htm

———. 2006a. *UNFPA on the Report of the Secretary-General on the Flow of Financial Resources for Assisting in the Implementation of the Programme of Action of the ICPD.* Document E/CN.9/2006/5, 39th Session of the Commission on Population and Development, Statement by Ms. Ann Pawliczko, 3 April, New York.

———. 2006b. *Global Population Policy Update* 64. New York: UNFPA, 1 June. Accessed 28 May 2007 at http://www.unfpa.org/parliamentarians/news/ newsletters/issue64.htm

———. 2005a. *Reducing Poverty and Achieving the Millennium Development Goals: Arguments for Investing in Reproductive Health and Rights: Reference Notes on Population and Poverty Reduction.* New York: UNFPA. Accessed 29 July 2007 at http://www.unfpa.org/upload/lib_pub_file/450_filename_ReducingPovert y1.pdf

———. 2005b. *Financial Resource Flows for Population Activities in 2003.* New York: UNFPA. Accessed 29 July 2007 at http://www.unfpa.org/upload/lib_pub_ file/526_filename_resource_flows_2003.pdf

———. 2005c. *The World Reaffirms Cairo: Official Outcomes of the ICPD at Ten Review.* New York: UNFPA. Accessed 29 July 2007 at http://www.unfpa.org/upload/ lib_pub_file/404_filename_reaffirming_cairo.pdf

———. 2005d. *The ICPD Vision: How Far Has the 11-Year Journey Taken Us?* New York: UNFPA. Accessed 29 July at http://www.unfpa.org/upload/lib_pub _file/594_filename_IUSSP%20icpd-vision.pdf

———. 2005e. *Child Marriage Factsheet.* New York: UNFPA. Accessed 18 March

2006 at http://www.unfpa.org/swp/2005/presskit/factsheets/facts_child
_marriage.htm

_____. 2004a. *Investing in People: National Progress in Implementing the ICPD Programme of Action 1994–2004*. New York: UNFPA. Accessed 24 July 2007 at http://www.unfpa.org/upload/lib_pub_file/278_filename_icpd04_sum mary.pdf

_____. 2004b. *The State of World Population: The Cairo Consensus at Ten: Population, Reproductive Health and the Global Effort to End Poverty.* New York: UNFPA. Accessed 4 March 2006 at http://www.unfpa.org/swp/2005/english/ch5/chap5_page3.htm

_____. 2004c. Glion Call to Action on Family Planning and HIV/AIDS in Women and Children. 2004. Glion, Switzerland, 3-5 May.

_____. 2003. *Achieving the Millennium Development Goals: Population and Reproductive Health as Critical Determinants.* Population and Development Strategies 10. New York: UNFPA.

_____. 2002. *Financial Resource Flows for Population Activities in 2002.* New York: UNFPA,. Accessed 29 July 2007 at http://www.unfpa.org/upload/lib_pub_ file/359_filename_financial_resource_flows.pdf

_____. 1998. *Indicators for Population and Reproductive Health Programmes.* New York: United Nations.

UNFPA/UNAIDS/NIDI. 2006. *Resource Flows Newsletter,* January. New York: United Nations.

United States Agency for International Development. 2006a. Health. Accessed 3 June 2007 at www.usaid.gov/our_work/global_health

_____. 2006b. Family Planning. Accessed 2 June 2007 at www.usaid.gov/our_ work/global_health/pop/indes.html

_____, Asia and the Near East. 2007. *Background on the Rural Expansion of Afghan Community-Based Health Care Program.* USAID Asia and the Near East Website. Accessed 20 April at http://www.usaid.gov/locations/asia_near_east/ afghanistan/health.html

U.S. General Accounting Office. 2005. *Food and Drug Administration: Decision process to Deny Initial Application for Over-the-Counter Marketing of the Emergency Contraceptive Plan B Was Unusual.* Report to Congressional Requesters. Washington, D.C.: GAO.

Valente TW and Davis RL. 1999. "Accelerating the Diffusion of Innovations Using Opinion Leaders." *Annals of the American Academy of Political and Social Science* 566: 55-67.

Van Balen F and Inhorn MC. 2002. "Introduction—Interpreting Infertility: A View from the Social Sciences." In MC Inhorn and F Van Balen (eds.), *Infertility Around the Globe: New Thinking on Childlessness, Gender, and Reproductive Technologies.* Berkeley: University of California Press.

Van Dalen HP and Reuser M. 2006. "What Drives Donor Funding in Population Assistance Programs? Evidence from OECD countries." *Studies in Family Planning* 37, no. 3: 141–54.

Van Damme L, Ramjee G, Alary M, et al. 2002. "Effectiveness of COL-1492, a Nonoxynol-9 Vaginal Gel, on HIV-1 Transmission in Female Sex Workers: A Randomized Controlled Trial." *The Lancet* 360: 971–77.

Van Der Maas PJ. 2003. "How Summary Measures of Population Health Are Affecting Health Agendas." *Bulletin of the World Health Organization* 81, no 5.

Vogel CG. 2006. "The Changing Face of Foreign Assistance: New Funding

Paradigms Offer a Challenge and Opportunity for Family Planning." *PAI Research Commentary* 1, no. 8.

Walker D, Campero L, Espinoza H, et al. 2004. "Deaths from Complications of Unsafe Abortion: Misclassified Second Trimester Deaths." *Reproductive Health Matters* 12, no. 24: 27–38.

Weigman R. 2005. "The Possibility of Women's Studies." In EL Kennedy and A Beins (eds.), *Women's Studies for The Future: Foundations, Interrogations, Politics.* New Brunswick, N.J.: Rutgers University Press.

Westoff C, Kerns J, Morroni C, et al. 2002. "Quick Start: Novel Oral Contraceptive Initiation Method." *Contraception* 66, no. 3: 141–45.

White House, Office of the Press Secretary. 2001. *Restoration of the Mexico City Policy, Memorandum for the Administrator of the United States Agency for International Development.* Media release, Washington, D.C., 22 January. Accessed 29 July 2007 at http://www.planetwire.org/wrap/files.fcgi/1177 _bush_mexico_city_memorandum.htm

Women's Link Worldwide. 2007. "Excerpts of the Constitutional Court's Ruling That Liberalized Abortion in Colombia." Colombia Court Ruling C-355/2006. Accessed 25 July at http://www.womenslinkworldwide.org/pdf/ pub_c355.pdf

_____. 2006. "Colombia's Highest Court Rules in Favor of Easing One of World's Most Restrictive Abortion Laws." Media release, 10 May. Accessed 25 July 2007 at www.womenslinkworldwide.org

_____. 2005. "Constitutional Challenge to Colombian Abortion Law Launched." Accessed 25 July 2007 at http://rs6.net/tn.jsp?t=scjlsjbab.0.bhimsjbab .5cvjg8n6.2985&p=http%3A%2F%2Fwww.womenslinkworldwide.org%2Fco_ lat_colombia.html

World Bank. 2007. *Population Issues in the 21st Century: The Role of the World Bank.* Washington, D.C.: World Bank. Accessed 22 July at http://siteresources .worldbank.org/HEALTHNUTRITIONANDPOPULATION/Resources/281 627-1095698140167/PopulationDiscussionPaperApril07Final.pdf

_____. 2005. *World Bank Development Data 2005.* Washington, D.C.: World Bank. Accessed 5 March 2006 at http://devdata.worldbank.org/hnpstats/ HNPDemographic/year5/WLD_POP.xls.

_____. 2000. *The Nature and Evolution of Poverty.* World Development Report 2000/2001. Washington, D.C.: World Bank.

_____. 1993. *Investing in Health: The World Development Report.* Washington, D.C.: World Bank.

World Health Organization. 2007. "The Partnership for Maternal, Newborn and Child Health." Accessed 25 July at http://www.who.int/pmnch/en

_____. 2006a. *Defining Sexual Health: Report of a Technical Consultation on Sexual Health, 28–31 January 2002.* Geneva: WHO. Accessed 15 November 2007 at http://www.who.int/reproductive-health/publications/sexualhealth/defin ing_sh.pdf

_____. 2006b. *Sexual and Reproductive Health of Women Living with HIV/AIDS: Guidelines on Care, Treatment and Support for Women Living with HIV/AIDS and their Children in Resource-Constrained settings.* Co-produced with UNFPA. Geneva: WHO. Accessed 24 July 2007 at http://www.who.int/reproductive-health/docs/srhwomen_hivaids/text.pdf

_____. 2006c. *Engaging for Health: 11th General Programme of Work, 2006–2015: A Global Health Agenda.* Geneva: WHO. Accessed 2 June 2007 at http://www.who.int/gpw/GPW_En.pdf

_____. 2005. *World Health Report 2005: Make Every Mother and Child Count.* Geneva: WHO. Accessed 28 May 2007 at http://www.who.int/whr/2005/en

_____. 2004. *Reproductive Health Strategy.* Department of Reproductive Health and Research. Adopted by 57th World Health Assembly, May. Geneva: WHO. Accessed 29 July 2007 at http://www.who.int/reproductive-health/strategy.htm

_____. 2003a. *Contraceptive Implants Come of Age.* Progress in Reproductive Health Research 61: 2–5. Geneva: WHO.

_____. 2003b. *Safe Abortion: Technical and Policy Guidance for Health Systems* Geneva: WHO. Accessed 29 July 2007 at http://www.who.int/reproductive-health/publications/safe_abortion/safe_abortion.pdf

_____. 2002. *Defining Sexual Health: Report of a Technical Consultation on Sexual Health, 28-31 January 2002.* Geneva: WHO. Accessed 2 June 2007 at http://www.who.int/reproductive-health/publications/sexualhealth/defining_sh.pdf

_____. 2001a *Reproductive Health Indicators for Global Monitoring: Report of the Second Interagency Meeting.* Document WHO/RHR/01.19, 17–19 July 2000. Geneva: WHO.

_____. 2001b. *Transforming Health Systems: Gender and Rights in Reproductive Health.* Geneva: WHO. Accessed 30 April 2007 at http://www.who.int/reproductive-health/publications/transforming_healthsystems_gender/index.html

_____. 1998. *DALYs and Reproductive Health: Report of an Informal Consultation.* Geneva: WHO.

_____. 1994. "Global Policy Committee of the World Health Organization." WHO Position Paper on Health, 2 May, Population and Development, Cairo 5-13 September.

_____. 1987. *WHO Global AIDS Strategy.* Document WHA40.26, WHO, Geneva. Accessed 29 July 2007 at http://www.who.int/entity/bloodsafety/en/WHA40.26.pdf

WHO Commission on Social Determinants of Health. 2007. WHO Commission on Social Determinants of Health website. Accessed 24 July 2007 at http://www.who.int/social_determinants/en

WHO Department of Child and Adolescent Health. 2004. *Children and Young People are at the Centre of the HIV/AIDS Epidemic.* WHO, Geneva. Accessed 18 November 2006 at http://www.who.int/child-adolescent-health/HIV/HIV_epidemic.htm

WHO Department of Reproductive Health and Research. 2006. *Reproductive Indicators: Guidelines for Their Generation, Interpretation and Analysis for Global Monitoring,* Geneva: WHO. Accessed 1 May 2007 at http://who.int/reproductivehealth/publications/rh_indicators/index.html

WHO Global Health Workforce Alliance. 2007. Global Health Workforce Alliance—Because They Save Lives Website. Accessed 24 July at http://www.who.int/workforcealliance/en/index.html

WHO Special Programme for Research and Training in Tropical Diseases. 2007. TDR Home Page Website, UNICEF, UNDP, World Bank, WHO. Accessed 24 July at http://www.who.int/tdr

WHO Task Force on Post-Ovulatory Methods of Fertility Regulation. 1998. "Randomized Controlled Trial of Levonorgestrel Versus the Yuzpe Regimen of Combined Oral Contraceptives for Emergency Contraception." *The Lancet* 352, no. 9126: 428–33.

_____. 1993. "Termination of Pregnancy with Reduced Doses of Mifepristone." *British Medical Journal* 307: 532–37.

WHO and Program on International Health and Human Rights, Harvard School of Public Health. 2001. *Using Human Rights for Maternal and Neonatal Health: A Tool for Strengthening Law, Policies and Standards of Care.* Geneva: WHO. Accessed 25 July 2007 at http://www.who.int/reproductive-health/gender/country.html

WHO, UNAIDS, and UNFPA. 2004. Position Statement on Condoms and HIV Prevention, July. Accessed 29 July 2007 at http://data.unaids.org/una-docs/condom-policy_jul04_en.pdf

Worthington T and Kjaerby AM for All Party Parliamentary Group on Population, Development and Reproductive Health. 2004. *The Missing Link! Parliamentary Hearings Linking Sexual and Reproductive Health and HIV/AIDS.* Hearing Report. All Party Parliamentary Group on Population, Development and Reproductive Health, London.

Yamin AE and Maine D. 1999. "Maternal Mortality as a Human Rights Issue: Measuring Compliance with International Treaty Obligations." *Human Rights Quarterly* 21, no. 3.

Contributors

Alaka Basu is Associate Professor of Demography in the Department of Sociology and Director of the South Asia Program at Cornell University and a Visiting Associate Professor of Demography at the Harvard School of Public Health. She is a distinguished researcher and writer in the fields of population studies, gender and development, family planning, reproductive health, health, culture and behavior. She holds many board-level appointments in national and international organizations, including the Governing Council; International Union for the Scientific Study of Populations; the Board of Directors of the Population Association of America; the Board of Trustees of the Population Council; and the Panel on Population Projections for the National Research Council, National Academy of Sciences. Professor Basu earned her Master of Science in Medical Demography from the London School of Hygiene and Tropical Medicine, a Master of Science in Biochemistry from the University of London, and a diploma in Journalism at the Bombay College of Journalism, University of Bombay.

Marge Berer, M.A., is cofounder and editor of the international peer-reviewed journal *Reproductive Health Matters*. She has worked as a writer and activist in the field of reproductive and sexual health and rights in the United Kingdom and internationally since 1978. She was a Visiting Fellow at the Harvard Center for Population and Development Studies from 2002 to 2005. She has chaired the Steering Committee of the International Consortium for Medical Abortion since 2002, was the first Chair of the Gender Advisory Panel of the WHO Department of Reproductive Health and Research/HRP (1996-2001), and has served as an expert consultant to the World Health Organization and other international organizations. Ms. Berer is editor/coauthor of a book on HIV/AIDS and sexual and reproductive health, and author of numerous published articles, conference presentations, and book chapters on reproductive health and rights. Prior to founding *Reproductive Health Matters*, she worked for the National Abortion Campaign and then the Women's Global Network for Reproductive Rights. She has been involved in organizing a number of international conferences, workshops and seminars on reproductive health and rights, most recently on promotion of condoms and on medical abortion and second trimester abortion.

Kelly Blanchard, Sc.M., is President of Ibis Reproductive Health. Ibis's mission is to improve women's reproductive autonomy, choices, and health worldwide by conducting original clinical and social science research, leveraging existing research, producing educational resources, and promoting policies and practices that support sexual and reproductive rights and health. Her recent research has focused on contraception, including emergency contraception, medical and surgical abortion, and female-controlled HIV prevention methods, including microbicides and cervical barriers. She has authored or coauthored more than forty articles on reproductive health in developing and developed countries. Prior to joining Ibis, Ms. Blanchard worked at the Population Council as a Program Associate, where she managed a growing program on reproductive health in South Africa and the Southern Africa region. In 2006, she received the American Public Health Association Section on Population, Family Planning and Reproductive Health's Outstanding Young Professional Award.

David E. Bloom, Ph.D., is an economist and demographer and the Clarence James Gamble Professor of Economics and Demography at the Harvard School of Public Health. In January 2003 he was appointed Chairman of the School's Department of Population and International Health. Prior to joining the public health school faculty in 1996, he served on the public policy faculty at Carnegie-Mellon University and on the economics faculties at Harvard University and Columbia University. At Columbia, he was Professor of Economics and Department Chairman from 1990 to 1993. From 1996 to 1999 he served as Deputy Director of the Harvard Institute for International Development. Professor Bloom has worked extensively in the areas of labor, population and health and has been retained as a consultant to various public and private organizations, both in the United States and throughout the developing world, including Indonesia, China, India, Sri Lanka, Pakistan, South Africa, Jamaica, and El Salvador. He has taught numerous courses on labor economics, development economics, global health and population, and statistics and econometrics at both the graduate and undergraduate levels, and has published more than two hundred articles, book chapters, and books.

David Canning, Ph.D., is an economist and Professor of Economics and International Health at the Harvard School of Public Health. His research focuses on the role of demographic change and health improvements in economic development. Before taking up his position at the

Harvard School of Public Health, he held faculty positions at the London School of Economics, Cambridge University, Columbia University, and Queen's University Belfast. He has served as a consultant to the World Health Organization, World Bank, and Asian Development Bank. In addition, he was a member of Working Group One of the World Health Organization's Commission on Macroeconomics and Health. He is currently deputy director of the Program on the Global Demography of Aging and heads the economics track of the doctoral program in Population and International Health.

Rebecca Firestone, Sc.D., M.P.H., is a recent graduate of Harvard School of Public Health. Her research interests are in the areas of sexuality and reproductive health, HIV/AIDS, maternal and child nutrition, and social inequalities in health. She served as the editorial assistant for the production of this volume in her capacity as research assistant and coordinator of the Group on Reproductive Health and Rights at the Harvard Center for Population and Development Studies. She has over a decade of experience with policy advocacy, program evaluation, and organizing in the field of reproductive health and rights with organizations such as the Center for Health and Gender Equity and the Program for Appropriate Technology in Health. She has long-term research and programming interests in Southeast Asia, particularly Thailand.

Françoise Girard is Director of the Public Health Program at the Open Society Institute, where she was also Regional Director for Southern Central and Eastern Europe and Haiti in the 1990s. A lawyer by training, Ms. Girard has worked many years as an advocate for women's health, gender equality, and sexual rights, with a focus on advocacy and policy development with UN agencies and at UN conferences (ICPD+5, Beijing+5, Special Session on HIV/AIDS and on Children, ICPD+10, 2005 World Summit). From 1999 to 2003, she was Senior Program Officer for International Policy at the International Women's Health Coalition. She has also served as a law clerk to Justice Charles Gonthier of the Supreme Court of Canada. She has contributed articles to *International Family Planning Perspectives, Reproductive Health Matters, Journal of Women's Health and Law, Populi,* and *QCQ,* among others. Her other publications include "Global Implications of U.S. Domestic and International Policies on Sexuality."

Sofia Gruskin, J.D., M.I.A., is Director of the Program on International Health and Human Rights, and Associate Professor in the Department of Population and International Health at the Harvard School of Public Health. Her work emphasizes the conceptual, methodological, policy, and practice implications of linking health to human rights, with particular attention to HIV/AIDS, women, children, gender issues, and vulnerable populations. She has extensive experience in research, training, and programmatic work with nongovernmental, governmental, and intergovernmental organizations in the fields of health and human rights around the world. She is the principal investigator for several UNAIDS, WHO, and UNFPA sponsored projects intended to strengthen the health and human rights research and policy agenda—particularly in the areas of HIV/AIDS, sexual and reproductive health, child and adolescent health, and gender-based violence. Ms. Gruskin is associate editor for *American Journal of Public Health* and *Global Public Health*, and lead editor of the volume *Perspectives on Health and Human Rights*. She was Chair of the UNAIDS Global Reference Group on HIV/AIDS and Human Rights (2003-2006) and editor of the international journal *Health and Human Rights* (1994-2006). She serves on numerous national and international boards and committees, is a permanent member of the NIH Behavioral and Social Consequences of HIV/AIDS study section, and within the Harvard School of Public Health serves as codirector of the Interdisciplinary Concentration on Women, Gender, and Health.

Joan Kaufman, Sc.D., is founding Director of the AIDS Public Policy Project at the Mossavar Rahmani Center for Business and Government, Harvard University's Kennedy School of Government, Lecturer on Social Medicine at Harvard Medical School, Senior Scientist at the Heller School for Social Policy and Management, Brandeis University and China Team Leader for the International AIDS Vaccine Initiative (IAVI). She was the Ford Foundation's Reproductive Health Program Officer for China from 1996 to 2001. She spent the 2001-2002 academic year as a Radcliffe fellow at Harvard University and was a 2005-2006 Soros Reproductive Health and Rights Fellow. She is a member of the Gender and Health Equity Network, a three-country study of gender, governance, and health planning for which she directs the China case study. She was a Lecturer on Population and Reproductive Health at Harvard School of Public Health (1990-1999) and Senior Associate at Abt Associates Inc. (1992-1996), developing and directing projects on HIV/AIDS, sexually transmitted diseases, and other public health problems. She was the first international UNFPA program officer for China, from 1980 to 1984. She holds a doctorate in population and international health from Harvard School of Public Health. She has published widely on reproductive health, AIDS, health systems and health sector reform, gender issues, and population policy, often with a focus on China.

Frances Kissling is former president and CEO of Catholics for a Free Choice in Washington, D.C. From her work with family planning clinics in the 1970s to her leadership in the feminist religious and international reproductive health movements, she has been working to improve women's lives for over 30 years. She has published articles and op-ed pieces in the *Times of London, New York Times, Los Angeles Times, Washington Post, The Nation, Boston Globe, San Francisco Chronicle, Christian Century, Christianity & Crisis,* and the *Journal of Feminist Studies in Religion.* She gives frequent speeches and is often interviewed by international media. Active in international public policy issues, she was a prominent participant in the UN conferences in Cairo and Beijing. She was a 2007 Fellow at the Radcliffe Institute for Advanced Study at Harvard University and is currently a visiting scholar at the Center for Bioethics at the University of Pennsylvania.

Heidi Larson, Ph.D., is an associate research professor of International Development at Clark University and a research associate at the Harvard Center for Population and Development. She is a specialist in risk analysis and is currently working on a book on risk and rumor in global health, analyzing the rumor-driven polio vaccine boycott in Nigeria, along with other examples of managing public questioning and rumors in public health. Heidi has served as a senior adviser to the UN and other international organizations on a number of public health issues, including AIDS, TB, and child health and vaccines, particularly focusing on the socio-cultural and political determinants of health, including the role of religion and belief systems. She has also advised on anticipating and managing organizational risks and rumor. Heidi is currently coordinating a UNAIDS-commissioned initiative called aids2031, which is bringing together economists, epidemiologists, and biomedical, social, and political scientists to map future options for the AIDS response. 2031 will mark 50 years since AIDS was first reported.

Tom W. Merrick, Ph.D., works with the Learning Program on Population, Reproductive Health and Health Sector Reform at the World Bank Institute. Prior to joining the World Bank Institute in 2001, he served as Senior Adviser for Population and Reproductive Health for the Human Development Network at the World Bank, where he worked for nine years. He has served as President of the Population Reference Bureau and as Director of the Center for Population Research at Georgetown University, where he also chaired the department of demography. He also worked as a Demographer/International Economist for the United States Agency for International Development offices of Population and Program and Policy Coordination from 1968 to 1971. His teaching experience includes positions at the University of Pennsylvania, Georgetown University, and the University of Minas Gerais in Brazil, where he taught and conducted research as a Ford Foundation advisor.

Michael R. Reich is Taro Takemi Professor of International Health Policy, and Director of the Takemi Program in International Health at the Harvard School of Public Health. He has written widely on international health policy and politics, including various aspects of global pharmaceutical policy. He received his Ph.D. in Political Science from Yale University in 1981, and his M.A. in East Asian Studies and B.A. in Molecular Biophysics and Biochemistry, also from Yale University. His recent books include *Getting Health Reform Right: A Guide to Improving Performance and Equity* (coauthor), *Wounds of War* (coauthor), and *Public-Private Partnerships for Public Health* (editor). He has served as Director of the Harvard Center for Population and Development Studies.

Laura Reichenbach, Sc.D, M.P.A., is currently Senior Researcher at the Population Council, Islamabad, Pakistan, and formerly a Research Scientist at the Harvard Center for Population and Development at the Harvard School of Public Health. Her research is in the field of reproductive health, including gender issues of the health workforce, issues related to priority setting, resource flows, and policy processes, and the interlinkages between population, development, and poverty. Her work on reproductive health has involved field experience in a number of developing countries around the world including Bangladesh, where she is currently based and conducts research.

Mindy Jane Roseman, J.D., Ph.D., is Academic Director of the Human Rights Program at Harvard Law School, and a Lecturer on Law. Before joining HRP, she was Senior Research Officer at the International Health and Human Rights Program, François-Xavier Bagnoud Center for Health and Human Rights, and an Instructor in the Department of Population and International Health at Harvard School of Public Health. There she researched and reported on a range of health and human rights issues, with special focus on reproductive and sexual rights, including HIV and AIDS, and women's and children's rights. Before coming to Harvard she had been a staff attorney with the Center for Reproductive Rights in New York, in charge of its East and Central European program. After graduating from Northwestern University Law School in 1986, she clerked for Judge John F. Grady, Chief Judge, U.S. District Court, Northern District, Illinois. She also holds a doctorate in Modern European History with a focus on the history of reproductive health from Columbia University. Her publications include *Beyond Words: Images from America's Concentration* Camps (coauthored) and *Women of the World (East Central Europe): Laws and Policies Affecting Their Reproductive Lives.* Her current research projects include a history of the eugenics and human rights movements in France.

Bonnie Shepard, M.Ed., M.P.A., is a Senior Planning and Evaluation Specialist at Social Sectors Development Strategies, Inc. and a consultant, writer, trainer, and researcher on topics related to sexual and reproductive health and rights, and women's rights. She has concentrated on Latin American programs for most of her career, first at Pathfinder

International in the 1980s, and then at the Ford Foundation Andean Region and Southern Cone office in Santiago, Chile, from 1992 to 1998. She was Senior Consultant to Catholics for Free Choice for its Latin American Program from 2000 to 2004, providing technical assistance in strategic planning, program design, and evaluation. As a consultant to UNICEF in two regions, UNFPA, and the Bill and Melinda Gates Foundation, she has concentrated on strategic assessments of reproductive health and youth/adolescent programs. Her recent book *Running the Obstacle Course to Sexual and Reproductive Health: Lessons from Latin America* includes an in-depth study NGO networks, and analysis of the political and cultural barriers faced by a popular sex education program in Chile.

George Zeidenstein is Visiting Distinguished Fellow at the Harvard Center for Population and Development Studies, where he has been teaching and mentoring graduate students since 1993. Before that, he was President and a Trustee of the Population Council for seventeen years. Earlier, he worked on a wide spectrum of international development issues with the Ford Foundation and the Peace Corps, including several years of residence with his wife and their two children in Nepal as Country Director of the Peace Corps and in Bangladesh as Resident Representative of the Ford Foundation. He has been decorated by the governments of Finland and Senegal for his international development work. He is author of a recently published memoir of his early life entitled, Lifelines. During his first ten years of professional life, he practiced corporate and securities law in New York City.

Index

Acknowledgments

This volume has had a long gestation and exists solely because of the hard work and innovative thinking of a number of people. While we the editors take complete responsibility for all errors and any misrepresentations in the book, we are pleased to have the opportunity to acknowledge those who are responsible for its successful apparition.

This book would never have been possible without the longstanding interest and support of the Group on Reproductive Rights and Health, Harvard Center for Population and Development Studies. Many of the contributors were active participants in the Group and helped craft the early ideas for this book. The Group also generously assisted the process by providing lunches and other sustenance. Special thanks are due to Michael R. Reich, former Director of the Center who unquestioningly supported the Group, and believed in us, even as he periodically challenged us to push our analyses further. His advice and comments throughout the writing of the book and in its final production have immeasurably improved the book.

The contributors to this book first provided their thoughts in oral form and agreed to commit them to paper. Many attended one or both of the authors' meetings we held over the course of the book's development. We are grateful to each author for their participation and responsiveness in the book production process. Marge Berer, Sofia Gruskin, Joan Kaufman, Michael R. Reich, and George Zeidenstein deserve special mention for their willingness to comment and critique various chapters.

Rebecca Firestone, now a freshly minted Doctor of Science from the Harvard School of Public Health, may not have entirely known what she agreed to when she averred some interest in assisting us on this book. Her insights, disposition, and expertise have also ensured a level of excellence, without which, this volume would not have attained. We have tried to show our appreciation along the way, picking up the lunch check perhaps once. We hope these words convey our immense gratitude.

We would like to thank Judith Helzner, Director, and Ann Blanc, Program Officer, Population and Reproductive Health, John D. and Catherine T. MacArthur Foundation, who provided financial support for the production and distribution of this volume. The staff at the MacArthur Foundation rode the administrative vicissitudes of the Office of Sponsored Research with great aplomb. Mark Pachucki, a Ph.D. candidate in the Department of Sociology at Harvard University, devoted an entire summer to a social networking study of the field of "global" reproductive health and rights. We thank him and the respondents of this study. This exercise was in response to the MacArthur Foundation's request as part of the grant that supported the production of volume. Nathaniel Rosenblum and Olivia Rater also provided assistance in the social network study.

The book could not have been produced without the assistance of the staff at the Harvard Center for Population and Development Studies and the Harvard Initiative on Global Health. We would like to recognize the good humor and patience of Panka Deo, Sue Carlson, Jahan Habib, Jennie Bell, and Jeannie Millar.

Jessie Evans's patience and care in revising citations, checking for omissions, and formatting the bibliography truly deserves an Olympic medal; Deborah Gesensway's thoughtful editorial interventions have spared the reader many redundancies. Shaina Trotta and Shannon Philmon provided us crucial assistance in the final days of text production. We would also like to recognize the Human Rights Program at Harvard Law School for its many indulgences.

We would like to thank editor in chief Peter "patience of Job" Agree and the outside readers at University of Pennsylvania Press for their constructive criticism and support of this book.

Finally we want to acknowledge our families, whom we have at time neglected and strung along, as six months stretched out into a year and beyond. Noah Rosenblum encouraged us to rewrite grants and chapters when our enthusiasm was flagging; Nathaniel Rosenblum's good natured nudging kept our priorities in reasonably good order. Greg Chen exhibited unending patience and uncomplainingly provided extra childcare on nights and weekends over the many months it took to put this book together. Natalie, Alexandra, and Evelyn Chen were extremely patient with an often distracted mom and provided welcome and wonderful interruptions throughout the process. We are eternally grateful for all their love and support, and it is to them that we dedicate this book.